NURSING MANAGEMENT AND LEADERSHIP IN ACTION

NURSING MANAGEMENT AND LEADERSHIP IN ACTION

LAURA MAE DOUGLASS, R.N., B.A., M.S.

Formerly Chairman, Division of Nursing, Point Loma College,
San Diego, California

EM OLIVIA BEVIS, R.N., B.S., M.A., F.A.A.N.

Professor and Coordinator, Medical College of Georgia
School of Nursing, Graduate Satellite,
Savannah, Georgia

THIRD EDITION

The C. V. Mosby Company

ST. LOUIS • TORONTO • LONDON   1979

THIRD EDITION

Copyright © 1979 by The C. V. Mosby Company

All rights reserved. No part of this book may be reproduced in any manner without written permission of the publisher.

Previous editions copyrighted 1970, 1974

Printed in the United States of America

The C. V. Mosby Company
11830 Westline Industrial Drive, St. Louis, Missouri 63141

Library of Congress Cataloging in Publication Data

Douglass, Laura Mae.
    Nursing management and leadership in action.

    First ed. published in 1970 under title: Team
leadership in action; 2d ed. (1974) under title:
Nursing leadership in action.
    Bibliography: p.
    Includes index.
    1.   Nursing service administration.   2.   Leadership.
    I.   Bevis, Em Olivia, joint author.   II.   Title.
[DNLM: 1.   Leadership.   2.   Nursing, Supervisory.
WY105   D737t]
RT89.D67   1979   658.4   78-31960
ISBN 0-8016-1441-4

GW/M/M   9   8   7   6   5   4   3   2   1   03/D/326

To
Clara Ash and Kathleen Holloway
whose real contribution to my career can never be fully acknowledged.
L. M. D.

To
Ada Fort and Lois Wilder
for their continuing affection and encouragement.
E. O. B.

PREFACE

Many things have happened to nursing in the years since this book was first published in 1970 under the title *Team Leadership in Action*. Rapid changes are sweeping all the health-related disciplines. Nursing is attempting to devise care delivery systems that will better meet the needs of health consumers and provide continuity, comprehension, and quality. New practice modes are marked by autonomy, authority, and accountability. Nurses practice some form of collaborative care in most areas of the country, and more and more agencies and individuals are structuring delivery systems that will provide the client with better services and the nurse with greater challenge and satisfaction. Consequently, this book has enlarged its focus from leadership to the broader spectrum of leadership and management in nursing. Principles of leadership and management apply regardless of the specific nursing care delivery system in use at a given agency.

Schools and agencies that teach nursing management and leadership principles for utilization in nursing practice in any type of delivery mode will produce a more flexible and skilled nurse.

Except for the broadened focus of the book, the basic intent has not changed. The book still attempts to help nurses learn the functions that make the delivery of nursing care work. Management and leadership activities, whether used in team nursing, primary nursing, functional nursing, or case nursing, require the skills discussed here. Every nurse practices leadership by the very nature of nursing, and most nurses are called on to be managers at some level, for decisions must be made and problems solved whether they concern one or many patients or nurses.

Education of nurses has traditionally emphasized the study of knowledge and skills of patient care and assumed that the graduate could function in management and leadership roles with minimal preparation. This preparation was expected to be provided by the employer, who in turn anticipated that the graduate would be able to function in a leadership capacity from the first day of employment with only brief orientation to agency routine and policy. Lack of sufficient leadership preparation has resulted in the nurse's frustration and disenchantment with leadership activities and in disillusionment on the part of the employer whose expectations have not been met. Nurses are promoted through the bureaucratic hierarchy to lower, middle, and higher management positions on the basis of nursing care skills rather than administration and managerial knowledge and ability. Efforts to remedy this situation are being exerted by individuals, schools of nursing, professional organizations, and employing institutions. This book is designed to assist in this effort.

One goal of nursing education is to teach the use of foresight. Anticipating the result of behaviors and the effective use of self requires the ability to predict outcomes and therefore to behave in a way that will produce the desired results. This book is an attempt to elaborate a framework for staff nursing that will enable the nurse to mobilize all available resources for the benefit of those who need health service. Other goals are to offer the nurse-leader/manager a body of knowledge that will supply a conceptual framework of administrative principles for use by the nurse-leader/manager, to provide a practical method for the use of these administrative principles in day-to-day nursing activities, and to promote a cognitive habit that will transform the nurse using these knowledges and methods into an effective leader and manager. These objectives are met through a consideration of the staff nurse as a leader and manager and through the formulation and utilization of principles necessary for effective functioning.

In Chapter 1, a conceptual framework for the book presents the basic hypotheses on which the book is based. Subsequent chapters deal with management, teaching and learning, effective communication, delegating authority, evaluation, changing, and leadership.

No attempt has been made to cover the entire field of the subjects implied by the chapter headings. We have carefully selected material that we consider to be most useful to nurses. The book continues to be designed for use by students, staff nurses, supervisory staff, teachers, and independent nurse practitioners.

We are grateful to family, friends, and colleagues who gave their understanding, support, and time so that this book could be written. We are especially grateful to our students, whose need inspired the book and whose studies helped us to grow.

Laura Mae Douglass
Em Olivia Bevis

CONTENTS

NURSING MANAGEMENT AND LEADERSHIP IN ACTION

1
CONCEPTUAL FRAMEWORK FOR THE NURSE-MANAGER AND LEADER

All nurses today function as leaders and managers. Health agencies in every setting and of every type expect nurses to be leaders of patients, nursing teams, health teams, and community groups and managers of workers, environments, budgets, time, and equipment.

Leadership and management are learned behavior patterns. To function effectively the nurse must acquire fundamental principles that make management and leadership a learned process rather than a series of duties described and listed in a policy manual. Principles of effective management and leadership and their use can be learned by both the student and the experienced nurse. The knowledge, skill, and experience of every nurse can be organized so that the quality of management and leadership ability is improved. The development of management and leadership ability may be achieved through the following:

1. Formulating principles of management and leadership based on a sound body of knowledge (input)
2. Utilizing these principles systematically to solve problems (operation)
3. Obtaining evaluative information (feedback)

Learning principles of management and leadership through the traditional cognitive methods is insufficient. The terms "management" and "leadership" imply behaviors; they imply interaction with people. The term "manager" implies systematic operations. Therefore the knowledge and skills of management and leadership must be acquired where people work together, where behaviors and operations can be practiced.

This chapter establishes the conceptual framework from which the remainder of the book derives its form and structure. Basically the authors and readers must be able to meet on conceptual and theoretical common ground. John Stuart Mills' admonition, ". . . above all, to insist upon having the meaning of a word clearly understood before using it, and the meaning of a proposition before assenting to it,"* clearly bespeaks the obvious need to set about a simple but scholarly task. That task is one of coming to grips with key concepts and hypotheses (meanings and propositions) prior to elaborating ideas that are both consequences of and

*From Mills' inaugural address as Rector, University of St. Andrews, February 1, 1867.

1

subsequent to theoretical or conceptual constructs. Meanings and propositions will be provided for management and leadership; for the nature of roles and role assumptions; for theories generally, with particular emphasis on predictive theories or predictive principles; and for problem solving and decision making.

DEFINING LEADERSHIP AND MANAGEMENT

June Bailey and her associates at the University of California, San Francisco, defined leadership as follows:

> Within the conceptual framework of the Power/Authority/Influence Model, we define leadership as a set of *actions* that influence members of a group to move toward goal setting and goal attainment. Inherent in the *actions* are situational variables; personal, organizational, and social power bases; formal and functional bases of authority; and accountability. Other elements in the spectrum of leadership actions are sound managerial and human relations behaviors and the use of influence strategies that will promote a willingness to follow so that individual and organizational goals can be achieved. Thus, leadership is viewed as multidimensional, encompassing the wise use of power, managerial functions, and human relations processes.*

Leadership can be defined by the behaviors manifested by leaders, by characteristics, or by role enactment. Leadership that is defined only by leadership behavior becomes nonfunctional; in other words, behavior alone cannot be operationalized. If, as is hypothesized, leadership is a learned behavior and therefore can be taught, then it follows that leadership must be defined in some way that makes it feasible to operationalize the definition. For this reason, Dr. Bailey's definition is a highly pragmatic one. Fig. 1 is a model of the interactive flow of the components of leadership as defined. Note the set of actions (processes), the organizational structure (human relationships), and the task (goal setting–goal attainment functions) are all placed within the context of the characteristics and values of the leader and the led, and all the foregoing are placed within the larger context of the external environment.

Management is the manipulation of people, environments, equipment, budgets, and time. It involves many of the same skills as leadership but has a wider range of function, a wider variety of roles, and a more legitimate source of power and authority. In any organization or agency, management involves the following:

1. Planning and providing professional services within the mission and goals of the agency
2. Providing for the continuity of those services
3. Providing for the quality control of those services
4. Managing the budgets and business and financial arrangements that make the services possible
5. Safeguarding the legality of the services
6. Coordinating the environmental services such as equipment, housekeeping, maintenance, and parking
7. Ensuring that support materials, supplies, and services are available

---

*From Claus, K. E., and Bailey, J. T.: Power and influence in health care: a new approach to leadership, St. Louis, 1977, The C. V. Mosby Co.

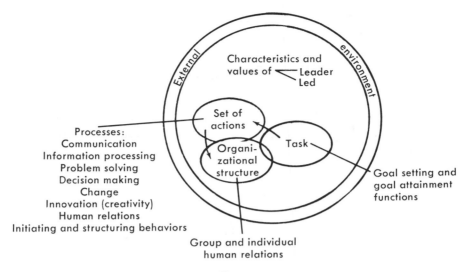

Fig. 1

8. Providing for the improvement of the quality of services through educational programs, library, and information

In addition, management is directly involved in the logistics of nursing care. This means (1) purchasing supplies and materials; (2) transporting these supplies and materials to the areas where they are needed; (3) maintaining storerooms (central supply rooms—CSRs) and supply depots where adequate materials and equipment are on hand; and (4) coordinating dietary, housekeeping, laboratory, and medical services so that nursing services dovetail with them.

Good managers are better if they are also good leaders; however, good leaders may or may not have managerial knowledges and skills. Many of the processes that leaders and managers use are the same. However, most of the functions that managers carry out are not ordinarily functions of the nurse-leader. Traditionally, nursing leadership has been the term used for lower level management—team leaders, assistant head nurses, and staff nurses. Middle management—head nurses and supervisors—have generally been referred to as supervisory personnel, and their roles and functions have been differentiated from those of lower management or nurse leaders. Upper level management—directors of nursing service and their assistants—have usually been referred to as administrators, and their roles and functions have been covered in books on nursing administration. In essence, all managers, regardless of their level or functioning, utilize similar processes. This book concentrates on the common elements of all managerial levels.

Leadership can be assumed. In some groups, it tends to shift from person to person, depending on such relative factors as the area of expertise needed, the energy level of the participants, and the charisma of the people involved. Leadership can be an opportunity of the moment, a dynamic thing that shifts from one person to another as the situation and circumstances demand. Management, on the other hand, is a legitimately designated position. Managers obtain their authority from two sources: supervisors and subordinates. Managers are some-times elected by the people they lead; however, they are always confirmed in their position by the people who employ them and pay their salaries. Sometimes managers are not elected by the people they lead but are imposed from above. This does not relieve these managers of the necessity to constantly validate their power base with those they manage. Managers who are not cognizant of the two sources from which their power is derived will fail to meet the objectives of one group or another and will therefore jeopardize the whole enterprise or their own positions in the organization.

For convenience, the components of leadership and management behaviors have been grouped and dealt with in this book in a variety of ways in appropriate places. Information processing, problem solving, and decision making are covered in the chapter on conceptual framework. The section is labeled problem solving–decision making and includes goal setting and goal attainment. Informa-tion processing encompasses problem solving and learning and is treated here as predictive principle formation. Even though information processing is a larger process than that of formulating predictive principles, the limitations of the book preclude inclusion of the whole subject.

Management principles are covered in Chapter 2; communications, human relationships, and the use of these processes in such contexts as conferences and group dynamics are covered in Chapter 4; initiating and structuring behaviors are dealt with in Chapters 3 and 5; and change and innovation are discussed in Chap-ters 6 and 7. It becomes clear that the complete separation of processes into exclusive categories is an artificial and sometimes arbitrary division. Each of the processes listed as sets of actions in the definition is used interrelatedly with each other process. *Management and leadership involve the ability to use the processes of life to facilitate the movement of a person, a group, a family, or a community toward the establishment and attainment of a goal. Nursing management and leadership involve the ability to use the processes of life to facilitate the move-ment of a person, a group, a family, or a community toward the establishment and attainment of goals pertaining to health.* This includes the manipulation of all factors related to goal pursuit and attainment.

PROCESS—A THEORY ABOUT THE NATURE OF THINGS

Inevitably, words must be used to define other words, and in the definitions of both management and leadership the words "process" and "processing" are used. The word "process" has become popular in education and in nursing during the last twenty years. People refer to *process* teaching, *processing* information, the *process* of problem solving, nursing *process,* and so on. One has but to connect the various ways the word is used and examine the context of its use to observe that the common denominator of meaning is flow, or, as Alfred North Whitehead labels it, flux.* Process is change toward an objective using feedback. Change—flow, flux, dynamics—is in the nature of all things. Some things flow more

---

*Whitehead, A. N.: Process and reality, New York, 1929, Macmillan Publishing Co., Inc.

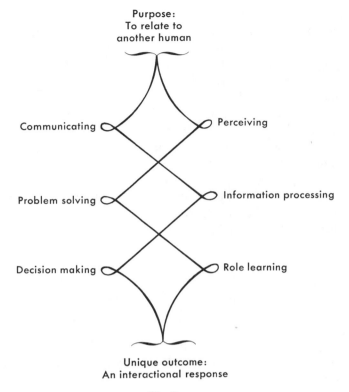

Purpose:
To relate to
another human

Communicating

Perceiving

Problem solving

Information processing

Decision making

Role learning

Unique outcome:
An interactional response

Fig. 2

rapidly than others; the flow of time, measured by the rising and setting of the sun, is more rapid than the flow or change of granite. But even granite, that symbol of permanence, decomposes and crumbles; thus it becomes part of the flux of nature.

Each change, each product of flux, is new and unique from its antecedents; therefore flux is the creative thrust of life. This creativity—uniqueness—comes about from the interaction and the mutually inclusive nature of processes. The result of interaction is that each process does indeed affect the "new" product. Take, for instance, the processes included in the definitions of leadership and management. The process of relating to other humans includes elements of the process of communicating (see Fig. 2). One cannot communicate without processing information; for example, "to relate to" means (1) to perceive; (2) to validate, classify, sort, and interpret the perceptions (which is one way to process data); (3) to solve problems by thinking of alternative responses to the perceived messages; (4) to weigh the consequences of each possible response; and (5) to choose a response and respond to the other human being. Thus in a single encounter in reacting to another human being, the processes of communication, information processing, problem solving, and decision making have all been used to initiate and structure one unique, new, transient act or behavior. Fig. 2 depicts how single processes interact, intertwine, and combine to produce a single new episode—a unique act or behavior. *A process has purpose, organization, and outcome. The purpose is the goal; the organization is the way in which many components or other processes unite to produce the unique outcome. The whole of the three components flow inexorably into the next life episode.*

One of the most common examples used to illustrate the nature of processes is the phenomenon of human reproduction. The purpose of reproduction is to continue the species. Each reproductive episode or successful birth produces a new, unique human being; yet siblings are created from the same antecedents or ancestors. The antecedents or ancestors combine in uniquely organized ways and provide endless genetic combinations to produce an infinite number of possible products, or children—each child different from his sibling.

This concept of flux and flow and the unstoppable nature of this flow are beautifully expressed in the *Rubaiyat* of Omar Khayyám. The entire work is an expression of the flux of life. Captured in these few lines is part of that expression:

> The Moving Finger writes; and, having writ,
> Moves on: nor all your Piety nor Wit
>   Shall lure it back to cancel half a Line,
> Nor all your Tears wash out a Word of it.

A process, to summarize, is the phenomenon of life that hypothesizes that each thing has a purpose, an organization, and an innovative outcome and that each innovative outcome is a result of many unique factors combining purposefully. All managers use process. They combine many factors in ways that produce desired results.

LEARNING LEADERSHIP AND MANAGEMENT ROLES

Leadership and management roles, like other roles, comprise an organized set of behaviors assigned to or assumed by a person. The role of leader can be assumed, but the role of manager is always assigned. The management position can be attained by job description, but the role of leader is often attained by the power that knowledge and skill generate, by assumption of the role, or by investment of power by others. The leadership role is interactional in nature and cannot be learned or enacted out of the social context of complementary roles. In other words, every leader, to be a leader, must have someone, some group, to lead. The role of being led is the role that complements the role of leader. A leader not only must learn the leadership behaviors that enable the assumption of the leadership role, but the leader must also learn the role of the led. Only through learning the complementary role of the led can a leader know and enact the leadership role appropriately.

A role is learned using an entire role set, which includes the role of *leader or manager,* the *complementary* role, and the *audience* (interested others). The complementary role of the led creates the expectation of leadership behavior. Every patient who is led by a nurse has certain behavioral expectations for the nurse, which are communicated in overt and covert ways. The patient may communicate to the nurse-leader the expectation that the nurse will act as information giver, disciplinarian, nurturer or mother figure, authority person, teacher, decision maker, or advocate or will display any number of other behaviors or functions. The better the nurse-leader knows the complementary role of the led, the better the nurse will be able to perform the leadership role.

The audience, or interested others, performs vital functions, even though this group is neither the leader nor the led. For the nurse-leader role the audience may be families, supervisors, administrators, patients, or colleagues, depending on who plays the complementary role of the led. For instance, if the patient is in the complementary role of the led, then families, supervisors, administrators, and colleagues will be the audience. The audience performs the following functions: (1) creates the social reality of the role; (2) gives cues for leadership behaviors, expectations, and role enactment; (3) provides social reinforcement through praise, approval, participation, and rewards; and (4) contributes to the maintenance of the leadership role behavior.

Roles can be either ascribed or achieved. *Ascribed* roles are those roles people are born to or are granted through socialization. The roles of son, daughter, or child are examples of ascribed roles attained through the process of socialization. *Achieved* roles, on the other hand, are roles one aspires to or earns. The role of nurse, for example, is an achieved role. One sets out to learn the nurse role; similarly, one sets out to learn the leader role. Achieved roles are more complex than ascribed roles in that they are superimposed on the ascribed role. Women nurses bring to the role learning of the nurse-leader characteristics and behaviors of the ascribed roles of women in this society—mother, daughter, sister. Similar superimposition of achieved role of nurse-leader on ascribed roles of men—father, brother, son—exists for men nurses.

One of the obvious problems of learning a professional role, such as nursing, is that role preconceptions of anticipatory socialization are simpler and more stereotyped than the reality of the role. The person aspiring to the role of nurse can envision a Sue Barton or a Cherry Ames, both highly stereotyped misconceptions of reality. Therefore a conflict arises because preconceived role expectations do not conform to the complex reality of the role as it must be enacted. Further complications arise when previous learning of ascribed roles conflicts with the learning needs of the achieved roles.

This pyramiding of roles (see Fig. 3) produces highly complex identity and behavioral learning situations. A clear picture of the various roles being played in one life episode enables the player to establish role priorities or role combinations compatible with role expectations of the audience and complementary role players.

According to role theorists, roles must be learned as a Gestalt, or as a whole, total, organized pattern—including both the cognitive and behavioral components. Learning bits and pieces of a role can occur as separate learning episodes, but the success of role enactment depends on the learner's ability to integrate the total set. In other words, learning bits and pieces must be followed by learning the interrelationship of these bits and pieces and insights and behaviors with the total field, or pattern. The implication of this statement for learning leadership and management roles is that this learning must occur in a manner that facilitates

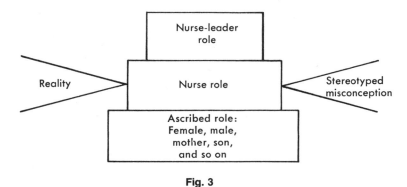

Fig. 3

interaction, either real or simulated, with all characters: leader, led, and audience. Learning each of these roles independently will not result in the ability to enact successfully the leadership role. Practice, with coaching, in situations in which all elements of the leadership set of behaviors occur is necessary for the leadership role to be achieved.

DEFINING ROLES*

The concept of roles in nursing has been defined in a variety of ways but has usually focused on describing the actions nurses perform. As the nurse's responsibilities have changed and expanded, so have the activities, so that descriptive definitions no longer serve the purpose of facilitating role enactment or of making role change. A brief discussion of definitions of role will demonstrate the differences and will highlight the implications the definition has for the nurse's ability to function in a role or to make role change.

Normative definitions. Defining roles using normative criteria means roles are viewed as fixed and standardized. Rules or expectations for behavior associated with a given position or office govern the individual's way of functioning. Cultural norms, the result of values and attitudes ascribed by society, act as a guide for the conduct of the occupant of the role. These same values and attitudes assign roles a status; the rights and privileges that constitute the status of the role must be assumed by the occupant of the role if an overt expression of the rule is to fit the expected norm.

Defining the nurse's role using normative criteria means the nurse's performance is determined by prescribed societal expectations and attitudes. The nurse who deviates from this view may find it difficult to enact the role. For example, men are readily accepted in the role of physician but are sometimes labeled "gay" or "queer" in the nurse's role. Assertive women nurses are often labeled "castrating"; nurses with organizational skills are seen as cold and impersonal; and nurses who cry are viewed as "out of control." In each of the examples, the behaviors labeled were not part of the cultural norm for the nurse role. Labeling is used

*This section is from Bower, F. L.: Nursing process roles and functions of the nurse. In Bower, F. L., and Bevis, E. O.: Fundamentals of nursing: concepts, roles and functions, St. Louis, 1979, The C. V. Mosby Co., pp. 178-181.

in an attempt to explain deviant behavior. In time and with change in societal attitude and expectations, these behaviors may be accepted as the norm.

Role congruency, the compatibility of one role with another, is more likely to occur when role definitions are normative. The "role taker" simply follows the prescribed and predetermined set of expectations. He accepts the expected role behaviors and the rights and privileges that accompany the role and performs accordingly. The role taker knows what to do, and the reciprocal role enactors get what they expect. There are no role conflicts, discrepancies, or role strains. Of course, role change is difficult. In fact, role change depends on the redefinition of the role by *others*.

Perhaps one of the reasons role change for the nurse has been so difficult is that most people have viewed the nurse role from a normative stance.

Situational definitions. Another way to define role is to use situational criteria. A situational definition of role refers to the pattern or type of social behavior that is appropriate in terms of the demands and expectations of the situation in which the role is enacted. Like normative definitions, situational definitions are based on norms, but in this case the norms are set in relationship to the particular set of circumstances of the situation. Defining the nurse's role using situational criteria means the nurse's performance is prescribed and performed in light of its fit with the situation. The nurse in the hospital setting may act quite differently with the client and his family than when in the client's home. In the hospital the nurse is "at home" and has many resources, whereas in the home the nurse is the "visitor" with a very different set of resources.

Acute situations demand role behavior different from that of nonacute ones. In acute situations the nurse's performance may be very different from that when there is time to seek the help of others. For instance, in situations where childbirth is imminent the nurse delivers the baby. If time allowed, that same mother-to-be would be referred to a physician.

Role congruency with situational definitions is variable. Since all those involved in the situation take their cues from "what is happening," conflict could occur if two people responded to the same "cue." Conversely, the situation could define exactly who is to do what. For example, a cardiac arrest in a coronary care unit precipitates actions by nurses and physicians in very definite ways.

Role change with situational definitions is easy. Since the situation defines the performance, the players act in a variety of ways. There are no set norms or prescribed performance expectations—no limits on what the players are sanctioned to do. Unfortunately, this means many persons can decide to perform the same act. The nurse practitioner's role can be defined situationally, since the nurse practitioner and the physician may perform the same act, depending on the situation.

Personal definition. Using a functional perspective to define roles means roles are defined by what players do. Roles are not defined by norms or situations but by how an individual performs when given a particular function to accomplish. Role is the manner in which a person actually functions. Role is influenced by factors other than the stipulation of the office. Role performance has important consequences for the functioning of the group in which the role is performed and important personal consequences for the individual who performs it. Unlike the other definitions, which define role in terms of demands and expectations, functional definitions of role are concerned only with what functions the role player performs. For instance, a coordinator coordinates, teachers teach, and planners plan.

Nurses' roles are often defined in functional terms. Such labels as facilitator, leader, change agent, listener, validator, assessor, data gatherer, and evaluator are used to describe the many nursing roles nurses play. Most recently, nurses have assumed the role of consumer advocate. If nurses' roles were to be defined functionally, the list would be long and encompassing.

In a traditional sense, congruency is difficult with functional definitions, since distinct differences in roles are lacking. Roles overlap as people acting in different positions play the same role. Congruency does occur if there is agreement among the role players that there are no distinct standardized rules to follow or limits on what they can do. A role diffusion results, with functions being enacted by the one who accepts the responsibility, regardless of position or status.

This molding of roles across positions has implications for role learning. Individuals do not have rules of behavior for performance or specified expectations as models for role enactment. Role-specific behaviors are nonexistent. The role aspirant must learn the new role by learning the appropriate role behavior. Appropriate role behaviors are learned in the context of acting out what is *thought* to be appropriate rather than what *should* be done. There are trial and error attempts in role taking. Some individuals find this freedom to determine roles to be stimulating and challenging. For others, it is anxiety provoking.

Functional definitions of role tend to facilitate role change. Since there are no prescribed expectations, the individual is free to try new behaviors. The usual constraints of culturally accepted norms are not present, so the individual defines role by the behavior displayed. This means roles are shared by persons of different status groups and positions. For example, the nurse, physician, psychologist, and psychiatrist diagnose; the administrator, dietician, physical therapist, and nurse are planners; the teacher, student, lawyer, and nurse evaluate. It is possible that people in all these positions are fulfilling many of the same roles. Their differences are not delineated by what they do (functional roles) but by what position they occupy (teacher, physician, nurse, etc.).

Interactional definition. From the standpoint of an interactional definition, roles become more than a prescription for the behavior expected of a person occupying a given position. Role is conceptualized as a constellation of behaviors that emerge out of an interaction between self and others. Role identification becomes the function of how others act and not merely the behavior of self. The individual acts out the role based on the purpose or meaning assigned to the behavior as it relates to the relevant others. For example, the role of nurse may be meaningless or misinterpreted unless it is reciprocated by the role of client. Therefore the interactional concept of role permits the perception and enactment of role as reflective of the other role in the situation.

The interactional concept of role does not deny that certain patterns of behavior are perceived as appropriate for a person occupying a particular position, nor does it imply an expectation-conformity model is incorrect. It does suggest, however, that these approaches are incomplete, since they describe only one of the several bases on which interaction can proceed.

Similarly, role learning and role conflict are viewed in a somewhat different light by the interactionist. Roles are not learned as rules of behavior for performance in isolation. Roles are learned in pairs. In the process of learning a role the role taker learns the role of the relevant other. Thus the recruit in the process of learning the nurse's role is also developing some sense of the behaviors, expectations, attitudes, and desires of the client role.

Role conflict in an interactional framework consists of making compromises so that viable relationships with relevant others can be maintained. Unlike the other definitions of role, the role enacter in an interactional sense does not have to abandon one role in favor of another. The individual is able to shift, alter, and utilize different behaviors within and between role enactment so that conflict is avoided or resolved without too much difficulty.

•   •   •

Although the four definitions presented here offer different views of the concept of role, there are three basic similarities in all the definitions. Individuals assume roles (1) in social locations, (2) with reference to expectations, and (3) with behavior related to the nature of the expectations.

These four definitions of role enactment (normative, situational, personal, and interactional) are presented with the realization that the nurse performs many roles and that role enactment, role change, and role conflict depend on the frame of reference of those who work with or influence the nurse's scope of practice.

THEORIES—THE BASIS OF LEADERSHIP AND MANAGEMENT ACTIVITY*

A theory is an invention of man. Man theorizes to explain or speculate about what something is; what it is like or what its characteristics and attributes are; how something exists in relation to other things; what circumstances or conditions will make things behave in certain ways and what will prevent them from behaving in certain other ways; and, finally, how they can be used in life situations. In other words, a theory enables the nurse-leader/manager to work with others in speculating about problems, to devise hypotheses about alternative solutions to those problems, and to develop ways to test those hypotheses in nursing actions.

The word "theory" can be used in many different ways. People use "theory" to separate the cognitive components from the practical or activity components of a discipline. Sometimes "theory" is used to indicate the speculative as opposed to the proved; sometimes it is used to refer to guesses or hypotheses about how simpler concepts or laws relate to one another; sometimes it is used to mean predictions about how things are going to behave; and sometimes it is used to pre-

---

*This discussion on theory is adapted from Bevis, E. O.: Curriculum building in nursing: a process, ed. 2, St. Louis, 1978, The C. V. Mosby Co.; and derived and synthesized from the works of Dickoff, James, and Wiedenbach; Gagne; and Abdulla and Levine (see bibliography).

scribe ways to make certain behaviors occur. "Theory" has many definitions because it is a complex phenomenon, and all the definitions or meanings just listed do refer to one or more of its aspects (sometimes referred to as levels). Theories evolve through a hierarchy of serial levels. They are still theories, regardless of their level of development. An analogy to this phenomenon of theory levels can be found in Erikson's theory of human development. Human development theory maintains that success in life or human maturity is attained when each central task of development is accomplished, at least in part, in its proper order. Further, full maturity is not attained until these tasks of development are minimally accomplished. In the same manner the attainment of the highest level of theories depends on the successful completion of each prior level of that theory. *Skilled leadership and management exploit a given theory or hypothesis by testing out in practice the validity of the prediction.*

The four levels or phases of theories in practice disciplines

Four stages of development are necessary for a theory to reach its full maturity and thus be optimally useful in nurse management practice. These theory levels are labeled (1) factor isolating, (2) factor relating, (3) situation relating, and (4) situation producing. Basically, nurse management practice relies on the third and fourth levels of theories. The third level of theories is *predictive* theory, and the fourth level is *prescriptive* theory. These two levels enable the nurse to formulate action hypotheses and to construct or prescribe ways in which one can create the environment or the series of events that will allow the prediction (action hypothesis) to come true. However, since a theory to be workable—to have reached its full maturity and have some chance at validity—must have evolved through the prior levels of development, the nurse needs to have a working knowledge of all four levels of theories. In this way, nurse management action hypotheses (or predictive principles) have a much higher validity and reliability than those formulated in the limbo of the third and fourth levels, without reference to or cognizance of the prior two levels.

James Dickoff, Patricia James, and Ernestine Wiedenbach's classic article in *Nursing Research** provides the best source for a clear explanation of theory levels. Presented here is a highly simplified summary of the levels of theory in practice disciplines, as presented in their article.

Level I—Factor-isolating theories. Level I has two activities: (1) naming, or labeling, and (2) classifying, or categorizing.

NAMING. The function of the naming stage is to allow an idea or object to be perceived and talked about or referred to. Once something is named, it is mentionable. One must isolate identifying aspects or factors to recognize that a thing is what it is and not something else—thus the title of this level: factor-isolating theories. Names may be assigned for a variety of reasons: (1) the order of discovery (such as the Caribbean hurricanes—Angela, Bob, Carol, Don); (2) the discoverer or inventor (such as Cushing's disease or Bowman's capsule); (3)

---

*Dickoff, J., James, P., and Wiedenbach, E.: Theory in a practice discipline. Part I. Practice oriented theory, Nurs. Res. **17**(5):415-35, 1968.

function (such as heart-lung machine or walkie-talkie); (4) similarity to other things that have previously been identified and named (such as kidney basin or kidney bean); and (5) description (such as the black-backed three-toed woodpecker).

CLASSIFYING. The second activity in level I is classifying. Classifying is sorting, categorizing, or grouping things according to some commonality. Classifying by commonality requires that the factors or attributes of an object, idea, or thing be *isolated*. The second activity is not possible without the first, that of perceiving and naming, having occurred. Categorizing requires one to identify what something is and what it is not. Categories can be grouped just as single items can be grouped. Grouping or categorizing is possible because of some common denominator or unifying factor. Thus a hierarchy of categories is formed. (*Acute inflammatory response* is a large category that contains subcategories such as *fever* or *local edema*.)

Level II—Factor-relating theories. Level II also contains two activities: (1) depicting, or describing, and (2) relating factors. This level of theory building depicts or describes how one, single, named and classified thing (factor) relates to another single, named and classified thing (factor); thus the title of this level: factor-relating theories. For example, a description of the face requires communication of how the eyes sit in relation to the nose, mouth, ears, and forehead. This level of theory describes relationships to other factors. In other words, it is a "natural history" of any given subject. Any descriptive science, such as anatomy, is an example of factor-relating theory.

Level III—Situation-relating theories. Level III is concerned with causal relationships. It relates one situation to another in a way that allows for prediction. One of the essential ingredients of this level is causal-connecting statements that give a basis for prediction. Prediction is a statement of causal or consequential connections between two states of affairs or two concepts. This level of theory reveals what conditions, circumstances, or behaviors (for example, the cost in time, energy, effort, pain) will promote or inhibit the occurrence of an event or consequence. Dickoff, James, and Wiedenbach consider this level of theory building to be of "incredible importance" to practice. Predictive principles, the format for this book, are in reality third-level theories. They are guides for developing realistic alternatives for nursing actions and are essential to the judgments and decisions of leadership and management. Simply stated, third-level theories tell you that if "A" occurs, "B" will occur. Third-level theories explain what promotes, speeds up, has a catalytic effect, slows down, inhibits, highly correlates with, or prevents something from happening. Promoting or inhibiting theories indicate under what circumstances things will occur and with what speed and effort.

Level IV—Situation-producing theories. Level IV, the final level of theory building, comprises prescriptive theories; it is the level at which theories come to maturity. This level of theory indicates how one arranges the environment and circumstances so that the desired goal is achieved. Situation-producing theories have three aspects—goal, prescription, and survey list.

GOAL. The goal aspect is the simple establishment of a goal. It is the primary act of any problem-solving organism. The nurse-manager and leader is a goal-oriented human whose behavior is geared toward helping others in goal identification and attainment.

PRESCRIPTION. The prescription aspect is a diagram or road map of the specific activities and directions that, when completed, will produce the results predicted in level III (predictive theories) and achieve the desired goal. Prescriptions can be the actual directions for carrying out a plan necessary to achievement of a goal. Both leaders and managers provide prescriptions. The prescriptions of leaders involve lower level—usually direct client care level—work. The prescriptions of managers involve manipulations of all factors enabling successful direct client care.

SURVEY LIST. The survey list contains the dimensions, knowledge, and other resources that might be helpful in structuring or completing the activity and provides the basis for judgments about alternatives in achieving the established goal. Managerial level survey lists are more extensive and far-reaching, involve many other people and departments, and include financial as well as environmental and staff considerations. Leadership level survey lists involve resources and factors directly related to client care.

Summary on theorizing

This book uses as its format predictive theories. Instructions in the construction and use of predictive theories are provided for the nurse learning leadership and management. These instructions will show how second-level theories are used in constructing third-level theories. Problem solving is also one of the primary conceptual constructs of this book. Subsequent discussions will show how problem solving and decision making are, in essence, fourth-level theories. Problem solving produces the judgments and decisions necessary to select the series of actions that will achieve the desired result. In other words, the final act of problem solving is the selection of the series of actions or behaviors (prescriptions) that will produce the desired situation as predicted in the third level of theory building.

PREDICTIVE PRINCIPLES

Utilization of predictive principles in problem solving is based on a knowledge and understanding of theory levels and problem solving. Understanding the composition of a predictive principle and the actions involved in using it is to acquire a *working definition,* or a definition that can be made operational. Real understanding of a definition comes when one has acquired the ability to use the definition in suitable activities. Some activities requiring the use of the definition of a predictive principle are identifying principles either in the literature or in use, constructing specific principles using the component parts (lower level theories) appropriately, and using principles in solving problems.

The following section begins with a working definition of a predictive principle and proceeds through the use of principles in solving a problem. This is designed to guide the nurse to an increased understanding of principles and enables the practitioner to use principles in activites that require leadership.

Definition

For use in this book, *a predictive principle is defined as a set of circumstances, conditions, or behaviors that produces a given, definable outcome*. A principle expresses relationships of conditions, circumstances, or behaviors to predictable consequences. A predictive theory is a nursing action hypothesis. Predictive principles differ from facts or concepts in that a fact or concept need only be valid, whereas a predictive principle, in addition to being valid, must predict outcomes. Principles are derived from authoritative sources or through scientific observation, experimentation, or compilation of data. Predictive principles are third-level theories.

The predictive relationships that exist between the circumstances, conditions, or behaviors and the predicted outcome or consequence of those circumstances, conditions, or behaviors can best be articulated by the use of an active verb or verb clause that is causal connecting in a predictive way.

Predictive relationships may also be shown in two other ways:

1. "If-then"—if this happens, then this will happen.
2. Proportions—the greater this, the greater or less that.

Cause and effect relationships can be stated in future perfect ways because predictions are, in essence, an educated guess about what will happen in the future.

The following is an example of the definition in use. The example provides four different ways to state the same prediction and is fragmented into its component parts for illustrative purposes. In this book the word "valid" is used to mean empirically true, that is, that available evidence supports rather than refutes the predicted outcome.

EXAMPLE 1

Circumstances, conditions, or behaviors	Active verb phase	Given, definable outcome
A. Having knowledge pertinent to the current situation	assists the leader in making	valid judgments and decisions
B. The leader who has knowledge pertinent to the current situation	will be able to make	valid judgments and decisions
C. If the leader has knowledge pertinent to the situation	then he will be able to make	valid judgments and decisions
D. The greater his knowledge about the situation	the more likely the leader will be to make	valid judgments and decisions

Henceforth, for the purpose of brevity, the "circumstances, conditions, or behaviors" referred to in the preceding definition shall be known as the *CCB triad;* the "given, definable outcome" shall be known as the *predicted outcome* or the PO.

Developing principles

In the development of principles three separate stages of cognitive activity are required. These three stages are also the first three levels of theory building.

1. Identifying or accumulating facts and experiences or isolating and classifying factors (level I theory)
2. Depicting and describing factors or experience commonalities and relationships (a high-order conceptualization and level II theory)
3. Relating circumstances, conditions, and behaviors (situations) to consequences (level III theory)

Facts and theories can be fairly easily and rapidly identified and acquired through processes that enable and promote recall. Experiences (mental, emotional, and physical) allow for the further acquisition or retention of facts through the usage of learned material. Acquisition of facts could include such information as anatomy, physiology, or hospital or agency structure.

When facts begin to form a pattern and are applicable to several experiences, they become the second stage of cognitive activity, the formulation of concepts. For use in this book, *a concept is a classification of experiences that have similar properties:* the recognition of commonalities for the purpose of useful classification. Concepts can be communicated to others. They can be converted into words or phrases that represent the ideas, objects, characteristics, or behaviors held together in groupings by the commonality. Concepts are the way people categorize experiences so that mental filing systems have organization. Concepts grow and enlarge as the number and variety of an individual's experiences increases. As examples, a compilation of facts, experiences, and observations concerning anatomy and physiology and the perception by the individual form the basis for the concept of pain. Facts related to hospital or agency structure serve as a basis for the formation of the concept of hierarchy. This activity is level II of theories.

The third stage in the development of principles is relating concepts to predict outcomes. This is a complex, but useful, thinking process because predictive principles show the relationship between concepts. *A predictive principle shows the relationship between the concept(s) drawn from the CCB triad and the concept(s) of the predicted outcome.* The concepts of *motivation* and *learning* will be used for illustrative purposes.

Motivation is a condition and is an example of a concept used as a CCB triad. Learning is an outcome and is an example of a concept used as the predicted outcome. Many discussions of the relationship motivation has to learning can be found in the literature. An observer of the learning process quickly recognizes that there is an inherent relationship between motivation and learning. The effect these two concepts have on each other can be expressed in a principle. The principle's components are separated in example 2.

EXAMPLE 2

CCB triad	Active verb phase	PO
Being motivated	influences	learning

This principle is simple and direct but lacks specificity and direction. The use of qualifiers gives principles increased usefulness. This is illustrated in the following way:

EXAMPLE 3

Having qualifiers	CCB triad	Active verb phase	Qualifiers	PO
Being highly	motivated	influences	the rate of	learning

In the examples used thus far the CCB triad has always been on the left and the predicted outcome on the right. This is not necessary to the construction of a principle. To change the order of the concepts one need only change the orientation of the active verb phase. The order of the concepts used in example 1 can be reversed as follows:

EXAMPLE 4

PO	Active verb phase	CCB triad
Valid judgments and de-cisions	result more frequently when the leader has	knowledge pertinent to the current situation

The definition of a principle and the examples of principles used imply that the CCB triad with its qualifiers describes the environment, activities, knowledge, skills, or state of being necessary to make the predicted outcomes occur. The CCB triad is the concept subject matter and contains the necessary qualifying descriptions for the formation of principles. The CCB triad and its qualifiers can be positive or negative.

It is important to know what will produce, aid, ensure, or promote a desired outcome; however, it can be equally useful to know what will inhibit, prevent, or block a desired outcome. In the four examples given the principles have been positive in nature. Negative CCB triads indicate what will not achieve the predicted outcome and, therefore, are used to formulate negative principles. These are inhibiting theories in level III of theory building. The following states the principle in example 1 negatively:

CCB triad	Active verb phase	PO
Lack of knowledge pertinent to the current situation	inhibits the leader's ability to make	valid judgments and de-cisions

The active verb phase may also contain qualifiers. These are words that relate the CCB triad to the predicted outcome and may also tell who, how far, how much, how often, or what action takes place. Some words that indicate positive action are *facilitate, precipitate, aid, result in, determine, assist, influence, promote, ensure, contribute to, enhance,* and *enable.* Note that most of the action words suggested have limitations by definition. For instance, *facilitate* means to "make easy or less difficult," whereas *ensure* means to "make certain." The difference is important because the choice of the connecting action words helps to determine the validity of the principle. Some action words that indicate negative action are *inhibit, prevent, discourage, negate, invalidate, obviate, preclude, deter,* and *damage.* Active verbs, in addition to indicating the positive or negative direction of the activity, can, with qualifying phrases, indicate person. *Person* is the one who perpetrates the activity, for example, the nurse-leader, the learner, the patient, the ancillary worker, the student, or the group. It is not essential that person be indicated but to do so promotes clarity and specificity. The following illustrates how different active verbs and persons alter the principle:

EXAMPLE 5

CCB triad	Active verb phrases and person(s)	PO
Having knowledge pertinent to the current situation	(a) ensures that the leader makes (b) aids the group in making (c) promotes the making of (d) facilitates the making of (e) results in the group's making (f) helps the nurse-leader to make (g) enables the group to make	valid judgments and decisions

Example 5 indicates the variety of ways cause-and-effect relationships of a principle may be linked together. Choices depend on the situation under consideration.

Clarity is achieved through accurate, concise statements of principles that are positive instead of negative, are logical in their sequence, and contain connecting words and phrases that produce valid principles.

The Appendix contains detailed directions for formulating predictive principles. Nurses attempting to improve their leadership and management skills will find predictive principle formulation a valuable tool for acquiring and storing knowledge in a form useful for rapid decision making. Knowledge storage and retrieval in the form of facts makes no use of the practice implications. Predictive principles tie facts and experiences to practice consequences and thus are more useful to nurse practitioners.

The Appendix also contains a few common construction errors made by the novice in predictive principle formulation.

USING PRINCIPLES IN NURSING PROCESS

Nursing process, in essence, is dealing appropriately with nursing problems to bring about effective solutions. Organizing ideas and facts into predictive principles enables the nurse-leader/manager to have a clear, categorized fund of knowledge for immediate use in solving nursing problems. However, the acquisition of a body of knowledge in the form of practical and usable predictions is only part of the problem facing the nurse who wishes to be a proficient leader and manager. Predictive principles will have relevance only for the nurse who judiciously applies them to identified problems. Predictive principles are guides for developing realistic alternatives of action. The use of predictive principles is a process that requires (1) identification of the real problem; (2) selection of the appropriate, valid, and relevant principle(s); (3) identification of alternatives for action sequential to the selected principle(s); (4) the ability to select one or more of the alternatives; and (5) the ability to prescribe the ways and means to actualize the alternative selected.

Initially this is a slow, laborious process, but through repeated application to various types of problems the process becomes a behavior habit. Habits of thinking beget habits of behavior. Habits are developed after thoughts or activities are repeated in the same pattern or way until the behaviors become customary. Habits are characterized by automaticity (without deliberation). Any skill, whether it is intellectual or manual, involves habits. (Even bed making was a slow process for the nurse at first.)

The mechanics of problem solving (nursing process) using predictive principles is a habit, not a reflex. Reflexes are inborn and inherent in the nervous system of the being; habits are learned. The answers to problems or possible alternatives of action do not materialize automatically; it is the *process* of arriving at the best possible alternatives that becomes the habit. When this process becomes habitual, the nurse-leader/manager will automatically use the predictive principles approach to nursing process when faced with nursing problems. This means that each step in the process may lose its identity, become blurred, and may not be conscious; nevertheless, the process takes place. Arriving at this degree of skill requires consistent, repeated, conscious practice with positive reinforcement of successful use of the process.

Acquiring skill in problem solving must be reconciled with the needs of patients and the demands of agencies for ongoing nursing services. Nurses cannot cease activities or leave patients or team members in suspended animation and adjourn to the library to read about a topic and formulate principles. Real nursing problems, whether obvious or obscure, usually require some immediate action. Formulating and acquiring a list of principles, learning an organized methodology for problem solving, and enlarging the problem-solving tool chest and the critical thinking necessary to select the most effective nursing interventions are skills that must be learned initially in situations that permit time and freedom to err. One effective method is to allot a specified interval when the involved personnel are relieved of nursing responsibilities and can work through the nursing process. Reality can be preserved by using problem situations observed in practice by the involved nurses.

Learning nursing process by using real problems in the class or conference room is a simulated problem-solving situation. Simulation, for the purpose of learning the role of problem solver, allows for the practice of skills in a safe, non-threatening environment. Neither the nurse nor the patient or client can be severely damaged in a simulated environment. Mistakes in judgment, errors of commission or omission, are without deadly consequences. Yet, actual practice, an essential ingredient for learning any role, can be available. In the simulated learning situation, coaching can take place, complementary roles can be learned, the audience (classmates) can participate, and competence in decision making and other leadership skills can be acquired. However, although competence can be gained in simulated situations, only reality enactment of the role can provide confidence in the nurse for that role.

After knowledge of principles and their use in solving nursing problems has been acquired, nurse-leaders can apply this knowledge to solve obvious nursing problems within the real situation with success and without disruption of necessary activities. The solving of complex or obscure problems frequently takes time and involves groups of people. The results of this group effort are (1) an increased awareness by the nursing group of nursing problems, (2) increased quality of nursing services for patients, (3) broadening and deepening of the individual care giver's group nursing skill, and (4) utilization of each care giver's potential contribution to patient care. Management problems are handled by individual managers or committees, depending on the circumstances, the urgency, and the complexity of the problem.

Problem solving is a process. A process is an organization of many components, parts, other processes, and tasks to achieve an explicit purpose. The outcome of this combination of many factors is one unique episode, act, task, factor, thing, person, or process. The discussion of the processes of problem solving will be clearer if problems are divided into two categories—obvious and obscure. *Obvious* problems are problems open to view. In nursing, they usually originate from procedures, schedules, timing, machinery, and work loads. *Obscure* problems are most frequently problems of behavior, communication, or interpersonal relations. Obscure problems are usually complicated by emotional overtones and loss of objectivity. In general, the more human interaction in an event or situation, the more difficult the identification and solution of the problem. Even overt problems may be difficult for the nurse-leader to identify because of strong distracting stimuli or inattention to or breakdown in the processes preliminary to identifying the problem.

The processes that produce clear and accurate problem identification are the same for both obvious and obscure problems; however, the steps for identifying obscure problems may be much more protracted than those used when identifying obvious problems.

Problems are continually being solved by every individual. It is impossible to go through life without some kind of successful problem solving, either conscious or unconscious, formal or informal. Problem solving is one of the most important elements of leadership and management. It becomes increasingly important that nurses enter the practice of nursing prepared to engage in an organized problem-solving process. One of the basic tenets of any group practice of nursing is that groups collectively are more productive, more efficient, and more effective than the sum of their individual members. The inclusion of other nursing care givers in problem solving whenever possible or appropriate ensures group commitment to the solution. This activity also improves esprit de corps, taps the abilities of each individual member, and gives the group the benefit of diverse thinking. The group process is slow at first but functions more rapidly as the group gains skill in problem solving together.

Problem solving has two aspects that nursing leaders and managers must utilize: (1) the tools or heuristics of problem solving and (2) the facets or phases of problem solving.

Problem-solving heuristics

Problem-solving heuristics are tools, techniques, or devices people use to solve problems. Whereas problem-solving facets or stages are aspects of problem solving (such as assessment, problem identification, and data gathering), problem-solving heuristics are the activities one uses in each facet to complete the tasks appropriate to that facet. For instance, some tools one might choose to use for assessment are looking, observing, questioning, or assuming. For problem identification, one might use the activities of guessing, supposing, analyzing, categorizing, synthesizing, or generalizing. Characteristically, every nurse-leader and every person being led has favorite problem-solving tools. Some people are impulsive and just *leap in;* some *think the problem through* from the beginning to the conclusion; and some *work backward* from a possible solution to the necessary supporting data. Some people tend to *meditate* or *cogitate* over problems; others let an idea *incubate* and come to a decision without conscious thought ("sleep on it"). The wider the range of problem-solving heuristics available to the leader/manager, the more likely he will be to have at his disposal tools that will enable him to arrive at adequate decisions. No one heuristic or device is better than another; each has its use, depending on the group, the leader, the problem, and the situation. Every leader/manager must take inventory of his problem-solving tools, especially those he uses most frequently. He needs to watch and talk with others to find out what tools others use. By adding to his own tool chest and helping others add to theirs, he will expand his problem-solving skills and be more effective in facilitating the problem solving of others. Interaction Associates* has developed a list of problem-solving tools in common usage and has developed ways and means for facilitating the expansion of the tool repertoire for problem solvers.

Facets or phases of nursing process

Nursing process has four phases, facets, or stages. The term "facets" is used here because the terms "phases" and "stages" communicate an order to the sequence of activities. Although listed here from problem identification to the judgment or decision, actual nursing process is seldom followed in that set sequence. The human mind tends to work backward and forward between aspects of problem solving until completion or decision is reached. The development of data, alternatives, and other considerations throws light on aspects of the problem previously developed, so that the whole changes; this flux is the process nature of problem solving. Each facet of nursing process contains the tasks necessary for successful completion of that facet. No facet is static; each facet is dynamic, for information uncovered in one facet may alter the significance of information uncovered in previous facets.

The following four facets of nursing process are in sequential form, and the tasks necessary to each facet are given. The following nursing problem is considered throughout to illustrate the use of this process.

Problem: An aide on a nursing team failed to give oral care to the patients assigned to him.

PROBLEM-SOLVING FACET I: PROBLEM IDENTIFICATION (ASSESSMENT)

Following are the tasks involved in problem identification:
1. Observe an event or situation.

*Strategy notebook, San Francisco, 1972, Interaction Associates.

2. Obtain relevant, valid, accurate, detailed descriptions from appropriate people or sources.
3. Write a description of the situation.
4. Discard irrelevant or questionable data.
5. Isolate the tentative problem and state it concisely.

Task 1—Observe an event or situation. The first task of the problem identification facet is the recognition that a problem needs to be identified. It seems unnecessary to say that one must have a problem before the problem can be solved, but it is an important maxim. Problems, by definition, are a question or a perplexity. This means a process, activity, or normal progression of events has been interrupted, altered, or disturbed in some way. It means someone believes that the situation is not optimal or that expectations have not been met.

Nursing students are often given case histories of patients with directions to identify the nursing problems. In reality, these students are being asked to identify areas of nursing care necessary to the health of the patient. Specific problems cannot be identified without an event or situation in which a team leader's normal expectations have not been met:

> While functioning as a leader of a team of nursing personnel on an acute medical care unit, the nurse notes that an aide on the team is not giving oral care to the patients assigned to him.

The team leader having observed this event or situation proceeds to task 2.

Task 2—Obtain relevant, valid, accurate, detailed descriptions from appropriate people or sources. Accurate descriptions and observations are the forte of nursing; however, continued practice and study in this realm are necessary for maintaining and improving skill. Teaching observational skills to all nursing care givers will result in increasingly better nursing care. After one nurse-leader had repeatedly sensitized the ancillary personnel to accurate descriptions, an aide was asked in casual conversation if she had seen the director of nurses' new car. The aide answered that she had. The nurse-leader inquired about the color of the car. The aide responded that it was "blue on the side toward me." Although the aide's answer was facetious, this kind of cautious accuracy will increase the speed and validity of solving nursing problems through accurate and objective observations and reports.

Good results can be obtained by the nurse-leader/manager if effective interviewing skills are exercised. Descriptions of situations collected from all individuals concerned can become confused and subjective if inappropriate questions are posed. Desired information can be obtained if the nurse-leader/manager asks such questions as "What happened?" "What preceded the event?" "What followed then?" "What else was going on while this was occurring?" "How did you feel about the incident?" Further data can be obtained by leading statements such as "Tell me more about that," "Help me to understand the events." Sometimes simple listening postures and sounds are enough. Oh? Yes? And then . . .?

Open-ended questions and statements such as these will assist the nurse-leader/manager and those involved to separate feelings from facts, achieve objectivity, and formulate a more vivid description of the problem.

For example, the nurse-leader/manager gathers the following descriptive information from appropriate sources:

1. There are twenty patients assigned to the nursing team on the given day; all but five are seriously ill.
2. Basic technical care to be administered to the twenty patients includes ten complete bed baths, five partial bed baths, five showers, and twenty beds to be changed; seven patients must be fed their meals.
3. One nurses' aide scheduled to work on the team failed to report to work because of illness. A replacement was not available.
4. Some team members had complained of overwork and expressed feelings of injustice.
5. The aide not giving oral care has been employed in this health agency for one month.

Task 3—Write a description of the situation. The nurse-leader/manager will find it helpful to take notes on the descriptions of the event as reported by all those concerned with the problem situation. Summarizing the descriptions in a short, concise, clear paragraph that contains all relevant material will aid the nurse-leader/manager in clarifying the event. When events are in written form, it is much easier to identify material that does not contribute to the description of the problem situation. Writing helps to crystalize thinking and is a valuable step in problem identification. A paragraph description of the problem situation is written here:

An aide who has been employed one month is not giving oral care to patients assigned to him. Team members feel overworked with one unreplaced absent member. There are twenty patients, ten who need complete care and seven who need feeding.

Task 4—Discard irrelevant or questionable data. Data that are irrelevant or of questionable use in identifying the problem may be of considerable use when gathering data for the solution of the problem. Superfluous material in the descriptive situation increases the confusion and difficulty of isolating the problem. These same data may be helpful at a different stage of problem solving. Here is the described situation with noncontributory material deleted:

An aide who has been employed one month is not giving oral care to patients assigned to him.

Task 5—Isolate the tentative problem and state it concisely. Problem identification is a dynamic, not static, process. As information is gathered subsequent to the implementation of principles, it may become necessary to alter the original identified problem so that reality and accuracy are preserved. Identified problems should always be considered tentative or subject to change by the group or leader. When identified problems are labeled "tentative," there is greater willingness on the part of those participating in problem solving to change the identification of the problem. Groups and individuals can change the identified "tentative" problem with less embarrassment and fewer feelings of inadequacy than they can a "definite" problem.

The temptation for the beginning problem solver is to put conclusions about why the aide is not giving oral care into the statement of the problem. Following are two possible erroneous statements of the problem:

1. Aide not giving oral care because he resents his work load.
2. Aide inadequately oriented to ward routines and does not know he should give oral care.

Such guessing wastes time in idle speculation and leads to a search for substantiation of the hypothesis rather than selection of the appropriate principles and consequent activities necessary to the efficient and objective solution of the problem. Problems are easier to solve if stated as questions. Following is a concise statement of the problem:

How to ensure that oral care is given to patients.

PROBLEM-SOLVING FACET II: SELECTION OF APPROPRIATE PRINCIPLES (THEORIZING)

Following are the tasks involved in selecting the appropriate principles:
1. Determine topic(s) or area(s) of principles relevant to the subject.
2. Formulate the principles of the determined area or topic from authoritative sources appropriate to the tentative problem, or select appropriate list of principles from a cumulative file.
3. Select the specific principles applicable to the problem based on validity, relevance, and practicality.
4. List principles in the order they may be used most effectively.

Selection of appropriate principles depends totally on the proper identification of the problem. Principles useful to the solution of the problem will be selected only if the correct problem has been identified.

Task 1—Determine topic(s) or area(s) of principles relevant to the subject. Selection of the topic or subject of the principles is done by determining the subject area to which the problem relates. For example, if the nurse-leader/manager concerned in this situation had identified the problem as "inadequate orientation," his principle area would have been "teaching-learning." Had he identified the problem as "resentment of work load," his principle area would have been "team spirit." However, the identification of the failure to carry out properly a job assignment clearly put the area of necessary principles as "delegation of authority."

Task 2—Formulate the principles of the determined area or topic from authoritative sources appropriate to the tentative problem, or select appropriate list of principles from a cumulative file. Nurse-leaders/managers who utilize the principles method of problem solving accumulate large numbers of principles from which to draw. If the leader or group has no list of principles for the area selected, the principles will have to be compiled as discussed earlier in this chapter. However, if a list has been compiled, it should be examined for inclusiveness. If additional principles are needed, they must be formulated from authoritative sources and added to the list.

Nursing problems frequently require the utilization of principles from several subject areas. In the interest of simplicity a problem has been chosen that can be satisfactorily solved using principles from one subject area. The following is a partial list of principles of delegation of authority from Chapter 4.

1. Written descriptions of policies, procedures, and/or guidelines by which an employee can handle situations when they occur promote ease of operation for the care giver and control of the authority delegated by the nurse-leader/manager.
2. Member participation in the formulation of policies, job descriptions, and procedures increases member cooperation.
3. The philosophy and policies of a health agency determine the pattern of the nursing care delivery system to be provided.
4. Guidelines, such as established channels, methods, and provisions for communication within an agency, enable the nurse-leader/manager to delegate tasks and authority appropriately.
5. Clear lines of communication promote morale among organization members and enhance goal accomplishment.
6. A sufficient number of prepared personnel allows effective delegation of authority to meet organizational and patient needs.
7. Matching the abilities of the care givers to the jobs to be done increases work productivity and individual job satisfaction.
8. Assignments that have clearly defined standards and goals provide a basis for measurement of outcome.
9. Frequent comparison of actual performance with criteria determines the quality of care and the level of actual performance.

Task 3—Select the specific principles applicable to the problem based on validity, relevance, and practicality. It is apparent that only selected principles within an area apply to a given problem. Some problems may require the use of only one or two principles for a solution to be reached; others may require many principles. The number of principles selected depends on the nature of the problem.

After careful consideration the nurse-leader/manager decides that the problem can be solved using principles 1, 4, 5, 7, 8, and 9. Principles 2, 3, and 6 are not relevant.

The nurse-leader/manager will evaluate each principle selected using the criteria of validity, relevance, and practicality. Principle 5 will be used as a model.

PRINCIPLE: Clear lines of communication promote morale among organization members and enhance goal accomplishment.

This principle is valid because if lines of communication are not clear or are not followed, mistrust develops rapidly in a group and morale decreases. For example, if the delegator has been unaware of the activities of each nurse's aide, all team members might have been confronted for an explanation of the lack of good hygienic care. The use of this haphazard approach not only may offend the workers who are doing their jobs correctly but also may cause the team member involved to feel justified in offering retaliatory remarks such as "You should have known that these patients were mine; you assigned them to me, so why didn't you come to me for an explanation?" The new employee may also feel insecure in his position and therefore take other means of self-defense; these usually involve "grapevine" activity that undermines the nurse as an effective leader and manager.

The principle is relevant, for if the team leader knows to whom the responsibility for the patients involved is delegated, immediate personal contact can be established with that particular team member. The nurse-leader/manager can then obtain immediate feedback about what is going on and why it is occurring.

The principle is practical because it will work at the time and place needed within the natural limits of the situation.

Task 4—List principles in the order they may be most effectively used. Principles show outcomes, and outcomes usually have a logical, necessary, desirable sequence. For example, the nurse-leader/manager has channels-of-communication guidelines established by the agency; using those guidelines ensures that actions are within designated authority. Using established, designated lines of authority the nurse-leader/manager must take steps to ensure that the job descriptions, policies, and procedures include the assigned tasks and are available to each aide. The process of arranging principles in their logical order of use continues until all selected principles are arranged in an ordered sequence. The order in which the principles selected for the example problem can be most effectively used is as follows:

1. Guidelines such as established channels, methods, and opportunities for communication within an agency enable the nurse-leader/manager to delegate responsibility appropriately (4).
2. Written descriptions of policies and procedures by which an employee can handle situations when they occur promote ease of operation for the team member and control of the authority delegated by the team leader (1).
3. Frequent comparison of actual performance with assignment determines the level of actual performance (9).
4. Clear lines of communication promote morale among organization members and enhance goal accomplishment (5).
5. Matching the abilities of the team members to the jobs to be done increases work productivity and individual job satisfaction (7).
6. Assignments that have clearly defined standards and goals provide a basis for measurement of outcome (8).

Flexibility in both selection and order of application of principles is important. The result of an action dictated by a principle may necessitate substitution of one or more subsequent principles. The nurse-leader/manager familiar with all the important principles of a given area or topic finds flexibility easy to maintain.

PROBLEM-SOLVING FACET III: DETERMINING ALTERNATIVES FOR ACTION (PLANNING)

Following are the tasks involved in determining alternatives for action:
1. Determine all alternative courses of action that are a natural consequence of each principle.
2. Determine who will select the course of action.
3. Select the courses of action to be instigated and establish a serial order for implementation.
4. Evaluate selected alternatives for practicality. This requires determining if the proposed courses of action are:
   a. within the philosophy of the agency

    b. supported by the administration

    c. reasonable investments of time, energy, equipment, and money

    d. technologically current, yet within the abilities of the group

    e. assessed for safety and risk probability

    f. legally and morally acceptable to the nurse, group, and patient

    g. planned in conjunction with those who are most concerned with the problem (physician, patient's family, social services, occupational therapy, physical therapy, or rehabilitation personnel)

Facet III is a planning facet. Determining alternatives for action is a selective process in which one deliberates about the principles and the possible courses of action that arise from the principles, determines who must select the course of action, and attempts to establish the best *order* for implementing actions. Facet III is not the facet in which intervention behaviors occur; it is the facet in which plans, preparations, and decisions about intervention are made. Rapid judgments and decisions can be made by the nurse-leader/manager, or discussions may be held with appropriate people.

Task 1—Determine all alternative courses of action that are a natural consequence of each principle. Since a "principle" is by definition a circumstance, condition, or behavior that produces a given definable outcome, activities are the natural extension of a principle. The activity consequence of a principle can take any number of forms, depending on the specific problem and ramifications of that problem. Consideration of a variety of alternative courses of action increases the probability of choosing a workable course of action. However, any activity considered must comply with the dictates of its antecedent principle.

In the example used here the following principle has been selected as the model: *Clear lines of communication promote morale among organization members and enhance goal accomplishment.* This principle indicates that the existence of "clear lines of communication" is a condition necessary to maintenance of morale and accomplishment of goals. Clear lines of communication can be achieved in a variety of ways, depending on the people and circumstances involved. Behaviors that lead to clear lines of communication are tailored to each problem or situation.

Following are some suggested alternatives for establishing clear lines of communication in the example situation:

1. Go immediately to the aide and ask for a conference.
2. Wait until there is a natural pause in his work and ask him to come for a conference.
3. Wait until his work is over for the morning and request a conference.
4. Go to the aide and tell him you wish to speak to him as soon as he is free.
5. Give him a note asking him to come and see you as soon as possible.

The best way to establish clear lines of communication depends on the people involved and the circumstances. The nurse-leader/manager must consider all alternatives and select the best for each situation.

Task 2—Determine who will select the course of action. Selecting the course of action to be taken may not always be the responsibility of the nurse-leader/manager. If the situation involves policy, procedure, patient safety or treatment, or cultural, religious, emotional, or interpersonal matters, the nurse may be compelled by policy, law, safety of the patient, or good judgment to involve other people in the selection of the appropriate course of action. In this example the *nurse-leader/manager* will be the one to choose the alternatives to be used.

Task 3—Select the courses of action to be instigated and establish a serial order for implementation. As shown in task 1, each principle has one or more courses of action. In task 3 the nurse-leader/manager must select the most effective actions from the list suggested in task 1. When the decision is made concerning the available alternative to be used, the order in which the courses of action are to be actualized must be determined. These activities are nursing action prescriptions and are in part level IV of theory building. The selected courses of action derived from the selected principles and arranged in the appropriate order for this situation would be as follows:

1. Seek out the aide in question.
2. Arrange a meeting in private with the aide.
3. Gather data that would determine the aide's:
    a. level of understanding of role
    b. ability to fulfill expectations
    c. reaction to the incident
    d. rationale for omission
4. Request the aide to give oral care to patients assigned to him (providing necessary assistance, teaching, and supervision).
5. Evaluate overall patient assignment to ensure continuing orientation and practice commensurate with experience and ability of all personnel.
6. Establish time for future conference.

Task 4—Evaluate selected alternatives for practicality. Practicality is an important consideration. Prescribed action must be possible within a given framework at a specific time and place. "Common sense" or intuition is not sufficient. Social, physical, and biologic science factors must be considered when testing principles for practicality. The practicality of any plan of action can be assessed through the use of the following criteria:

a. *Within the philosophy of the agency.* If the selected alternative is not within the philosophy of the agency, it is inappropriate for the nurse-leader/manager to pursue that particular action. Policy is not the same as philosophy, but it reflects philosophy. For example, the philosophy of an agency may state that basic nursing care is to be provided or administered to every patient. Policy would then dictate that the one assigned to give care would follow through with the commitment.

b. *Supported by the administration.* Administration and high level management backing usually implies that policies and procedures have been formulated and that orientation has been provided. In the situation under question the nurse's aide, although a new employee, would have been exposed to appropriate procedure through in-service programs and supervision and would have had an opportunity to review the procedure manual any time a need was felt.

c. *Reasonable investment of time, energy, equipment, and money.* Nurses have responsibilities for providing care to patients. Regardless of the agency involved, each patient is entitled to receive services according to his needs and according to the commitment of the agency to meet those needs.

The nurse-leader/manager need not expend time and energy to determine whether the service of oral hygiene should have been administered. All data support the need for this service. The next logical step is to investigate equipment. Were supplies available for the administration of oral hygiene? If not, why not? If so, why were they not used? The economic factor could play a part in this situation, depending on the philosophy of the institution. The health agency might expect each patient to provide his own equipment. If so, does the patient have supplies? When the institution provides equipment, supplies cannot be considered always available or unlimited in number. These are areas in which energy need be expended. The nurse-leader/manager should have someone available to check nonnursing details, but in every case the responsibility for determining facts lies with the delegator of authority.

When emergencies arise, such as a reduction in the number of personnel, some goals are sacrificed and priorities among patients' needs are established. The authority figure will have the knowledge necessary to make judgments about the importance of oral hygiene in providing for the needs of an ill patient.

The leader of the nursing team will seek out the nurse's aide to find answers about why oral hygiene was not administered to the patients assigned to him.

d. *Technologically current, yet within the abilities of the group.* The field of technology includes scientific knowledge and mechanical and procedural skills. The investigator must know if the nurse's aide failed to administer oral hygienic care because of a lack of knowledge or skill. If lack of knowledge or skill is the reason, remedial steps are in order. The leader knows there has been a breakdown in initial or continuing orientation.

There is a lag between current technology and workers' knowledge and abilities to implement technology. The field of oral hygiene has moved away from a simple gargle or a few strokes of a brush into a procedure that depends on knowledge of anatomy and physiology, bacteriology, and dental hygiene. Patients have a right to the most technologically advanced care available, and nurses and employers need to keep abreast of advancements in order to provide the best care possible.

e. *Safety assessed and risk probability established.* Safety is always a primary consideration in selecting nursing interventions. Safety cannot be assumed for any act that has inherent risk. When selecting a realistic, usable alternative of action, one must consider what the gains and losses will be for patient, family, nurse, and hospital. Weighing risks and ascertaining the alternative that gives greatest benefit to the recipient of the action, with the least possibility of damage, can become quite complicated. The process can be compared to item pricing. If one goes out to buy a pair of shoes, one wishes to know how much quality and service can be obtained for how much money. All shoes cost something. The question becomes "Is the expected purchase worth the price?" There are times when the contemplated actions are simply not worth the risks involved, whether a health and safety risk or a social-interpersonal risk.

In the situation under consideration the team leader, in telling the aide about the omission of mouth care and asking for clarification, risks several things, among which are the following:

1. Offending or embarrassing the aide
2. Damaging rapport or relationships
3. Being placed in the vulnerable position of being asked why oral hygiene is important

If the omission is allowed to continue and nothing is done, the nurse-leader/ manager risks the following:

1. Reinforcing unacceptable behavior by silent consent
2. Allowing patient health, hygiene, and comfort to suffer
3. Criticism from team members who do give mouth care

Implementation of alternatives for each principle carries with it risks that must be evaluated. Actions and interventions will then be actualized in full knowledge of the risks, and preparation can be made in anticipation of consequences.

f. *Legally and morally acceptable to the nurse, group, and patient.* Since nursing practice is governed by local, state, and federal regulations, most personnel are aware of basic laws concerning the practice of nursing. There are ample sources of reference if legal or moral issues become a question.

In the nursing situation posed the nurse-leader/manager must be convinced that the nurse's aide did not omit oral hygienic care because of laziness. Serious moral and legal implications are presented if negligence is established. The supervisor of care realizes the possibilities of infection, malnutrition, and other problems that can occur as a result of omission of this important part of care.

g. *Planned in conjunction with those who are most concerned with the problem.* Many alternative solutions to problems involve members of other disciplines, whether the problem be patient centered or organization oriented.

In the nursing situation under discussion the nurse's aide may need additional classes with the in-service education department, more supervision from the nurse-leader/manager, or participation in group discussion with members of the nursing team. All three alternatives may be desirable.

PROBLEM-SOLVING FACET IV: IMPLEMENTING INTERVENTION (INTERVENTION)

Following are the tasks involved in implementing intervention:

1. Assume the responsibility for coordinating or implementing activities.
2. Determine what must be done to establish authority to implement the plan.
3. Establish time and place for follow-up, reassessment, and evaluation of activities.
4. Carry out plans.
5. Reassess, evaluate, follow up, and revise plans according to data.

Facet IV is the action facet. All work prior to this phase has been in preparation. Facet IV is that phase in which the nurse-leader/manager and the nursing group have responsibility for actualizing the philosophies, objectives, principles, and plans that have been previously determined. Facet IV is equivalent to the situation-producing theories (level IV) of theory building. They are prescriptive theories, which include prescription, implementation, and evaluation of a nursing intervention.

Action requires not only implementing behaviors but also concurrent evaluation of the effectiveness of the action. Formalized reassessment depends in part on data gathered during action. The following tasks of facet IV are the crux of the problem-solving process and the proof of the validity of all foregoing facets.

Task 1—Assume responsibility for coordinating or implementing activities. A responsible leader and manager is essential to smooth implementation of alternatives. Often intervention activities occur over a period of several weeks. Patient problems are seldom solved quickly, and interdepartmental problems within an agency require continued effort; these activities require a manager who will be responsible for seeing that efforts are ongoing. This does not imply that the nurse who assumes this responsibility will do all the work. It implies only that the manager will see that the planned activities are carried out.

The nurse-leader/manager in the problem example is the organizational person most familiar with the situation and nearest to the level of operation. The responsibility for implementation and follow-through belongs at this level. Frequently nurse-leaders/managers "pass the buck" for any number of reasons to those who might assume the responsibility for implementation. The head nurse or in-service education instructor is the most likely recipient of "buck passing" from lower level management. The nurse-leader/manager must fully assume leadership responsibilities and act with the authority of the role. Any activities relevant to patient care must be instigated and coordinated by the team leader or primary nurse.

Task 2—Determine what must be done to establish authority to implement the plan. To carry out a selected alternative the authority to implement an activity must be clearly established by going through the proper channels and lines of authority. Written memos are the best means of clearing channels or informing appropriate people, regardless of the friendliness of relationships with line or staff people, other departments, or physicians. Conversations, both in person and on the telephone, that establish the authority to implement should be followed by a memo referring to the phone call or conversation and summarizing the content. These memos should be kept for future reference. Trust and good relationships are maintained through the use of good business practices. Good records of memos reinforce memory and provide a reference source. Reliance on memory alone is a shaky foundation for any relationship because it permits misunderstanding to occur without revealing to the participants that a misunderstanding exists and, therefore, clarification is not possible. Memos reveal misunderstandings and allow the participants to clarify positions immediately. The memo also serves as a reminder of commitments or activities in progress. In this example, authority to act is invested with the position of team leader, and no other channels need be cleared.

Task 3—Establish time and place for follow-up, reassessment, and evaluation. Establishing a time and place for follow-up and reassessment is important to ensure continuing awareness of and continuity in handling the problem. Crisis situations invariably draw the strongest and most immediate response, and situations that have ceased to be crises are often delegated to places of less importance and are not followed through to completion. This practice increases the possibility that the same situation will again become a crisis. Planned follow-up establishes a system whereby further complications can be avoided and continued growth can be promoted.

Plans for follow-up and reassessment are most important when groups are involved in problem solving. Planning times for this important activity gives the group a sense of continuity. It provides target dates and motivates individuals to think in realistic terms about what they can contribute to such a conference. This activity not only underlines the importance of the planned intervention but also allows the group to evaluate effectiveness and further plan other activities or even reassess the problem (see principle 6, facet II, task 4, p. 26).

Task 4—Implement prescriptions. The problem is identified, the principles selected, the alternatives established and chosen, authority clearly defined, and implementation is under way. Nurse-leaders/managers who are implementing plans and are wary of forgetting a part of the planned implementation may wish to make a list. This list, if made, should be kept small and brief.

When groups are involved, roles need to be clearly defined in the perpetration of a plan of action so that each person knows what every other person is doing. If all are to participate, *how* each will participate needs to be discussed so that guidelines for action are established and each person can fit within the framework.

In the situation under discussion the nurse-leader/manager would find the appropriate aide, take him aside, and privately find out the information necessary. Basing actions on the findings of the interview, the leader would provide the necessary equipment, assistance, teaching, or supervision and arrange for the aide to give the oral care to the patients assigned to him. The team leader would arrange for further evaluation, assessment, and follow-up and evaluate the overall patient assignment.

Task 5—Reassess, evaluate, follow up, and revise plans according to data (evaluation). Task 5 occurs after the initial actions that deal with the immediate situation and is designed to determine if the problem has been adequately solved or if alterations in plans need to be made. Participation by all concerned is important to the success of this task. Retrospective as well as concurrent evaluation is necessary to the solution of any problem. The nurse-leader/manager's evaluation, together with the aide's evaluation, will serve as a guide to determine the relevancy and effectiveness of all the problem-solving steps. Revision of plans may be necessary because of further developments, such as more trust and better communications, additional data, or the rapidity with which the aide learns. Procedure manuals or orientation programs may need review, or patient assignments may need more planning. This information may not become apparent until follow-up conferences are conducted in which all people concerned honestly attempt to evaluate the entire situation. From such conferences may come continuity and progress for the entire unit or a redefinition of the problem and subsequent problem-solving activities.

CONCEPTUAL FRAMEWORKS—A GUIDE TO NURSING CARE DECISIONS

Conceptual frameworks were once the exclusive domain of nursing education. Graduate students were required to construct conceptual frameworks for papers, theses, and dissertations. Schools of nursing are required to have conceptual frameworks from which curriculum is derived in order to have a unifying mechanism and decision-making strategy for their plans for learning. With increasing frequency, health care institutions are formulating philosophies and conceptual frameworks to enable management to make decisions that are consistent with the philosophy, mission, and goals of the agency, responsive to the needs of the setting and clients, and consistent in the type and quality of health care desired.

The conceptual framework is an interrelated system of premises that provides guidelines or ground rules for making all nursing care and organizational decisions. It is derived from a philosophy and is the conceptualization and articulation of concepts, facts, propositions, postulates, theories, phenomena, and variables relevant to a specific nursing care system. It describes the relationships these concepts and theories have to one another and to the nursing care given in each agency. It is the structure that provides the map for all managerial and staff nurse level decisions. It is like the framing of a house in that it furnishes the specifications and the decision-making guidelines for the walls, rooms, forms, and functions of the house. The conceptual framework provides the perimeters (limits and constraints) and parameters (values) for nursing care, giving consistency and integrity to the entire nursing department. The conceptual framework of each department of nursing or health care agency differs, at least slightly, from that of every other agency, even though large areas of similarity may exist because of the nature of nursing.

Just as each person has a frame of reference that is influenced by his culture—his life experiences, ethnicity, philosophy, and personality—so each nursing service agency is influenced by its "culture"—its philosophical set, the clients it serves, the community it serves, and the type of nursing care it offers. These elements, when brought together, compose an implied and expressed value system and provide explicit decision-making rules for nursing care. According to Chater* there are three areas that provide concepts, theories, and decision-making guidelines (a conceptual framework) for curriculum building. These same three areas are useful for devising a conceptual framework for nursing practice. Progressive nursing care agencies such as the University of California Hospital at San Francisco, Nursing Service Department, have successfully used the Chater model for devising a conceptual framework for nursing service. The three

---

* Chater, S.: A conceptual framework for curriculum development, Nurs. Outlook **23:**428-433, July 1975.

areas that Chater recommends for inclusion in a conceptual framework are as follows:

1. Setting or context
2. Clients
3. Conceptualization of nursing practice, or the knowledge base

Fig. 4 is a diagram of the Chater model.

Much nursing literature, when referring to a conceptual framework for nursing, seems to refer only to the knowledge base, or conceptualization, of nursing practice. Most authors communicate concepts and theories relevant to this area to the exclusion of the other two factors represented in the Chater model, which are equally influential in nursing service decision making. Nursing service departments successful in the delivery of care are responsive to all three areas identified by Chater.

All nursing service departments operate under conceptual frameworks; however, some are clearly articulated, and some simply exist and are understood. The three areas of the Chater model may be applied in nursing process in specific ways, as shown here.

Setting

The setting of nursing practice refers to various things. One is the agency or institution that houses the nursing service department. The type of agency, the kinds of services offered, the composition of the sponsoring group, the budget constraints, and the philosophy, mission, and goals are the major elements for consideration about the sponsoring agency. A large teaching general hospital would have a mission, a philosophy, and goals different from those of a small specialty hospital such as eye, ear, nose and throat hospital. Parochial institutions such as Mount Sinai Hospital or Holy Cross Hospital would have philosophies and missions different from those of large, state-supported institutions. Health departments operate on a philosophical premise and have a mission different from clinics or general hospitals. These varying agencies focus on the following:

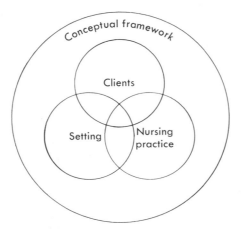

Fig. 4. The Chater model for conceptual frameworks.

1. What health problems they address
2. What ethnic and moral precepts or conditions are imposed by their funding source
3. The realities of the size and categories of their budgets
4. The type of health provided in their care systems

These factors dictate many of the service goals of the nursing department.

Another aspect of the setting component is the influence of those factors contributed by the community the agency serves. That community may be the immediate geographic area of the health agency; it may be a state or, in the case of some health agencies such as the National Institutes of Health at Bethesda, Maryland, it may be a nation. In the case of agencies such as the World Health Organization, it can be global. Factors that must be considered in the conceptual framework of any agency regarding its community or service area are as follows:

1. The politics of the area
2. State and federal regulations about practice and quality control standards
3. Geography of the area (climate, topography)
4. Types of industry and economic basis of the area

A third group of factors to be considered in the setting is the type of nursing care delivery system generally used in a geographical location. The nursing care delivery system is influenced by several factors:

1. The types and qualifications of the nurses available to fill positions
2. The character of nursing practice in the geographic area of the hospital, that is, what is acceptable nursing practice in the area
3. The structure of the health care delivery system within which the nursing department operates

The fourth factor involves the availability of professional nurses. The availability of people prepared as nurse specialists and nurse practitioners varies from one geographic area to another. The availability of people with baccalaureate and masters degrees varies from place to place, and the number of people available having special preparation in nursing administration varies, depending on the availability of these special educational programs. It is impossible to plan a nursing care delivery system that calls for many nurse practitioners, nurse specialists, or masters-prepared people in nursing administration when these people are not available. In most urban areas, people are available to fill special kinds of jobs requiring special education; however, in many of the rural or remote areas of the United States, nurses who have special training are not always available. Naturally the availability of highly trained people influences the kind of nursing care delivery system that can be implemented in an agency.

The type and kind of nursing practice in the geographic setting constitute a fifth factor. Some modes of nursing care delivery systems are more popular in some areas than in others. The four classical kinds of nursing care delivery systems—case method, functional method, team method, and primary nursing method—are used in various configurations throughout the country.

Case method is regaining a measure of popularity because of the increasing popularity in primary nursing. Many agencies that believe they cannot implement primary nursing do implement case method nursing instead and combine some of the aspects of case method nursing with primary nursing. This has caused a resurgence in popularity of the case method. The team method, used with varying degrees of success throughout the country, is still one of the more popular methods of nursing care delivery in use. It is usually mixed with some form of functional nursing and is seldom seen in its pure state. The functional method of nursing care delivery is probably the most common method in use and it requires the least amount of organization and planning.

That a particular kind of nursing care is popular in a geographic area does not necessarily mean that this mode of nursing care delivery will be chosen for every agency in that area; it simply means that nurses in the area may or may not be more familiar with one mode than another, and when switching to another mode of nursing care delivery, the degree of familiarity is a factor to be considered. If, in an area where functional nursing has been in use, team nursing or primary nursing is instituted, a much more extensive educational program must be planned to ensure success in the new delivery system.

The sixth factor about setting is the structure of the health care delivery system in the area of the nursing department. Some health care delivery systems, by their very nature, rely more heavily on the independence of nurses than do other health care delivery systems. Nurses operating with protocols function with a fair degree of independence in many clinics, health departments, and hospitals. (Protocols are medically endorsed procedures for health care that enable a nurse to order diagnostic or therapeutic regimens clearly specified in writing.) However, if the health care delivery system in an area is not structured to accommodate the degree of independence of practice desired by the nursing service department, plans may be thwarted. Sweeping changes in the health care delivery system may be beyond the energy level of nursing service departments; therefore nursing service departments may have to alter the degree of independence expected of its employees based on the structure of the health care delivery system in that area.

Clients

The Chater model for construction of a conceptual framework considers the character of the clients served. In order to structure the data about clients, one must determine the kind of people who will be or are being served by the agency, their needs, and their expectations and characteristics.

Some of the factors to be considered that will enable a clear statement of commitment to the group to be served are as follows:

1. Ethnicity of the population
2. Educational level—literacy rates
3. English language comprehension or foreign language usually spoken
4. Cultural mores and folkways
5. Values of the people
6. Economic level of the people
7. Ethnicity of the nursing staff and its ethnic congruency with clientele
8. Employment and unemployment rates
9. Age statistics
10. Health problems of the population

Each of these factors provides critical information that helps an agency determine its service commitments. Each influences the priority of problems, the management of budget, the planning of staff development, and the concentration of effort. These items and their impact on nursing care will not be discussed individually. However, an example of the impact of each of these items can be seen in item 10, the health problems of the population served.

Some health service areas have vastly different health problems from others. For instance, the San Francisco Bay area has exceptionally high rates of cirrhosis of the liver whereas the coastal areas of South Carolina and Georgia have exceptionally high rates of stroke. Parts of the Midwest have high rates of tuberculosis. Some agencies address particular health problems with greater vigor because they are special problems peculiar to the community in which the agency is placed.

Knowledge base

The knowledge base is what Waters* calls "the conceptualization of nursing practice." Each nursing service department needs a conceptualization of nursing practice to provide structure to the practitioner's role, the organization, and the client care approach. A conceptualization of nursing practice gives unity and integrity to nursing care. The conceptualization of nursing practice will dictate the way in which the nursing service department wishes nursing to be practiced. It will explain what happens to patients when they are nursed. According to Waters, a conceptualization of nursing practice has six aspects:

1. The goals of care
2. Who the clients are
3. What the nursing problems are
4. The types of nursing interventions that will be enacted
5. The settings of practice
6. The work role relationships

The kind of conceptualization of nursing practice chosen or devised by a nursing service agency dictates the content under each of these six areas.

Goals. If Dorothea Orem's framework for nursing practice is chosen, the goals of nursing practice will be self-care or self-help. If Sister Calista Roy's perception of nursing practice is chosen, the goals of nursing will be adaptation. If Dunn is selected as a component of the conceptualization of nursing practice, the goals of practice will be high-level wellness. An acute care hospital may have as its goal the return to optimal health, whereas a public health department nursing service may have as its goal a return to complete independence. A hospice for the terminally ill may have goals such as maximum comfort of its patients and death with dignity. Goals will vary according to the agency's philosophy, mission, and perception of nursing practice.

Clients. The kind of clients depends largely on the setting, that is, the kind of institution. Some agencies treat only pediatric clients, or only pregnant women,

---

*Waters, V.: Address: Conceptualization for nursing practice, presented at Workshop: Conceptual frameworks for nursing, Calgary, Canada, July 1975, Institute of Nursing Consultants.

or only people with eye, ear, nose, and throat conditions. The kind of agency will dictate the selection of clients that nursing service will address. The client's developmental level, ethnicity, and personality characteristics are factors that must be identified and described if the conceptualization of nursing practice is to be functional.

Problems. The kinds of problems nursing will address are an important aspect of the conceptualization of nursing practice and are derived from the mission of the agency as well as the philosophy and intent of the nursing service department. A nursing department that operates on the medical model will probably choose to address those problems centered around the medical diagnosis of the clients, for example, diabetes, fractures, congestive heart failure, strokes, pregnancy, or blindness. Nursing service agencies that are centered on the nursing problems will choose nursing's domain of practice as the area of problems for nursing service to address. These will be problems in mobility, self-help, communications, grief, sexuality, etc. Clarity in the domain of practice and the nursing care diagnoses enables nurses to function as nurses, rather than as "junior doctors," and to provide nursing diagnoses and nursing care prescriptions in keeping with the whole framework of the agency, thereby clearifying such things as the way nursing care can be evaluated, audited, and quality controlled. It is extremely important for nursing service managers to be clear about the kinds and types of problems their nurses may legitimately confront.

Intervention. The kinds of interventions legitimized by the conceptualization of nursing practice follow various formats. One is the focus of the intervention. Focus of the intervention may be prevention/care/cure/rehabilitation, or it may go into Leavell and Clark's three levels of prevention—primary prevention, secondary prevention, and tertiary prevention. Nursing services may choose to look at the divisions of interventions according to the 1965 AMA position paper, that is, care, cure, and coordination, or, may choose to devise a separate category system for practice interventions. Whatever the case, some agencies concentrate more on prevention than on care; for example, public health agencies tend to concentrate much more on prevention than on care. Some agencies are rehabilitation hospitals and concentrate on rehabilitation interventions. Most general hospitals concentrate on secondary prevention, or the care/cure aspect, with minimal emphasis on prevention and rehabilitation. Thus the emphasis on the kind of care is an important highlight to the conceptualization of nursing practice, since it enables nurses to know where the energy focus lies. Other things pertaining to intervention are the tools of the trade, that is, the processes, techniques, and concepts that nurses use to carry out their interventions. These would include such things as problem solving, systems theory, research, communications, stress theory, role theory, caring, teaching/learning, and maturational theory. These tools and processes tell the nurse which theoretical base will be used in practice to provide the basis for the vocabulary and jargon that will be used in making diagnoses, in writing nursing care prescriptions during charting, during nursing audits, in devising criteria for the evaluation of nursing care, or in any other communication.

Settings. Settings are the fifth item to be considered in conceptualization of nursing practice. Some agencies have a wider variety of settings than others.

All settings where nursing will be practiced must be listed and described in the conceptualization of nursing practice. Some agencies send nurses only into homes and clinics; other agencies have them in the structured environment of the hospital. Some hospitals have both clinical and home care follow-up and therefore have a wider variety of settings than those offering only acute hospital treatment. Some hospitals provide a variety of settings within themselves. Intensive care, rehabilitation, intermediate care, and ambulatory care are some of the work settings of hospitals. These settings require a wide variety of skills and will dictate such prerequisites as orientation programs, in-service education programs, and selection of employees.

Work role relationships. The work role relationship is one of the more difficult areas to deal with in any nursing care agency. Work role relationships are dictated not only by the conceptualization of nursing practice of the agency but also by the culture of the health care provider group in any given community. In some communities, work role relationships between physicians and nurses are easy and collegial; in others they are highly formal, hierarchical, and often patronizing. Nursing service departments that have a clear conceptualization of nursing practice and a clear articulation of the work role relationships expected of their employees can provide the support system necessary to enable nurses to act in colleague relationships with physicians. If the work role relationships of coordinator, collaborator, and colleague are supported by the conceptual framework, in-service programs can teach nurses these roles and how they may be developed in agencies where these roles will be new ones for nurses to assume. Work role relationships are, to some degree, influenced by the degree of independence supported by the nursing service.

• • •

In short, a conceptual framework gives structure to the practice of nursing, enables it to be carried forward by a whole group in a unified way, and provides a basis for talking about, as well as practicing, nursing care and guidelines for evaluating that care.

SUMMARY

This chapter provides the key hypotheses or theoretical constructs that form the premises on which the rest of the book is based. Management is, in the final analysis, the ability to bring together many areas of knowledge and skill into a unified set of behaviors that facilitate the movement of individuals, families, groups, and communities toward a goal. This role enactment presumes knowledge and skill in role learning and taking, in analyzing and organizing the components of life processes, and in theorizing, problem solving, and decision making. The ability to predict the consequences of a nursing act is one of the key cognitive processes of nursing problem solving. In other words, a predictive principle is a nursing action hypothesis and as such constitutes a limited nursing theory. The following five predictive principles summarize the conceptual framework of this book:

1. A clear operational definition of leadership/management facilitates role definition and enactment.

2. Eclectic selection and synthesis of the many components of the processes of life enable utilization of these components in a unique, effective leadership/management act conducive to an established goal.

3. Conscious role learning, role taking, and role enactment and a large role repertoire facilitate more effective and efficient role adaptation and perception and response to leadership/management role needs.

4. Skill in theory identification, selection, and building enables identification of the level at which individuals and groups are operating and facilitates the use of appropriate behaviors that will complete the theoretical progression toward a desired end.

5. Skill in the use of problem-solving facets and heuristics promotes more effective and appropriate decisions and ease in helping others in participatory decision making.

6. A clear conceptual framework provides cohesion, and decision-making guidelines for the management of the nursing enterprise.

BIBLIOGRAPHY
Books

Bevis, E. O.: Curriculum building in nursing: a process, ed. 2, St. Louis, 1978, The C. V. Mosby Co.

Bower, F. L.: The process of planning nursing care: a model for practice, St. Louis, 1979, The C. V. Mosby Co.

Bruner, J. S., Goodnow, J. J., and Austin, G. A.: A study of thinking, New York, 1956, John Wiley & Sons, Inc.

Burton, W. H., Kimball, R. B., and Wing, R. L.: Education for effective thinking, New York, 1960, Appleton-Century-Crofts.

Gagne, R.: The conditions of learning, New York, 1965, Holt, Rinehart & Winston, Inc., pp. 31-61.

Hughes, B. C.: Men and their work, New York, 1958, The Free Press, p. 120.

Leavell, H., and Clark, E. G.: Preventive medicine for the doctor in his community, ed. 3, New York, 1965, McGraw-Hill Book Co.

McDonald, F. J.: Educational psychology, Belmont, Calif., 1966, Wadsworth Publishing Co., Inc., pp. 48-67, 252, and 302

Sarbin, T. R., and Allen, V. L.: Role theory. In Lindzey, G., and Aaronsen, E., editors: The handbook of social psychology, ed. 2, Reading, Mass., 1968, Addison-Wesley Publishing Co., Inc., vol. 1, pp. 488-567.

Smuts, J. C.: Holism and evolution, New York, 1926, Macmillan Publishing Co., Inc.

Strategy notebook, San Francisco, 1972, Interaction Associates, Inc.

Tools for change, ed. 2, San Francisco, 1971, Interaction Associates, Inc.

Whitehead, A. N.: Process and reality, New York, 1929, Macmillan Publishing Co., Inc.

Periodicals

Arndt, C., and Laeger, E.: Role strain in a diversified role set: the director of nursing service. Part I. Nurs. Res. **19**:253-58, May-June 1970.

Arndt, C., and Laeger, E.: Role strain in a diversified role set: the director of nursing service. Part II. Sources of stress, Nurs. Res. **19**:495-501, Nov.-Dec. 1970.

Chater, S. S.: A conceptual framework for curriculum development, Nurs. Outlook **23**:428-433, July 1975.

Dickoff, J., James, P., and Wiedenbach, E.: Theory in a practice discipline. Part I. Practice oriented theory, Nurs. Res. **17**:415-35, Sept.-Oct. 1968.

Hall, J., O'Leary, V., and Williams, M.: The decision-making grid: a model of decision-making styles, Calif. Management Rev. **7**(2):43-54, 1964.

Schweer, M., and Gardella, F. A.: Planning, orienting, and preparing for a new kind of nurse leadership, Nurs. Outlook **18**(5):42-46, 1970.

Other

American Nurses' Association: Educational preparation for nurse practitioners and assistants to nursing: a position paper, New York, 1965, The Association.

Waters, V.: Address: Conceptualization for nursing practice, presented at Workshop: Conceptual frameworks for nursing, Calgary, Canada, July 1975, Institute of Nursing Consultants.

2 PREDICTIVE PRINCIPLES OF MANAGEMENT

DEFINITION OF TERMS
Definition of managerial terminology provides the learner with a basis for assimilating the concepts of management.

ORGANIZATIONAL STRUCTURE
Creation of an organizational system compatible with the philosophy, conceptual framework, and goals of the organization provides the means for accomplishment of purpose.

Understanding of the organizational structure as a whole facilitates development of roles and relationships enabling goal achievement.

Recognition of a dual pyramid of power between personnel employed by the organization and independent individuals authorized to practice in the agency assists the nurse-manager in coping with the dual forces.

OPERATIONAL STRATEGIES FOR EFFECTIVE MANAGEMENT
Awareness of management theories allows the nurse-manager to determine appropriate management styles for the work setting.

PLANNING PROCESS
The planning process that considers all ramifications to self, others, and agency in relation to past, present, and future increases the likelihood of successful implementation.

A statement of philosophy and conceptual framework for an agency, department, or group directs the individual involved in planning for achievement of purpose.

Management by policy, procedure, and method establishes the framework for conformity to preestablished regulations.

Management by objectives (MBO) provides a plan for the fulfillment of human needs and organizational purposes and goals.

STAFFING PROCESS
A statement of the philosophy and goals of the total health institution gives direction to the number and kinds of nursing services that will be provided in performing the mission of the institution.

Standards of care, clearly defined, allow for descriptions of personnel necessary for implementation.

Excessive turnover in nursing personnel causes the client to suffer loss of efficient and effective service and increases the cost factor.

A successful staffing process promotes job satisfaction.

Matching client need with personnel who are able to meet that need reveals the staffing pattern and schedule appropriate for the work setting.

Establishment of policies that ensure fairness, consistency, and professional development of human resources enables recruitment and maintenance of a sufficient number of qualified nurses.

BUDGETARY PROCESS
Participation by nursing personnel in planning and controlling the budget leads to cost consciousness, increased awareness of activities, and increased cost effectiveness.

A budgetary process that functions on a planned, continuous, and cyclic basis offers participants an effective way to operate efficiently and to provide information for making future key decisions.

COORDINATING PROCESS
Coordination of personnel and services through intradepartmental and interdepartmental activities brings about a total accomplishment far superior to that possible through fragmentation of individual effort.

The span of control directly affects the size and complexity of the coordinating function.

Activities directed toward regulating, preventing, correcting, and promoting coordination provide a comprehensive and efficient approach to management.

Review of the utilization of the nurse-manager's time provides a means for comparison of role expectation and fulfillment.

The presence or absence of conflict influences a nurse-manager's ability to coordinate activity.

CONTROLLING PROCESS
Contracting for accountability of services rendered identifies the scope and limitations of the nurse-manager's span of control and provides a guide for assessment of the degree to which the nurse-manager's responsibilities are being fulfilled.

Setting standards serves to clarify purpose and provides a gauge for controlling quality and quantity of services.

Consideration of structural, process, and outcome standards as interrelational and interdependent serves to keep the management process balanced and in perspective.

Management is considered both an art and a science. It is viewed as an integrated system in which human and technical resources are mobilized to produce desired outcomes. Management is seen as a process that meshes tested theories with findings discovered through trial and error in the work arena. Many health care organizations or components of these organizations managed by nurses do not have preparation in management. Therefore the organization and management of the delivery of health care services are hampered in keeping pace with clinical advances.

The term *"nurse-manager"* applies at every level in nursing, whether as staff nurse, head nurse, supervisor, or administrator, and varies from direct care of clients to responsibility for those persons providing direct care. Management usually refers to those in some position of authority who direct their energies to manipulating, directing, and coordinating people, environments, finances, time, and materials in ways that will accomplish purposes and goals. Staff nurses often function in lower managerial positions. The most effective managers are those who can use the scientific, technical, and behavioral modes to the best advantages for client, worker, and organization. The best workers are those who know the role of lower and middle managers so that they can better enact the role of the managed.

The purpose of this chapter is to present theories, systems, and predictive principles of management that will enable the nurse functioning at any level of management to confidently and successfully assume responsibility and accountability for the management of quality care.

DEFINITION OF TERMS

A health care delivery agency's primary function is to provide services to the client for disease prevention, health maintenance, diagnosis, treatment, cure, or rehabilitation. These agencies are of many types, with objectives and methodology depending on major purposes of the organization. Although differences do exist, all organizations provide for the managerial role. Labels ascribed in organizations often become blurred for lack of definition. Even with explanation, it becomes apparent that there is much overlap in function between managerial roles. The reader is encouraged to study the terminology so that positions within the work setting can be clearly understood.

PREDICTIVE PRINCIPLE: Definition of managerial terminology provides the learner with a basis for assimilating the concepts of management.

Organization: Purposeful structure and systematic arrangement of elements; can be applied to an entity such as a hospital or other health agency or to a process. The administrative and functional structure includes relationships of people, departments, and work to each other and to the whole. Organization enables the health care delivery system, or health agency, to implement its philosophy and achieve its purposes.

Administration: Comprehensive executive function; exercising organizational powers and duties, including setting goals, formulating policies, and establishing management procedures.

Administrator: One who performs the executive or power-laden role of formulating policy and establishing broad goals for implementation and monitoring the overall process of an organization.

Management: Process that takes place within the organization in accomplishing institutional goals and specific purposes through the use of interpersonal and technical aspects.

Manager: One who has the official authority and responsibility for overseeing and directing the work of others by virtue of his position in an organizational structure. A manager gets the work done at the right time by the use of manpower and material resources. Managers implement policy, plans, and directives by motivating and managing themselves and other individuals and groups to obtain the money, materials, and environment to meet successfully both agency goals and worker's needs. A manager has official authority and responsibility but may or may not have the power to establish goals for their immediate territories. Managers create and maintain an environment so that other people can work efficiently in it. In some settings the administrator and manager are one and the same.

Leader: One who uses the processes of life to facilitate the movement of one or more persons toward the establishment and attainment of a goal. The leader promotes a climate of cooperation and respect so that the follower(s) will want to be influenced by him. Leaders usually hold their positions more through characteristics and behavior than through official designation. A leader has some charisma that makes him followable. A manager, on the other hand, is official. He has a job description, designated responsibility, and a chain of command. A manager may be a leader and a leader a manager, but some managers are not good leaders and not all leaders are managers at all.

Levels of management: Organizational structure in nursing has levels. *Top-level management* positions are responsible for overall operation of the organization. These people are directors of nursing services, usually with policy-making power. *Middle-level management* positions usually direct the operation of several units within the organization. These people are often called supervisors and have the responsibility for coordinating activities and interpreting and implementing agency policy. *First-level management* positions direct the operation of one unit or a part of a unit within a department and are concerned with delivery of care to clients. This could be such persons as the head nurse, team leader, or primary care nurse. They have as their major purpose control of the work environment.

Centralization and decentralization: This is related to levels of management and refers to the kind of decision making done at each level. In a *centralized* structure, most major decisions are made at the top level. This system is congruent with the scientific method of bureaucratic control. Large organizations in which nearly every decision must go through many levels are highly centralized. Centralization also results from the design of the organization itself. When operations are highly specialized and departments finely subdivided, decisions must be made by higher levels in the organization and rigid rules and regulations employed. No manager, any more than a single employee, is in a position to be independent. Because only a small part of the total job is done by one member of a unit, upper levels of management must oversee all functions to ensure cooperation and coordination. Alternatively, in a *decentralized structure,* considerable planning and activities take place at the direct care-giving levels under the overall surveillance of the organization. Managers are considered resource persons for striving to achieve results rather than authoritarian decision makers operating at the apex of a hierarchical structure. Through decentralization the interrelated resources of environment, materials, and people are divided into subsystems performing a part of a task, and all efforts are integrated to achieve the goals of the subgroup.

Decentralization is dedicated to the concept that management belongs at the ground level. This grass roots approach is checked closely against policies and regulations of the total organization. Emphasis on decentralization places a high value on the assertion of independence, the willingness to make decisions and to act without constant consultation with superiors. Decentralization generates a sense of local control and encourages initiative and change. There is a danger in decentralization because it may lead to fragmentation of effort. Unless controlled, each unit could operate primarily in terms of its own subsystem rather than in terms of the needs of the organization as a whole.

ORGANIZATIONAL STRUCTURE

PREDICTIVE PRINCIPLE: Creation of an organizational system compatible with the philosophy, conceptual framework, and goals of the organization provides the means for accomplishment of purpose.

Organization comprises structure and process, which allow the health care delivery system to enact its philosophy and utilize its conceptual framework to achieve its goals. Organization refers to a body of persons, methods, policies, and procedures arranged into systematic process through the delegation of functions and responsibilities for the accomplishment of purpose. Organizations involved in health care delivery are many and varied. Most common are the hospital, which is the center of health care delivery in the United States, and health maintenance organizations. The latter are commonly referred to as "HMOs" and have been in existence for a number of years. The Kaiser-Permanente Plan in California and the Health Insurance Plan of New York are examples. The federal government has recently given backing to this system of care and has legislated monies and formulated guidelines to provide for an HMO option in public and private health insurance plans throughout the United States.

There are also nursing homes offering skilled, intermediate, and custodial care as well as group medical and nursing practices and clinics.

The degree of organization in health care delivery systems ranges from highly structured systems to loosely knit organizations bound by contractual and professional agreements. One of the more controversial aspects of leadership common to business, industry, government, education, and health care systems is the creation of the most effective organizational system for the enterprise.

Behavioral scientists such as Douglas McGregor, Frederick Herzberg, Rensis Likert, Chris Argyris, and Abraham Maslow suggest that the simpler the structure in organization, the better the outcome. They postulate that too much organization inhibits growth, creativity, and flexibility and often results in an authoritarian style of leadership. At the other extreme are countless organizations that have failed through too little rather than too much structure. The obvious goal is to develop an organizational policy that will allow structure to be designed to fit each particular setting, the unique clients served, and the type of care provided—in other words, the conceptual framework must be congruent with the organizational structure. This means the least structure possible to efficiently achieve goals.

PREDICTIVE PRINCIPLE: Understanding of the organizational structure as a whole facilitates development of roles and relationships enabling goal achievement.

Since the beginning of social structure, human beings have been organizing their activities and assigning the responsibilities for organizing to managers. Advances in medicine and science have extended man's life span, created empires, and produced large quantities of goods and services for almost every necessity and/or comfort. During the past years of social and technologic advancement and until recently little attention was devoted to the process of organizing systems and managing personnel and resources within a given environment.

Max Weber (1864-1920), a German sociologist often referred to as the father of organizational theory, is associated with the organizational concept of bureaucracy. He explored the concepts of hierarchy, specialization, rules, and impersonality that provide the basis for the classical principles known to organization.

The typical bureaucratic structure in health care agencies provides levels of control in pyramid form from the trustees and the administrator at the top of the pyramid, through the division and or department heads, to the various categories of hospital or health agency workers needed as a support system at the base of the pyramid. All regular activities are assigned to a position within the pyramid, and major directives are written and based on established policy. Personnel are selected on the basis of knowledge and expertise.

Health agencies (hospitals, clinics, health departments) are very complex social systems composed of clients, trustees or board of directors, administrative staff, health care providers, and support personnel. The governing board has the legal authority over and the responsibility for the institution or agency. The administrative staff has the responsibility for the institution or agency. Medical and nursing staffs make decisions regarding client care and treatment within the framework of policy and professional judgment. All share the same basic objectives, that of meeting the needs of the client.

The organizational structure (of an agency) usually indicates the various positions within the agency and the relationships of these positions to each other. The structure is designed to define the levels of management and to show the degree of centralization and decentralization of control for the coordination of all activities of the organization. Organizational structure provides a road map of who reports to whom (communication channels) and each person's specific responsibilities (job description).

The nursing services segment follows the same pattern of organizational structure as that established for the agency. Coordination is provided for all activities of nursing, with departmental units, numbers, and kinds of positions identified in accordance with objectives of the institution.

Although the typical health care organization is still organized along the traditional hierarchical lines, some are beginning to make adaptations that will more directly involve health professionals in the decision-making process.

PREDICTIVE PRINCIPLE: Recognition of a dual pyramid of power between personnel employed by the organization and independent individuals authorized to practice in the agency assists the nurse-manager in coping with the dual forces.

The organizational structure of the typical general hospital differs from the bureaucratic model of business and industry in that only those people who have their salaries paid by the hospital fit into the pyramidal structure and are subject to the controlling governing board. This generally includes all people with the exception of the private (nonagency-employed) physicians and some independent nurse practitioners who have been authorized by the hospital to practice in the institution. The independent nature of this arrangement creates some problems, as the organizational pattern is literally a dual pyramid, sometimes with conflicting goals.

In addition to the lines of authority usually existing in a hospital or health agency, there is a second pyramid of authority comprising professional people in the organization, such as physicians and nurses, who have little formal authority but who exercise a great deal of power.

Nursing tends to suffer most from this dual pyramid. Traditionally the nurse was the physician's helper, operating under the physician's orders and direct supervision. Physicians still perceive the nurse this way; yet in reality the nurse is the employee of the agency and is responsible directly to the agency hierarchy. The dual pyramid often places the nurse in a triple bind among agency, physician, and client. Only professional judgment helps the nurse clarify goals, chain of command, and legal responsibilities.

OPERATIONAL STRATEGIES FOR EFFECTIVE MANAGEMENT

PREDICTIVE PRINCIPLE: Awareness of management theories allows the nurse-manager to determine appropriate management styles for the work setting.

Organizational theory emerged in the literature just before the turn of the twentieth century. Scientific and technical theories were studied first, followed by a focus on behavioral management.

Scientific approach. Most literature dealing with scientific management focuses on management in the general industrial setting.

Frederick Taylor and the Gilbreths were the first to attempt the study of management on a scientific basis. In the early 1900s, these scientists studied industry at the worker's level to prove that methods could be used to identify the best ways to accomplish a task and that people in work situations were important factors in the search for efficiency. Taylor looked on workers as automatons, but he did recognize that individual differences existed and needed to be considered in the total work situation.

The basic criterion of the scientific approach is to achieve maximum output with resources available through *planning, directing,* and *controlling.* The four pillars of classical organization used in the scientific approach are (1) *division of labor,* almost always occurring where there are numbers of people attempting to provide a service; (2) *span of control,* referring to the number of people who can effectively be managed; (3) the *scalar process,* separating tasks vertically into managerial levels, recognizing that with more decentralized span of control, more levels are required; and (4) *structure,* referring to the basic orderly arrangement of functions between management and staff personnel.

All theories of scientific management present their major goal as that of organizing to produce maximal output. Certain common elements appear: (1) assumption of a hierarchical, bureaucratic model; (2) identification of the power structure with designated decision makers; (3) development of separate rules and regulations with detailed job specifications; (4) clear communication channels; (5) management by objectives providing the baseline for evaluation of outcomes; (6) equal treatment of all employees, with reliance on expertise relevant to each position; (7) a complete record-keeping system; and (8) a means for account-ability.

Scientific theories provide excellent guidelines for general management in any organization. However, because of the nature of the product in health care systems, there is need for adaptation. For example, delivery of care must always take into account the whole needs of the client, an area that presents difficulties in terms of maximal output with the least amount of services.

Behavioral approach. Behavioral science was begun seriously in 1927 with the Hawthorne studies. The first major attempt to understand the motivational processes of workers, it was geared toward the nonhuman element of work and was conducted by Elton Mayo, then at the Harvard Business School. Experimenters found that workers worked harder and increased their productivity when supervisory pressure was reduced and they had no one watching their every move.

Douglas McGregor produced *The Human Side of Enterprise* in 1957, having thirty years of behavioral science progress as a resource. He proposed a set of assumptions about the nature of people, labeling them "theory X" and "theory Y."

Theory X contained traditional assumptions that people (1) consider work as a job to be done with no thought of pleasure; (2) are naturally lazy and prefer to do nothing; (3) work mostly for money and status rewards; (4) are productive in their field because they fear being demoted or fired; (5) are children grown larger and are naturally dependent on leaders; (6) expect and depend on direction from above and do not want to think for themselves; (7) need prodding and praise; and (8) believe adults remain static and resist change.

Theory Y proposed that workers are emerging individuals who are dynamic, flexible, and adaptive. Assumptions included in this theory were that people (1) are naturally active and enjoy setting goals and striving for their achievement; (2) seek many satisfactions in work other than money and status, in that they take personal pride in a job well done, enjoy the people and process, and are stimulated to new challenges; (3) produce in their desire to achieve their personal and social goals; (4) are normally mature beyond childhood and aspire to independence, self-fulfillment, and responsibility; (5) need understanding of the work scene and are capable of assessing what needs to be done and are able to be self-directive; (6) understand and care about what they are doing and therefore can devise and improve their own methods of work; and (7) seek self-realization and are constantly striving to grow.

McGregor sought to prove the inherent complexity of human behavior and that people are not motivated by a single driving force. Instead, people move in and out of categories, seeking many satisfactions, and their needs change as they grow and develop.

In 1943 Abraham Maslow outlined the elements of his overall theory of human motivation. It was not until 1962 that he personally began to study industrial relations. According to Maslow, although external forces or incentives can have an effect on motivation, real motivation is not something that is externally produced or imposed on human beings. Motivation is the state of being stimulated to take action in order to achieve some kind of goal or to satisfy some kind of need.

Maslow's theory of personality and motivation classifies human goals according to a conceptual hierarchy of needs. He bases his theory on the following basic concepts about human behavior:

1. Man is a wanting person; as soon as one need is met, another need will emerge to take its place.
2. Satisfied needs do not motivate or cause behavior; only unsatisfied needs cause an individual to move.
3. Needs of individuals can be thought of in a hierarchy of importance, each with its own rank and level of importance to the individual.

Maslow defines five levels in the need hierarchy:

1. Physiologic, the most important to man, taking precedence over all other needs if unsatisfied. Needs such as air, food, water, sex, and sleep are examples.
2. Safety, which includes physical as well as emotional needs and reflecting the need to feel secure from harm at home, at work, or in any other activity.
3. Social, which includes a desire to belong, to be loved, and to be accepted in all environments.
4. Esteem, representing the desire for achievement and status, with the needs to feel good about one's self and to gain esteem from others.
5. Self-actualization, reaching the point that man has realized all his potential.

Maslow's theory relates to the work environment as physiologic needs are satisfied by remuneration earned from working and security and social needs are met through a feeling of belonging, friendships, and status. Organizations recognize that most people who work are no longer trying to satisfy primary or lower level needs. It is hoped that the work arena will provide opportunities for self-esteem and self-actualization.

In summary, the behavioral science approach stresses (1) the characteristics of a leader as a facilitator with respect to productivity and good management, (2) building morale and team spirit, and (3) motivation and self-development of employees through promoting work cooperation and communications. The premise is that when the employee is satisfied, the organizational goals will be met.

Although behavioral approach contains many fine elements, some limitations are present in the system. Not all employees respond well to the individualistic approach and therefore they may not produce the desired results. Assuming that each participant will exhibit initiative and creativity, there is no means provided for the manager to deal with noncompliance.

Technical approach. Technology calls attention to the need for tools and techniques that link the whole organization together. All approaches to management incorporate a degree of this element. The tools and techniques of management planning, budgeting, control systems, information systems, and even management by objectives are examples of linking technologies. The pragmatic approach views the content of the work as the most important aspect. Attention is devoted primarily to quality and quantity of nursing care, with little focus on organizational structure and behavioral concerns of the staff. With the technical or functional approach, job descriptions and procedure manuals are highly in evidence. The nurse-manager serves as a practicing role model and may be highly esteemed because of demonstrated competence.

Although there are definite advantages to a skill-oriented approach, there is danger in substituting the practical "how to do it" method for basic understanding of why these techniques are successful or unsuccessful. In addition, the technical approach assumes that every problem can be clearly defined and solved. A problem arises if the defined technique or skill does not have the right variables or if the formula for work production proves ineffectual.

Modified organizational-technical-behavioral approach. There is no one best way to organize and manage a health care facility or any part of it. Management is a process, with organizational, technical, and interpersonal aspects. To be effective, a nurse-manager approaches the task within the framework of the organizational structure, considers the tasks to be accomplished, and takes the human relations perspective into account. The nurse-manager will then attempt to incorporate the major advantages from each management system into the task of production through performance with other people.

PLANNING PROCESS

Health care facilities are in a particularly vulnerable position with respect to planning because they operate in an environment subject to social, economic, political, and technologic forces demanding almost continuous adaptation and change. Predictions cannot be made with assurance; however, planning must go forward. Planning can be defined as deciding in advance what needs to be done and how to do it. Planning includes the aspects of duration, function, and scope of operation. Planning involves analyzing relevant information from the past and present and using it to outline a course of action that enables goal achievement. The question facing the planner is "What has to be done today to be ready for tomorrow?" Planning in the simplest sense is a control system exerted before an action is taken. Planning is crisis prevention and is performed by all levels of management. Top-level administrators engage chiefly in long-range planning to achieve organizational objectives. This usually includes comprehensive planning that will take one or more years to achieve. For example, an agency may decide to plan for the opening of a kidney dialysis center or to add an entire floor to the building for treating geriatric clients. Plans at this level are usually broad in nature and general in terms. Any long-term plan must be flexible, permitting change as conditions dictate. Influencing factors might be financial implications, new knowledge, or a change in the law or regulations.

Concomitant with top-level management's concern for long-term planning is an interest in short-term goals. A well-run agency attends to policy, goals, and programs for implementation with a control system that sets target dates for assessment and accountability for both long- and short-range plans. Short-term objectives need to be replaced with new ones as soon as they are accomplished to ensure that efficiency and forward motion of the organization will occur. Similarly, the long-term plan cannot be alive, vibrant, and realistic except in account with the current progress. All objectives must fit into the overall philosophy, mission, and goals of the organization.

Planning is also engaged in at the middle and first levels of management within health care facilities. At these levels, planning is more operationally oriented, aimed at achieving specific tasks effectively and efficiently. Appropriate planning provides nurse-managers with the tools necessary to control rather than to react to change. It enables nurse-managers to avoid routinely making crisis or stopgap decisions. Planning also enables the nurse-manager to manage with efficiency rather than with fear.

PREDICTIVE PRINCIPLE: The planning process that considers all ramifications to self, others, and agency in relation to past, present, and future increases the likelihood of successful implementation.

Nurse-managers at lower levels formulate their own plans to assist them in (1) defining the nurse-manager's authority and responsibility when administering overall agency plans, (2) understanding interdepartmental relationships, (3) assessing interrelational activities, and (4) developing logical and organized plans in their own areas of responsibility. This deeper understanding of the organization reveals hidden strengths and weaknesses, uncovers previously unrecognized facets of the operation, and documents benefits to the nurse-manager, staff, and clientele.

Any consideration of the basic elements of planning as they relate to management of a health care facility, or any part of it, should include (1) assessment of conditions to determine if some changes need to be made to improve the environment or activities; (2) consideration of the time factor, analyzing the sequence of events in relation to points of time for degrees of accomplishment, keeping in mind short- and long-term planning; (3) collection of pertinent data from past and present; and (4) cognizance of how plans within the total health care agency relate to the plan under consideration.

If planning is to be successful, it is essential that plans be communicated to all who are affected by them. There cannot be a gap between the knowledge of top administration and that of middle- and first-level management with respect to plans. Effective planning takes place on the assumption that everyone who is affected is included in or informed of the process.

PREDICTIVE PRINCIPLE: A statement of philosophy and conceptual framework for an agency, department, or group directs the individual involved in planning for achievement of purpose.

The statement of purpose describes the reason for being. It is an explanation of the system of beliefs that determines the way the purpose is achieved. A philosophy addresses those issues about which the group is concerned and decisions are required. A good statement of philosophy is formulated when the nurse can supply positive demonstrations as to how the statement is actualized in the clinical setting. For example, if the statement is written "We believe that all persons should be admitted for treatment regardless of color or economic status," and it is discovered that delays occur with Blacks and nonpaying clients, the philosophy as written has little meaning. If the answer is that all eligible clients are admitted and treatment begun regardless of either of these contingencies, it is demonstrated that the philosophy has been put into practice.

A well-written philosophy stated in meaningful terms leads to the development of a conceptual framework, which in turn is a necessity for planning, organizing, implementing, and evaluating any operation (see Chapter 1, p. 33). A philosophy for a health agency, department, or group is a statement or system of beliefs about their collective concerns for man and their responsibility to serve him.

A philosophy can be defined as a system of values or beliefs. All individuals have a personal philosophy that motivates their actions and determines how they manage their lives. Likewise, a nurse-manager of an organization or any part of it serves as a guideline for determining the quality of service to be rendered. The manager's patterns of beliefs, attitudes, and values set the tone for all relationships with clients, personnel, physicians, and community.

It is the manager's responsibility to get in touch with his own feelings, to guide the staff in understanding the purpose and philosophy of the agency in which they function, and to help them identify what it is they believe about the provision of nursing services in their respective settings. The conceptual framework commits the agency to respond to setting, clients, and professional factors and provides decision-making guidelines for all agency operations. These commitments need to be periodically reviewed to determine what is worth preserving and what is not and to be sure the staff members adhere to what they believe in their everyday organizational life and service to the clients.

PREDICTIVE PRINCIPLE: Management by policy, procedure, and method establishes the framework for conformity to preestablished regulations.

Some agencies operate under the simple plan of establishment of policy, procedure, and methods. This plan is found primarily in hierarchical, bureaucratic structures. It is utilized in an effort to impose consistency throughout the organization and to avoid the time and cost of constant review of management at the lower levels of operation. Objectives are formulated at the top levels, and authority is delegated within a frame of policies and procedures devised by management.

Policy guides managerial thinking and action during the process of achieving objectives. It establishes broad limits and provides direction, but permits some initiative and individuality.

Procedures are plans that establish customary ways of handling specific, recurring activities, usually involving group effort. A sequence of steps or operations is established. Procedures provide the direction for carrying out policy. They also provide guidelines for taking care of commonly occurring events. An example of the procedures in health care agencies is the nursing procedure manual.

Methods are even more specific and detailed than procedures. They set up the manner and sequence of accomplishing recurring, individual tasks. Virtually no discretion is allowable. An example of method is the steps in assembling traction or in setting up an area for reverse isolation.

PREDICTIVE PRINCIPLE: Management by objectives (MBO) provides a plan for the fulfillment of human needs and organizational purposes and goals.

Peter Drucker, noted authority on management, introduced the phrase "management by objectives" in 1954 to demonstrate the central importance of establishing objectives before any undertaking. Through participatory goal setting, management attempts to create a climate conducive to achievement, motivation, and goal-centered behavior.

Management by objectives (MBO) is designed to minimize production efficiency problems facing health organizations by (1) integrating organizational objectives and individual needs, (2) changing traditional power structures from the top down through all levels of management by building intergroup teamwork, (3) adapting the institution to environmental elements (setting), (4) maintaining the institution's identity under constant change, and (5) providing for constant organizational renewal.

The thrust of the message of MBO is that every person in an organization has control that comes from internal rather than external forces and that specific, attainable, and measurable objectives are formulated by individuals concerned with actualization that coincides with the objectives of the organization.

MBO rests on a concept of human action, behavior, and motivation. Maslow's theory of motivation based on needs arranged in a hierarchy best exemplifies the concept. The implication for the manager is that he can help motivate the worker if he understands the need level at which the worker is operating.

The MBO system can be used by professional and nonprofessional employees alike. Objectives provide concrete and specific statements of the goals all participants wish to accomplish. They are action commitments through which the philosophy of the organization is sustained and the mission or purpose of the health agency will be achieved.

An effective, understandable procedure is necessary for an MBO system to be successful. There must be (1) establishment of goals, (2) planning for implementation, (3) implementation, and (4) evaluation.

Establishment of goals. A suggested procedure is that under the leadership of a nurse-manager, at a designated time each year, all nursing personnel share in identifying those items they believe should be improved for the delivery of care to clients, physicians, personnel, hospital department, and community. A two- or three-week period should provide enough time for all concerned individuals to provide input. Goals are established only after a thorough assessment of problems, needs, productivity, motivational levels, job satisfaction, employee attrition rate, client satisfaction, patient care audits, and patient care areas occurs to determine if various standards of care are met.

Items are then translated into goals that are considered important by all levels of the management system. Objectives should be challenging, yet realistic. Goals are reviewed and evaluated according to their (1) contribution to overall agency goals, (2) relationship to nursing care standards, (3) realism and feasibility in terms of time and resources (energy, cost, equipment, and personnel), and (4) priority of need.

The approved objectives are converted into long-term (a year or longer to complete) or short-term objectives (less than one year to complete).

Planning for implementation. Once objectives are established a plan of action must be initiated to determine the scope and complexity of the task and the range of activities required to accomplish goals. The format followed answers the following traditional questions: (1) who?—staffing; (2) what?—resources, money, equipment, etc.; (3) when?—time frame; (4) where?—in which setting; (5) how?—methods to be used; and (6) why?—significance of the goals.

If all phases are clearly defined and agreed on, progress will occur.

Implementation. The formulated plan of action is put into practice with participation by all personnel according to their assigned responsibilities. The goals and subgoals serve to indicate if the plan is on track and if each worker is doing his part. Each individual is accountable for the success or failure of goal achievement. The objectives are used as a means of upgrading individual skills and improving performance on a continuous basis.

Evaluation. In order for MBO to be effective, periodic evaluation is necessary to determine what is being accomplished. This is done through continuing observation and assessment, both formal and informal. The nurse-manager and participants will obtain a broad view of what is happening in relation to predetermined objectives.

During the evaluation process, consideration is given to questions such as the following:

1. Are the objectives being met, and if so how?
2. If they are not, what factors inhibit their accomplishment?
3. Should the objective(s) be abandoned or revised?
4. Is teaching, assistance, or encouragement needed?

Written evaluations are usually called for at least quarterly, with a year-end summary of accomplishments and problems. Such information contributes to a determination of goals for the next year.

Under a committed management the MBO system has great potential for developing more skillful and productive managers and participants and for improving organizational efficiency. As with any system of management, MBO has its limitations and strengths, all of which should be considered before embracing the plan.

Limitations of the MBO system. Problems with MBO are generally caused by weaknesses in the managers and are not inherent in the system. The system most commonly fails because of lack of participation and/or commitment, poor monitoring, ignored feedback, too little coaching and assistance, insufficient planning to reach objectives, overemphasis on objectives rather than perspective of the whole system, omission of review, and inability to delegate. There are, however, several assumptions made concerning the MBO system that need consideration:

1. The system presumes that participants will establish goals that are in the best interest of the institution it serves.

2. Some personnel seem unable to learn to manage with objectives. They fail either to define objectives in proper quantitative and qualitative terms or to conduct effective appraisals.
3. If too many objectives are formulated, personnel become overwhelmed.

Advantages of the MBO system. The major advantages of the MBO system are as follows:

1. Better planning occurs, in that the entire organization focuses attention on goal setting and plans to achieve those goals.
2. There is individual commitment and participation.
3. There are provisions for establishing motivation toward organization objectives, self-fulfillment, internal satisfaction, and successful accomplishment.
4. There is common ground and feelings of acceptance and security for widely different personalities.
5. There is recognition of the need to change traditional power structures through definition of the individual's authority, delegation, and self-control.
6. Authority is delegated along with responsibility.
7. Self-control replaces control imposed by outside forces.
8. Interaction among all branches of the organization is aided upward, downward, and laterally through a more effective communication system.
9. The organization maintains a clear identity under constant change, as objectives serve as a compass to properly direct effort and to offer standards for measuring progress.

Health organizations that have successfully implemented MBO agree that the benefits are many. The system allows for setting specific goals for a given time period by the persons engaged in the tasks, assessment, coordination, and collaboration between agency and personnel and affords a high-level sense of accomplishment by the membership.

STAFFING PROCESS

Staffing may be defined as the process of assigning competent people to fill the roles designated for the organizational structure through selection and development of personnel. Staffing is the most critical issue of administration because the quality of the participants' effort determines the degree of goal achievement. The issue of staffing is further complicated because it takes place in an ever-changing environment in which practices, task assignments, and responsibilities fluctuate.

An institution whose concern is the delivery of quality health care is presented with the problem of supplying sufficient human resources for the administration of that care. For most health care agencies, staffing constitutes 70% to 80% of the total budget, with nurses providing the major share of the personnel. When a nurse-manager is given responsibility over a particular part of an organization, staffing is one of the central aspects of this responsibility. Because there is limited research on the relationship between numbers and kinds of nursing staff and quality care, it is difficult to predict with assurance that whatever is done will produce desired results. However, there is enough sharing of theories and practice relating to matters of staffing to provide the nurse-manager with predictive principles that can be applied to the issue of staffing with a high degree of confidence.

PREDICTIVE PRINCIPLE: A statement of the philosophy and goals of the total health institution gives direction to the number and kinds of nursing services that will be provided in performing the mission of the institution.

Care-giving agencies have always existed for a purpose, but that purpose has not always been clearly defined. The health care industry is moving from an era of private accountability and responsibility to public accountability for quality, cost, and accessibility of care.

Before the numbers, kinds, and patterns of care can be established, the philosophy of a health care agency must be known. Ideally the nurse-manager and staff would have participated in the formulation of the philosophy and goals of the institution. Interaction and interrelationship among personnel within the organizational structure vertically and horizontally strengthen the probability that beliefs and values pertaining to the delivery of care will be actualized at all levels.

The written statement of philosophy and overall purpose is the basis for a conceptual framework and explains the rationale for the existence of an agency or department and serves as a basis for its mission and goals. A philosophy statement sets the character and tone of service and in effect, through the conceptual framework, gives direction to the quantity and quality of nursing services that will be provided in realizing the mission or purpose. For example, if the philosophy of an agency states that their mission is to provide holistic care to each client and the conceptual framework commits the agency to doing this through the system of primary nursing, provision must be made for employing nurses who view people as wholes interacting with their environments, families, and communities and who have the skills necessary to give comprehensive, high-quality care on a twenty-four–hour basis to a selected group of clients for their length of stay in the institution. Furthermore, consideration of staffing needs will have to include provision for coordination of efforts, continued staff development, and evaluation of care.

A written statement of philosophy provides the blueprint for all that follows in the effective management of an operation. Definitive goals and standards of care become a natural outgrowth of the statement of philosophy, purpose, and conceptual framework.

PREDICTIVE PRINCIPLE: Standards of care, clearly defined, allow for descriptions of personnel necessary for implementation.

Although each health care agency is charged with the responsibility for determining the level of service for their individual operation, there are many factors and constraints to be considered that influence the decision-making process.

In 1972 the U.S. Congress amended the Social Security Act and mandated the establishment of professional standard review organizations (PSROs) to review the quality and cost of care paid by Medicare, Medicaid, and Maternal-Child Health programs. The American Hospital Association (AHA) and the Joint Commission on Accreditation of Hospitals (JCAH) have established comparable programs for the evaluation of patient care.

Standards for organized nursing service have been developed by the Joint Commission for the Accreditation of Nursing Services, the National League for Nursing, and the American Nurses' Association. Care giving agencies must pay heed to all those bodies who control their operations.

Although standards of practice are either imposed or suggested by many bodies, nursing standards for the total enterprise for each level of operation need to be developed and tailored to fulfill the specific philosophy and purposes of the individual work setting, irrespective of any mandatory body. Standards of nursing practice have been established by the American Nurses' Association Congress for Nursing Practice and are available to any interested individual or group. They define nursing practice and provide models against which nurses can measure their practice. The American Nurses' Association has published standards of nursing practice, a general statement, and specific standards in each of the following areas: medical-surgical nursing, orthopedic nursing, maternal-child nursing, geriatric nursing, community health nursing, operating room nursing, cardiovascular nursing, emergency nursing, and psychiatric–mental health nursing. Guidelines such as these provide much help in facilitating the promotion of quality care because institutions can compare and contrast their own views and standards with those established by authorities to make sure that all important issues pertaining to the delivery of care have been included.

Nurses in an institution or agency can work through a nursing practice commission to set standards for practice and to plan for peer review. Everyone who is directly affected should be involved in the standard setting. Other knowledgable, talented, and experienced people should be sought to provide a foundation on which to build nursing standards. Setting of standards is a crucial matter, as everything that is done from the planning through the evaluation stage stems from these statements. When standards for the agency have been determined, nurses can gather together in their individual work settings and develop standards of care that relate directly to the needs of their particular kind of client.

PREDICTIVE PRINCIPLE: Excessive turnover in nursing personnel causes the client to suffer loss of efficient and effective service and increases the cost factor.

Excessive turnover in any group is potentially a problem, but it is especially so in nursing. Nurses provide most of the direct professional health service to clients. When this link is interrupted for any reason, the client suffers. The nursing profession is characterized by high mobility. Tenure of the majority of nurses in staff positions tends to be short. Studies of the turnover rate among nurses in hospitals reveal percentage rates averaging 3% to 5% per month, or from 36% to 60% per year. The rate is sufficiently high to warrant concern.

Another important issue involved with excessive turnover is the economic impact on employing agencies and thus the consumer. It is estimated that the cost of replacing one registered nurse ranges from $500 to $1400, depending on the variables that enter into the situation. Cost factors to be considered are advertising, interviewing, physical examination, orientation and training period, initial nonproductivity of the new employee, processing of papers, and cost of processing the employee who has left. Of course, there is no way to measure the cost of lessened efficiency and effectiveness of care created when an employee leaves.

A distinction must be made between unavoidable and avoidable turnover. Unavoidable circumstances refer to turnover because of illness, family responsibilities, beginning a family, or transfer of husband or wife. Avoidable turnover refers to situations in which the employing agency has failed to recognize or to meet the needs of the nurse.

PREDICTIVE PRINCIPLE: A successful staffing process promotes job satisfaction.

Job satisfaction studies have been conducted in business and industry since the early 1900s. Nursing became interested in testing for job satisfaction in 1940. Since that time, various studies by sociologists, psychologists, and nurses have investigated such major factors as hours of work, fringe benefits, income, environment, opportunities for practice of quality care, growth and advancement, social and organizational relationships, and participation in planning and development of the agency.

Most surveys reveal that nurses are more satisfied in agencies where the salary and benefits are reasonable. Among the findings the predominant indices to satisfaction are the presence of trust and open interrelationships among staff and within the organizational system, opportunity to participate in policy formation and standard setting, and sufficient staffing to allow for the administration of quality care.

Dissatisfaction arises when needs for satisfaction within the organizational social system are thwarted. Nurses indicate a willingness to cooperate in times of crisis, but they rebel when working conditions consistently overlook their desire for adequacy.

PREDICTIVE PRINCIPLE: Matching client need with personnel who are able to meet that need reveals the staffing pattern and schedule appropriate for the work setting.

After the preliminary work of developing the philosophy, conceptual framework, goals, and standards of care has been accomplished, an appropriate staffing pattern can be determined. The organizational structure will show the line of staff relationship of the personnel in the various departments. Also needed for successful staffing efforts are job descriptions that list the function and the various types and levels of personnel. (Refer to Chapter 4 for more detail.) Given this framework the nurse-manager will consider the following factors in the process of staffing: (1) the numbers and qualifications of personnel to meet the expectations of the institution, (2) circumstances peripheral to client needs and qualified personnel to meet those needs, and (3) assignment of staff for continuity of service and economical use of personnel.

Numbers and qualifications of personnel to meet the expectations of the institution

Traditionally, nursing administrators have used one or more counting methods for determining staffing patterns. These may consist of assessing the total client population of an agency or concentrating on a particular segment of services and dividing this number among the nursing staff available. This method assumes that the health care needs of the clients are identical despite diagnosis, treatments, and distribution by age group, sex, race, and socioeconomic factors. The system also assumes that all nursing staff members are equally competent.

Another counting method concentrates on activities or task performance. The number of direct and indirect nursing tasks is correlated with the amount of time spent on these tasks. This methodology is borrowed from business, where the study of work focuses on identification of tasks, work flow, work reorganization, reassignment, and work simplification. Task analysis is particularly useful in work of a repetitive nature, where conditions are standard and predictable. Although specific data are provided with the task analysis approach, there are issues left unanswered for nursing. Qualitative matters such as individual needs of clients, nurses fulfilling their roles to optimal capacity, and whether these tasks could be done better or equally as well by individuals with less preparation are cases in point.

Attempts to overcome these shortcomings in staffing have been made fairly widely by many nurse-managers through client care classification methods to determine the client's needs and then to match these needs with qualified personnel.

A *client care classification system* is an effort to quantify the nursing work load in terms of categories that are broadly identifiable. The classification system is based on the premise that better staffing patterns will be realized by adjusting staffing according to the number of clients needing certain levels of care. Client care classification may encompass any number of categories or levels of care. The most usual is three, concentrating on clients who need self-care, partial care, and complete care. Other terms used are essential nursing care, progressive nursing care, and comprehensive care. Specific criteria are described for each category or level of care, and a specific level of personnel is assigned for each category.

The problem of client classification is difficult because much overlap between classifications occurs. Several tools are used for data collection; direct observation, nursing audit, interviews with clients and staff, incident reports, and audit of charts are only a few.

The final step in the client care classification system is to predict the number of hours and the kind of personnel needed to meet the needs of clients in each classification or level. The general trend is to follow a ratio of five hours to the complete or comprehensive nursing care classification and one hour to the self-care or essential nursing care classification. Twenty-four–hour distribution of service is then taken into consideration. Variables to consider include the kind of care provided, when the bulk of service is rendered, and any special problems present that are unique to the work setting.

The ratio of registered nurses to nonprofessionals and proportions of staff on the various shifts are also considered in staffing. When careful attention is given to matching client need with personnel who are capable of supplying that need, efforts will be made to staff accordingly. With increased focus on classification of services, the nursing profession has been able to demonstrate the need to move toward greater registered nurse involvement in client care by all levels of nurses, including nurse-managers.

Both the American Nurses' Association *Standards for Nursing Services* and the Joint Commission on Accreditation of Hospitals emphasize the importance of the total concept of staffing. They call for sufficient numbers of registered nurses on duty at all times to provide clients with the nursing care that requires the judgment and specialized skills of the registered nurse. This standard is interpreted to mean that a determination of nursing personnel can be made only by evaluating the needs of the clients and the capabilities of the nursing staff assigned to a special area.

The goal of utilizing the professional nurse as fully as possible in performing only nursing functions has led to a reorganization of structure in nursing services to increase the proportion of personnel giving direct care to the client. Smaller spans of control through decentralization of services have helped to return the registered nurse to the bedside, planning and giving the care or directly supervising it.

A further delineation is needed between the registered nurses. If there is built into the system slots of various levels of nurses, for example, "AD RN," "BS RN," clinical specialists, or nurse practitioner, and various values are assigned to these differing classifications of personnel, then greater efficiency, more job satisfaction, and higher levels of productivity can be expected. The possible contribution and competency levels of personnel with different educational backgrounds vary greatly. The best approach is to review the classifications or levels needed by reviewing the job descriptions. This helps determine how much and what duties can be performed by one worker as compared to another. In agencies where workers other than registered nurses are utilized, the nurse-manager will look to see which activities can be performed best by licensed practical or vocational nurses and will determine those tasks that can well be assigned to a nurse's aide.

Circumstances peripheral to client needs and qualified personnel to meet those needs

There are many circumstances relating to the provision of quality care that may not have direct bearing on the individual need of the client or necessarily pertain to the competency of the nursing personnel but need to be taken into account when the staffing pattern is determined. The consistency of census is one problem. In some services, particularly where birthing and children are concerned, there is a great fluctuation in the census. Another issue is that of the physical layout of the area where excessive time and energy are required to cover the territory. Other circumstances that require consideration are use of automation through intercommunication systems and computerized control; employment of reusable versus disposable equipment; centralized or decentralized services; support staff; utilization of part-time nurses, students, or private duty nurses; and the size and involvement of the medical staff.

Assignment of staff for continuity of service and economical use of personnel

Basically a schedule for nursing staff needs to (1) adhere to the policies of the employing agency regarding utilization of professional nurse personnel and workers in different categories while ensuring appropriate balance of professional and nonprofessional staff, (2) provide for continuity of services, (3) seek to make effective and economical use of personnel, (4) consider vacations and other scheduled time off, (5) allow for adjustments in case of illness, emergencies, or changes in care needs, and (6) protect the rights of individuals against discriminating action because of sex, ethnic differences, or religious beliefs.

Scheduling may be performed centrally or at the departmental or unit level. There are advantages and disadvantages to each system. With centralized control the personnel can be distributed objectively in a more balanced manner among the nursing units, and understaffing or overstaffing can be handled to some degree. Centralized staffing is less time consuming. The one who determines the master schedule is in a position to know the overall staffing situation. Thus it is easier to make adaptations to unforeseen circumstances. Requests for special privileges are likely to be fewer than with the decentralized system.

Disadvantages of the centralized system are that opportunities for personal contact with employees is reduced, causing the one who plans the schedule to know little or nothing about the person scheduled on the time sheet. The maker of schedules may not have a true picture of the needs within each departmental unit.

Complete decentralization is uncommon. Total responsibility must be central for effective control.

With decentralization of schedules the nurse-manager at the middle or first level has opportunity to base the scheduling plan on knowledge of the clients and of the personnel assigned to that unit. The nurse-manager is more in control of the activities on the unit. The decentralized system poses some problems in that it is time consuming and sometimes provides inadequate coverage, as when there are not enough staff members on hand to cover unexpected absences or there is the need for additional help and individual employees are subjected to inequities in rotation and days off.

A common staffing pattern utilized by the nurse-manager is to plan a staffing schedule using the personnel assigned to a unit and to depend on additional help from other units for unexpected absences or emergencies, usually through the next one higher in authority. This staffing method works well if each nurse is expected to work a fair share of weekends, holidays, and unpopular work hours, such as evenings or nights. The approach to developing a time schedule often focuses on consideration of preferences of individual staff and the matter of seniority. Resultant inequities occur, with the newer or less experienced personnel being assigned to the undesirable shifts and most of the weekends and holidays. With this approach, little attention is given to the development of a schedule that is directed toward adequate and qualified nursing services on a twenty-four–hour basis.

Another staffing pattern considers the forty-hour, four-day workweek (Fig. 5). Advantages are that overlapping shifts provide for better coverage and client care, staff members have weekends off more frequently, there are decreases in absenteeism and in expenses related to overtime, and the system is cost effective. The main problems for the ten-hour day are fatigue and difficulty finding relief personnel to work an extended day.

Cyclic scheduling is one method of staffing that probably is the most valid and workable system for numbers of personnel. It involves the development of schedule patterns that are repeated at regular intervals. Schedule patterns for days and time off are established at a centralized level for a certain number of weeks, ranging from two to twelve, and are repeated within the given cycling period, while giving attention to the need for appropriate numbers and categories of personnel, continuity of client care, and establishment of work groups. Examples are given in Figs. 6 and 7.

In cyclic scheduling with a ten-hour day, four-day workweek, one plan is to provide every other weekend off, with single days off added to weekends (Fig. 8). No employee is scheduled for more than four consecutive ten-hour shifts in a row. All have at least fourteen hours free between any shift. Those who "float" are given a four-day weekend every six weeks. Likewise, it is possible to rotate shifts on a regular basis, usually every three months, if the staff is in accordance with the plan.

Cyclic scheduling of an eight-hour shift for a twelve-week cycle is particularly useful, because twelve weeks is easily divisible for days off and can be adapted uniformly to both large and small units. Each nurse has four weekends off, two of which are three-day weekends. The period also includes six single days off and five workweeks of six days each. The plan presented in Fig. 7 can be duplicated for the twelve-week span.

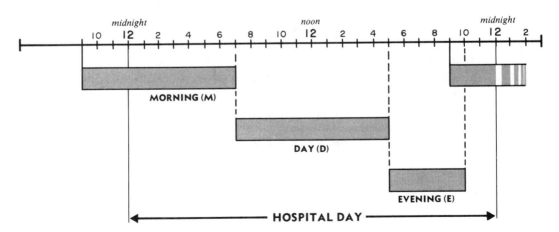

Fig. 5. Example of schedule for forty-hour, four-day workweek. (From Fraser, L. P.: The reconstructed work week: one answer to the scheduling dilemma, J. Nurs. Admin. **2:**12-16, Sept.-Oct. 1972.)

Elements:
Every third weekend off
Maximum days worked: 4
Minimum days worked: 3
Number of "split" days off each period = 2
Operates in multiples of 3, 6, 9, . . .
Schedule repeats every 3 weeks

☐ Scheduled day off

Position	Name	Week I S	M	T	W	T	F	S	Week II S	M	T	W	T	F	S	Week III S	M	T	W	T	F	S
Full time	R.N. 1																					
Full time	R.N. 2																					
Full time	R.N. 3																					
Total R.N.s on duty each day		2	2	3	2	2	2	2	2	3	2	2	2	2	2	2	3	2	2	2	2	2
Full time	R.N. 1																					
Full time	R.N. 2																					
Part time 32 hrs/week	R.N. 3																					
Total R.N.s on duty each day		2	2	2	2	2	2	2	2	2	2	2	2	2	2	2	2	2	2	2	2	2
Full time	R.N. 1																					
Full time	R.N. 2																					
Full time	R.N. 3																					
Full time	R.N. 4																					
Full time	R.N. 5																					
Full time	R.N. 6																					
Total R.N.s on duty each day		4	4	5	4	4	5	4	4	5	4	4	4	5	4	4	5	5	4	4	4	4
Full time	R.N. 1																					
Full time	R.N. 2																					
Part time 32 hrs/week	R.N. 3																					
Full time	R.N. 4																					
Full time	R.N. 5																					
Part time 32 hrs/week	R.N. 6																					
Total R.N.s on duty each day		4	4	4	4	4	4	4	4	4	4	4	4	4	4	4	4	4	4	4	4	4

Note: 8 hrs. of R.N. time saved per week by using part time R.N.s

Note: 16 hrs. of R.N. time saved per week by using part time R.N.s

Fig. 6. Example of cyclic scheduling using eight-hour day, forty-hour workweek. Master time schedule for three-week cycle. (From Eusanio, P. L.: Effective scheduling—the foundation for quality care, J. Nurs. Admin. **8:**12-17, Jan. 1978.)

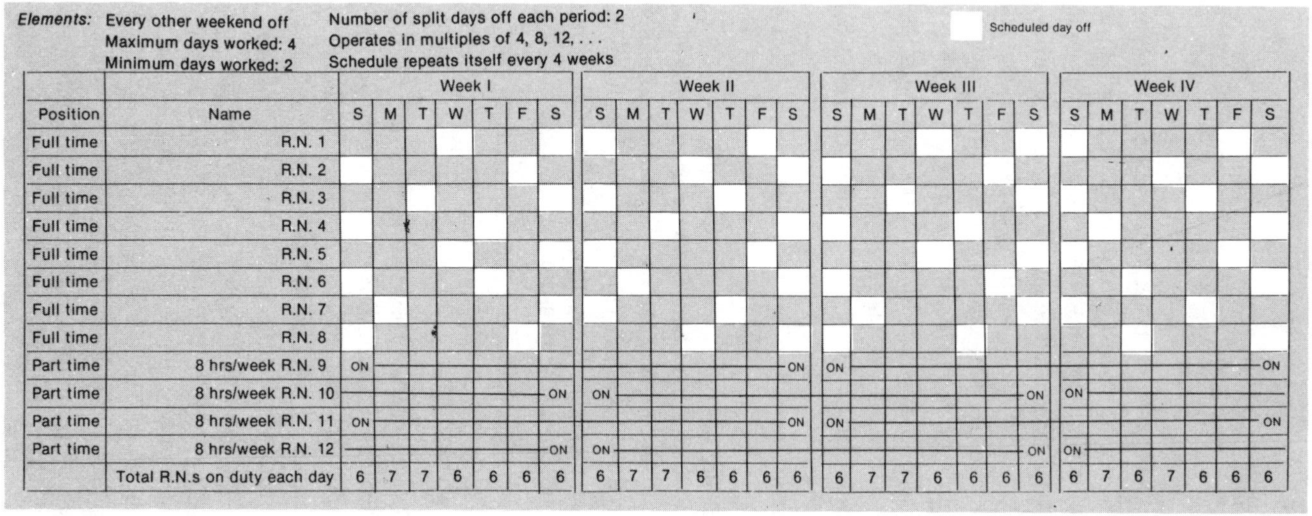

Fig. 7. Example of cyclic scheduling. Master time schedule for four-week cycle. (From Eusanio, P. L.: Effective scheduling—the foundation for quality care, J. Nurs. Admin. **8:**12-17, Jan. 1978.)

	S	M	T	W	TH	F	S	S	M	T	W	TH	F	S
Employee A	-	on	on	-	-	on	on	on	-	-	on	on	-	-
Employee B	on	-	-	on	on	-	-	-	on	on	-	-	on	on

Fig. 8. Example of basic ten-hour schedule for two-week cycle. (From Fraser, L. P.: The reconstructed workweek: one answer to the scheduling dilemma, J. Nurs. Admin. **2:**12-16, Sept.-Oct. 1972.)

The cyclic scheduling system lends itself well to the computer, thus saving manpower and providing for early printouts of the schedule. With the cyclic method a pool system of floating personnel is necessary to ensure assignment of an adequate number of personnel during each shift to any unit insufficiently staffed because of illness, absence, or emergency. If computers are not available, cyclic staffing sheets can be printed and names can be recorded manually.

The cyclic staffing system has a number of advantages:

1. A stabilized work force is provided, allowing personnel to synergize their efforts for the benefit of the clients.
2. A correct number and mix of personnel is provided with a minimum of floating personnel.
3. Time off is known well in advance so that workers can plan their personal lives.
4. "Good" and "bad" days off are shared by all.
5. A controlled maximum number of work periods before a day off is provided.

An added benefit to the nurse-manager is that the time spent on scheduling can be significantly reduced. Once the master plan has been developed, a person with less training can prepare and maintain schedules, freeing the nurse-manager for more direct contact with personnel and clients.

PREDICTIVE PRINCIPLE: Establishment of policies that ensure fairness, consistency, and professional development of human resources enables recruitment and maintenance of a sufficient number of qualified nurses.

There is really no beginning or ending to the staffing process. A stream of qualified personnel must be kept flowing into the health organization and through the various channels designed to develop and allocate human resources. No organization is static. At any given time, one can find employees leaving, and shortages occur at certain points and surpluses at others. Staffing is a composite of dynamic and persistent activities with which the nurse-manager must be concerned. Adequate attention to recruitment and maintenance of nurses will pay off in rewards of increased degree and retention and satisfaction among the staff employed. Retention of employees is cost effective. Every new nurse costs the agency time and money. Before staffing efforts can be successful, guidelines need to be established that provide a thorough and honest description of duties, responsibilities, and limits of authority of the position.

Prior to nurse employment, there needs to be an open exchange of information that will promote a better match between the nurse and the job. This can be done through interview, observation, and exposure to the work setting. The nurse-manager arranges a time for the prospective employee to tour the work area and to talk freely with the staff. Again, job descriptions are all-important. Detailed information about the duties involved in the job and the qualifications an employee must have to perform them are reviewed.

Formal induction of the employee is a crucial matter. This is the time when policies pertaining to salary, fringe benefits, retention, promotion, and tenure are discussed. It has been established by many authorities that although salary is important, compensation is not the major reason for nurses' satisfaction on the job. The underlying premise is, however, that the basic needs for security have been met.

The *wage and salary program* is the responsibility of the organization as a whole. However, the nurse-manager often plays a key part in making decisions about salary increases and about promotion for employees under his jurisdiction. Policies pertaining to the wage and salary program should address (1) differences in pay for various classifications of work, (2) a level of wage that is in reasonable alignment with the prevailing scale for institutions of similar nature in the same geographic location, (3) differences in preparation and experience of employees, (4) means for rewarding individual expertise and contribution through salary increment and/or promotion, and (5) a clearly defined procedure for offering complaints and grievances.

The nurse needs to know in advance of employment what avenue is used by the agency for wage control. The matter of bargaining with a union, a professional organization, individually or in subgroups within the agency may be a significant factor as to whether or not the nurse chooses to become aligned with the institution.

The *orientation period* is crucial to the retention and satisfaction of the employee. Progressive companies in industry have long recognized the need for properly introducing a new employee to his job. A study conducted by a large motor corporation proved to its satisfaction that employees who were provided adequate orientation to the job had a higher rate of retention, exhibited more positive work attitudes, and produced higher quality work.

Orientation is the formal process of familiarizing the new employee with the organization and his part in it. Not only does the program familiarize the new worker with the tasks he will be expected to perform, but also it provides him with information about the overall philosophy, conceptual framework, and objectives of the organization. A carefully planned orientation program helps the new employee to identify with the organization and its procedures, enables him to learn the unique ways the agency wants nursing roles and functions fulfilled, and gives him some feeling for the significance of the work he will be doing. The new employee is helped to overcome the fears and anxieties that are bound to arise in a new job. The orientation has the further benefit of helping the new worker gain acceptance by his fellow employees.

The time frame for orientation depends on such factors as (1) provision for employment of the individual while he is in the process of induction, (2) experience and competency of the employee, and (3) needs of the job to be filled. There is much controversy among nurse educators and nursing service personnel about the new graduate and the amount of orientation and on-the-job training required to fulfill expected work roles. It has been documented that a thorough orientation and time to adapt increases the level of performance of new graduates. Business and industry have long provided beginning and periodic orientation and retooling periods. More and more health care agencies find it cost effective to do so.

Of equal import is the problem of the large number of new graduates who leave hospitals after a year or two of employment. Reasons given for leaving are overwork, static environments, and inability to provide the quality of nursing care they find acceptable.

The educational process for nurses employed in an agency is another important factor leading to effective and efficient staffing and satisfaction of the employee. Even with excellent orientation, nurses can anticipate that jobs will change. With highly sophisticated professions such as medicine and nursing, there is a need for periodic updating of knowledge and skills. Many times both nurse-managers and staff alike are lulled into a false sense of security by the gradualness of change and are brought face to face with reality when they are confronted with a situation for which they lack coping skills. It is far better to anticipate the need for continued learning and to make the necessary provisions before a crisis develops.

There are three ways in which nurses maintain currency in their field. One is through on-the-job training, where each nurse is responsible for teaching part of his or her job. At this decentralized level the nurse-manager teaches staff, and staff help teach one another. A second approach is through a formal training department, usually called "in-service education," conducted at a centralized level. Depending on the size and purposes of the institution, one or more individuals are responsible for ascertaining educational needs and offering short-term programs to supply those needs. The focus of in-service education is specifically job related. Keeping current with new concepts, knowledge, and techniques that relate to health care and nursing activities is called continuing education (CE). Many states have legislated that a nurse must complete a specific number of hours of continuing education before each license renewal. This provides some impetus for nurses to avail themselves of ongoing education. Careful documentation of each educational experience assists in determining the extent of educational exposure needed for updating knowledge and skills.

The final phase of the staffing process is that of employee appraisal.* An employee appraisal is conducted for the purposes of assessing performance on the job and determining potential for development. The issue is discussed in relationship to the staffing process because retention, compensation, and promotion directly correlate with performance evaluation. Both formal and informal methods, ranging from verbal assessments to ranking methods, check lists, or rating scales, are used to determine proficiency. Performance, experience, and qualities of employees are reviewed and compared with the job description. Whatever approach is taken, it is important that the employee be apprised in advance of the procedure concerning methods used and frequency of evaluation. A planned

---

*Chapter 5 is devoted to evaluation, giving predictive principles for the management of ongoing evaluation and scheduled periods of summative review.

evaluation system helps the employee and nurse-manager consider all factors carefully, and it reduces the chances of personal biases. The employee appraisal allows the nurse-manager to scrutinize the work of the employee in terms of how well he is performing his job and also from the standpoint of what can be done to improve his performance. The nurse-manager may detect inadequacies in supervising and can improve his own performance.

BUDGETARY PROCESS

A budget is a plan that expresses the activities of a health care facility or unit in terms of dollars and covers a specific period of time. A budget is a forecast of anticipated operations. As such, it can never be definitive or absolute. The purpose of the budget is to set operating cost limits. It is a guide to performance, for although the budget includes costs of personnel, supplies, support services, travel, and buildings, it is essentially a commitment to the people who utilize the resources offered.

PREDICTIVE PRINCIPLE: Participation by nursing personnel in planning and controlling the budget leads to cost consciousness, increased awareness of activities, and increased cost effectiveness.

Operation of the nursing department or unit represents a large portion of a health agency's total expenses. Hospital management is becoming acutely aware of the importance of effective planning and the use of greater control in providing a sufficient number of appropriately prepared personnel and adequate facilities at minimum cost.

The effective nurse-manager recognizes that producing good nursing care can be strongly affected by the nurse's concept and practice of fiscal management. Nurse-managers who are aware of the procedure for budget planning and control can participate intelligently and can compete for the share of the budget necessary for their anticipated client care operation.

Successful planning for control of budget requires top-level management participation and approval. But all levels of management should understand and participate in both the planning and control phases as well, and a clear report system must be established, with specific target dates for accountability.

There are several advantages in involving nurse-managers in preparation of the budget. By looking intensively at activities and results from past expenditures, they are better able to modify future plans and objectives to increase cost effectiveness. Also, personnel who operate within a budget become cost conscious and begin to assign different priorities to the use of resources. They look for better and more efficient ways of delivering health care services to clients. In management by objectives, both setting of realistic objectives and the ability to obtain them are closely tied to budgets.

Nurse-managers who want to learn how to prepare and control budgets well may do so within the agency through guidance from experts, reading about budgeting process in material geared toward health care delivery system management, and taking courses of instruction concerned with budgetary planning. When nurses demonstrate their interest and competence in fiscal matters, they will have a better chance to be included in all aspects of the budgetary process, thereby becoming more efficient at realizing dreams and ideas about improved nursing services.

PREDICTIVE PRINCIPLE: A budgetary process that functions on a planned, continuous, and cyclic basis offers participants an effective way to operate efficiently and to provide information for making future key decisions.

The usual method for budget planning and monitoring the system is as follows: (1) determine requirements, (2) develop a plan, (3) analyze and control the operation, and (4) review the plan. The entire process functions on a continuous and cyclic basis, usually over a calendar year.

Determine requirements. Top-level managers usually assume responsibility for forecasting the needs for a new fiscal year. They do this by looking at major factors such as past experience and records, considering any changes such as closing or opening facilities or services, and studying anticipated population changes, needs for services, and any regulating changes that might occur as a result of policy change or legislation.

Ideally, these projections are reviewed with middle- and first-level managers to determine what the effect will be on departmental activity. It is at this time that needs for staffing, equipment, supplies, and facilities are scrutinized and requested. Once needs are assessed, cost studies of these needs are done; for example, the costs of supplies, manpower, equipment, and support services are estimated and allowances provided for the rate of inflation.

Develop a plan. Each manager, usually at the middle level, develops a budget for each quarter of the ensuing year, with the first quarter broken down into months. The established objectives are an integral part of the budget plan. The nurse-manager can set up simple graphs and charts to help control expenses on a day-to-day basis and contribute to cost containment. Business personnel are usually available to provide assistance in the formulation of such plans as needed. The astute nurse-manager will utilize this resource. Utilization of the support system of the budgetary department not only offers educational benefits, but the nurse increases his credibility in the eyes of the budgetary personnel, making routine inclusion of the nurse in the planning stage more feasible.

The items most common to health care budgets are personnel and operating expenses. Unfortunately, many nurse-managers deal only with the category of operating expenses. The significance of this matter is discussed under staffing.

Numbers and kinds of *personnel* and salaries and wages for each job classification reflect any anticipated changes in the upcoming year. These costs include employee payroll, provision for overtime, taxes, and fringe benefits. In order to accurately calculate these costs, the number of clients and the level and skill of the workers necessary to provide care for them must be determined. For example, for coverage to be sufficient it must be recognized that nurse, practical nurse, nursing assistant, and orderly ratios are directly related to the kind of care required by clients.

For *operating expenses,* each department or unit lists supplies by major types, determined on the basis of usage anticipated through the coming year rather than on purchases. Examples of items that may be included in the operating budget are medical and surgical supplies, repairs and maintenance, provision for depreciation and replacement, office equipment and supplies, and reference books and periodicals. Some operating budgets include appropriation for in-service education. Most budgets do not include consideration of utilities and housekeeping, as they are considered part of the indirect expenses. However, an accounting is shared with the nursing department or unit so that its members may be aware of the cost and assist with the control of these items to reduce waste and unnecessary expenditure.

Analyze and control the operation. Each level of management is held accountable for performance and corrective action. This accountability extends only to the costs the nurse-manager directly controls. The reporting system is based on the organizational structure of the individual agency.

The most effective system is to have a two-way flow of information between middle and top management with material distributed on a monthly basis for use in analyzing actual activity. The nurse-manager who has sufficient information can identify problem areas and unfavorable trends concisely and can initiate corrective action where necessary. If there are significant variations from the plan, an explanation indicating the nurse-manager's assessment as to possible causes of the expense variances needs to accompany the report. Of course, any noticeable deviation will be discussed with appropriate controllers at the time of the expenditure to determine if on-the-spot remedial steps are needed.

Review the plan. As the health agency and various components within the facility move through the fiscal plan for the year, each succeeding quarter is evaluated on the basis of current results. As each current quarter comes to a close, it is necessary to formulate a definitive plan for the upcoming quarter. Minor modifications are made in comparison with projections and actual occurrences. No major changes are made without going through the entire budgetary process.

• • •

Toward the end of the year the budgetary cycle is begun again. As the nurse-manager gains more experience with the planning cycle, more accurate forecasting results. An effective system of planning and controlling results in benefits of efficiency and cost savings, with provision of vital information necessary for making future key decisions. With such a plan the goal of providing quality care at minimum cost can be attained.

COORDINATION PROCESS

Coordinating is an essential part of managing. It is the orderly synchronization of individual efforts with respect to their amount, time, and directions, so that unified action is channeled toward the attainment of stated goals. The coordinating function helps the nurse-manager to ensure that all important activities are accounted for and assists in the identification of overlap, duplication, or omissions of function. Coordination pulls together all activities to make possible both their working and their success. In health care facilities, there is great diversity among workers and activities. To achieve coordination with minimal friction and maximal effectiveness, each member is helped to see how his work benefits the total enterprise.

It is important to keep in mind that the fundamental principles of management are interrelated. Philosophy, overall purpose, and conceptual framework affect planning, and planning affects organizational structure. Coordinating activities becomes a natural outgrowth of all these functions, for they are inextricably interwoven.

PREDICTIVE PRINCIPLE: Coordination of personnel and services through intradepartmental and interdepartmental activities brings about a total accomplishment far superior to that possible through fragmentation of individual effort.

Coordination of personnel and services within a health agency cannot be confined to a single area or a particular function. Overall collaboration must occur vertically and horizontally among departments to keep the viewpoint of management broad and to foster a desired balance among various, but interrelated, efforts. These controls provide a better means for (1) keeping the coordinating efforts adapted to the goals of the institution, (2) appreciating functions of other departments in order to better understand individual operations, (3) measuring the total effort of nurse-managers rather than assessing the work of a single manager, and (4) maintaining a control system for assessing the delivery of care to decentralized units.

Coordinated efforts at all levels can offer many benefits through planned and informal contact. Help can be forthcoming for problems with planning, staffing, and other aspects of nursing management. Greater knowledge and appreciation of the work of other nurses in the agency can be realized. Meeting with representatives from allied services can help to apprise the nurse-manager of the comprehensive range of services available that might better be utilized in coordinating work at the operational level.

By reaching out to others for information and support the nurse-manager becomes a more effective coordinator. Ongoing efforts can be improved. Accumulation of new knowledge will stimulate innovation of techniques. Behaviors will be changed, creating environments where work can be accomplished with efficiency and human satisfaction never before thought possible.

PREDICTIVE PRINCIPLE: The span of control directly affects the size and complexity of the coordinating function.

Span of control is a major concern in coordination because of the impact on how many and what categories of personnel are required to achieve the desired goals. There are some nurse-managers who have a centralized or wide span of supervision, ranging from coordination of all nursing services in an agency to responsibility for entire floors or clusters of units. Others manage groups of specialty areas, such as coronary care or maternal-child care.

An organizational approach that has received much attention, with varied results, is unit management. Unit management programs appoint a nonnurse unit or ward manager to relieve nursing personnel of many of their nonnursing activities and free them to provide client care. This concept, properly adapted to a hospital or agency setting, has been shown to be an effective productivity improvement technique for nursing, although it has not been proved cost beneficial for the hospital or agency as a whole. Unfortunately, if not properly implemented, the program can easily fail. In the majority of cases, unit management has been successfully implemented and its nursing benefits realized.

Decentralization in large-, small-, and medium-sized agencies is a valuable tool that allows nurse-managers to fulfill their responsibility for providing personalized competent care to clients through coordinated efforts. For best results, coordinating efforts should be made by a person at the lowest organizational level who possesses ability, desire, and access to relevant information and who is in a position to impartially weigh all factors. When a nurse-manager coordinates the unit within his realm of specific responsibility, all personnel can be supervised and are accountable to him.

PREDICTIVE PRINCIPLE: Activities directed toward regulating, preventing, correcting, and promoting coordination provide a comprehensive and efficient approach to management.

Managerial activities are varied and complex. The effective nurse-manager wants to (1) use planning strategies that will ensure smooth operations on the job while looking to the future, (2) organize the unit or department for maximum productivity, (3) utilize staff in a way that matches the tasks with talent, (4) delegate functions intelligently, (5) attend to employee needs and development, (6) motivate staff to perform to their maximum potential, (7) use leadership behaviors appropriate for the situation, and (8) adopt control methods that continually compare actual results with previously determined goals.

Skill and experience in problem solving and decision making are required for successful coordination. The heart and quality of operation are found in the nurse-manager's ability to assess needs for nursing service and to set in motion the activities that will meet those needs. In the decision-making process the nurse-manager recognizes the importance of assembling available information. The magnitude of data flowing through most agencies defies description, but it must be reviewed and processed. Provision of health care requires attention to the needs of daily living as well as the voluminous services necessary to prevent illness, promote and maintain health, and restore and rehabilitate the client. Data processing systems have had a definite effect on decision-making responsibilities. Computers can relieve nurse-managers of making decisions concerning staffing, budget, and some personal assignments, allowing the capabilities of the nurse to be used for more client-centered activities.

Another major approach in decision making is concerned with the communication system and the maintenance and improvement of human relations. The average nurse-manager spends a great amount of time in speaking, writing, reading, or listening. The ability or inability to communicate well with others and to determine which person or group should take part in the activities exerts a powerful influence on whether or not coordinative efforts are successful.

Although information gathering and communication are important, underlying the entire effort is a need to understand the policy-making and policy-implementing systems of the organization. The nurse-manager will understand how influence is exerted and will have a frame of reference for his coordinating activities.

Georgopoulos and Mann* have developed four types of coordination: (1) corrective, defined as those activities that correct an error or repair a malfunctioning or dysfunctioning system (this includes equipment or personnel); (2) preventive, which anticipates problems and coordinates efforts to prevent or reduce the impact of the problem; (3) regulative, defined as those coordinative activities that maintain the ongoing, day-to-day activities; and (4) promotive, interpreted as functions directed toward improving existing circumstances irrespective of identified problems. The basic premise is that there is a constant need for improvement. The most effective manager views coordination as an integrated system. If one phase of activity is weak or nonfunctioning, the output of the whole unit or department suffers. A successful coordinator translates his knowledge into practice.

Inclusion of preventive and promotional aspects in coordinating efforts provides higher quality care more efficiently and with greater cost effectiveness than if reliance is solely on coordination through regulatory and corrective activities.

PREDICTIVE PRINCIPLE: Review of the utilization of the nurse-manager's time provides a means for comparison of role expectation and fulfillment.

Using time effectively is a challenge to every manager. The nurse-manager in a health care facility is very often under pressure and is so involved in the day-to-day operation that he cannot see the relevant issues. The manager who has a heavy work load finds it difficult or impossible to stop what he is doing and take stock of the work process. He often conplains that his time is wasted on telephone calls and a myriad of other interruptions that keep him from doing his job. Surprisingly few nurse-managers can explain what their job is and how they spend their days. They move about exclaiming, "There never is enough time," or "I can't seem to get everything done." Each day they leave their jobs feeling frustrated that their work is unfinished. In contrast, observers might describe the manager as frittering away his time on trivial details.

For effective control, it is essential for a nurse-manager to recognize the importance of time-use control. Three approaches to improved time-use control by the nurse-manager can be employed: (1) use of assistants to protect him against time wasters, (2) primary use of manager time for major decision-making efforts, and (3) collection of time data on current activities, evaluation, and improvement of methods of time utilization.

A good assistant in the form of a ward clerk or secretary can help the nurse-manager save time. This assistant can take care of the endless paper work and the public, help in working out problems of other health professionals and ancillary personnel, and screen telephone calls. The key to relief through this avenue is in employing a capable person, training him well for the job, and then vesting authority in him to do his job without need for sanction from the nurse-manager concerning every detail.

*Georgopoulos, B. S., and Mann, F. C.: The community general hospital, New York, 1962, Macmillan Publishing Co., Inc., pp. 277-278.

The concept of using the major share of the nurse-manager's time for major decision making is sound in that he is employed for his expertise in managing nursing services and for his clinical expertise. It is logical to assume that the nurse-manager can better forecast the effect of alternatives in decision making when the major considerations are the care of clients and the implications of those decisions.

For a nurse-manager to recognize time-use controls in his work, he needs to collect the facts concerning his present time utilization. Keeping a daily log by 15-minute intervals is recommended for this purpose. The log should show what activity is performed, whether or not it is basic to his role, and the significance in terms of priority. Recording such information for a period of one month provides a reasonable sample. Study of such data could reveal that, in fact, the nurse-manager's time is put to good use and that he has an overload of responsibility. The data could also reveal what the time robbers are, what nonessentials should be eliminated, and what improvement can be made.

PREDICTIVE PRINCIPLE: The presence or absence of conflict influences a nurse-manager's ability to coordinate activity.

Conflict occurs where there is a struggle between interdependent forces. A controversy or disagreement exists in desires or opinions. Organizational conflict is both desirable and useful if maintained at a functional level. Most health care organizations experience a high level of conflict because there is much interfacing of roles and function, each dependent on the other. Clients are becoming very aware of their "rights" and of ways to achieve them. Nurses are giving more attention to such matters as patient advocacy, systems of care, salary, and benefits. Administrators, medical and nursing staff, and ancillary personnel are encountering an increasing amount of conflict as they seek to understand and to meet the expectations of the others. How conflicts in these kinds of interactions are managed determines positive or negative outcome. The good manager seeks to identify potential and actual points of friction in the organization and to determine whether they are the result of poor organizational design, personality problems, or problems with delegation and follow-up procedures.

Prior to the mid-1940s almost all management people looked on conflict as destructive and something to be avoided. Managers were trained to establish and maintain predictable patterns, with little or no allowance for individual reaction to the system. This traditional approach to social interaction has gradually given way to a recognition and acceptance of conflict as a way of life. The behavioral approach calls for rationalizing the existence of conflict, looking to the reasons why individuals and groups behave negatively, and focusing on the development of resolution techniques through which positive action can emerge.

Interactionists carry the behavioral approach even further. They recognize the absolute necessity of conflict to stimulate the search for new methods or solutions. They believe that conflicts are usually distributed along the continuum between a level of conflict that may be too high and require reductions and a level of conflict that may be too low and need stimulation before the individual or group becomes inept with regard to performance.

Human conflict arises at the intrapersonal, interpersonal, and intergroup levels. *Intrapersonal* conflict is that dissention within one's self regarding a troubling issue. Examples might involve a nurse who has seen a peer give a wrong medication and who has not reported the incident or one who consistently gives less than adequate care to clients for lack of sufficient staff and supplies.

Interpersonal conflict happens between two or more persons. Common examples are those differences of opinion between nurse-managers and members of the work force. The group, for instance, may believe it necessary to meet a client's need by assigning someone to be at his side constantly; the nurse-manager may think this action unnecessary. Or several members in the work group may perceive that one member is failing to carry his load.

Intergroup conflict takes many forms, depending on the interdepartmental interaction. Dissention commonly occurs between care givers and servicing units such as the dietary department, laundry, pharmacy, or x-ray department. Conflict is also an ever-present possibility between nursing units or nurse and physician groups within the organization.

Sources of conflict usually focus on role expectations, value systems, and communications. Characteristics of social relationships that are associated with various kinds or degrees of conflictive behavior are as follows:

1. Unclear boundaries of responsibility (job descriptions, assignments)
2. Conflicts of interest (nurse-manager interested in providing comprehensive care to the clients through primary care system and staff preferring functional system)
3. Communication barriers causing misunderstandings (evening versus night shift; language problem)
4. Dependency of one party or group on another (client at the mercy of staff for positioning; nurses waiting for housekeeping services)
5. Organizational structure related to the number of organizational levels and the number of job specialties represented (aide, LPN/LVN, ADRN, BSRN, nurse specialists, or nurse practitioners) and the degree to which labor is divided in the organization
6. Decision-making process (nurse-manager "tells" staff what they will and will not do about all activities)
7. Need for consensus (all parties believe they must agree on all decisions)
8. Behavior regulation (arrive at work on time, take breaks on schedule, adhere to a dress code)
9. Unresolved prior conflicts (resentful RN member who was not chosen to become nurse-manager; attitudes about what kind of care should be given versus what care is given)

These situations need not lead directly to conflict, but they have a high potential for doing so, thus influencing the coordination of activities. The direction taken depends on the perception of the conditions that exist and the attitude of the persons involved.

Not all conflicts are the same kind. There are basically those forms of conflict that follow definite rules (competitive) and those that are typically associated with angry feelings (disruptive). A third kind of conflict (constructive) uses open and honest dialogue to examine ideas until decisions are produced that are satisfying to all the participants.

American society generally subscribes to *competitive* behavior. A misinterpretation of Darwin's notion of survival of the fittest has led to individuals and groups competing with each other from the time they are able to react until life ends. Successful people, or "winners," receive the prize, and failures, or "losers," suffer the pain of defeat. It is argued that competition strengthens performance and increases cohesiveness within each individual group, and this does happen. After the competition is over, however, only one person or group is the winner and likely to remain satisfied and cohesive. The defeated individual or group may seek an opportunity for retaliation.

Consider the following situation. Two nurse-managers share a concern about a more than usual degree of dissatisfaction expressed by clients on their evaluation of care received during hospitalization. A plan was formulated and put into effect by the nurse-managers whereby evaluation forms would be tabulated, compared, and posted publicly in the agency's newsletter. Each group was presented the plan and agreed to work hard to "win." But the competitive scheme backfired. The winning group enjoyed having their achievements published as being the "best" care givers and felt cohesive and positive about their efforts. The "losers" were saddled with a label of failure and inadequacy, when in fact they believed they had provided excellent care that was not recognized for a number of legitimate reasons. This competitive situation ceased to be motivating and moved into disruptive conflict.

In *disruptive* conflict the intent is on reducing, defeating, harming, or doing away with the opponent. In the foregoing situation, members of the "losing" group shared their disgruntled feelings with each other interdepartmentally, during breaks, and in their daily on-the-job contacts. They used such tactics as rationalization ("If they had as difficult patients as we had to cope with, the results would have been different"), accusation ("They must have set the patients up to responding well for them"), and blame ("If so-and-so had worked harder, we would have gotten higher marks," or "If the administration had sent us enough help, we would have won").

In both competitive and disruptive conflict, there exists a win-lose situation, for only one person or group can emerge the victor.

There is a great deal of consistent evidence to suggest that cooperative effort results in reduction of conflict and therefore becomes *constructive*. When interdependent individuals cooperate in working toward the goal of quality client care, there is greater interest in the task, production is increased, and the clients and workers are more satisfied.

Strategies used by nurse-managers to handle conflict are either restrictive or constructive. The *restrictive* procedure is aimed at creating a situation where there are as few differences as possible or where differences exist, they are not recognized. Soothing platitudes are offered: "We don't need to worry about that; it doesn't matter." The staff are picked because they agree to be followers of direction. "Whatever you say" depicts the general attitude. Were this situation totally possible, individual and group actions would be quite predictable. One danger of smoothing over conflicts is that individuals and groups could fall into complacency. If everyone agrees to the same thing with no challenge, little thinking is going on, and quality of service rapidly deteriorates. More important, the soothing strategy is short lived, as strife will emerge in one form or another and must be handled.

Repression is another restrictive strategy. It is a "put-the-lid-on" approach. Leadership is aimed at punishing those who disagree and rewarding those who comply. The repressive climate overly stresses the organizational values of cooperation and framework, facing the danger of stifling individuality and creativity. "Those are the rules," "Do it because I say so," and "What you think doesn't matter" describe the prevailing attitude. The environment is so tightly controlled that latent ideas are curtailed. One problem with repression is that resentments are generated, and the workers punish or retaliate in ways such as procrastinating, doing a poor job, or taking sick leave.

The use of confrontation can also be restrictive in nature if the competitive "win-lose" approach is taken in which the individual or group seeks to gain as much as possible. Reaching a solution to a problem by an arbitrary decision, compromise, or majority vote results in losses for both sides. With this "lose-lose" strategy, differences are not dealt with and may fester again at other places, at other times, and in other forms.

Facilitating dispute resolution through the strategy of participative or integrative decision making takes a *constructive* approach. Participative effort implies the expectation of a "win-win" outcome or acceptable gain to both parties or groups.

Thomas Jefferson articulated the notion that power can be participated in by all the people in the social system. In 1820 he said, "The only safe depositor . . . is in people themselves." In the participative model, employers and workers try to produce the best result for all. It is a "both/and" system rather than an "either/or" system, thus creating a "win-win" possibility. The participative group requires (1) clear definition of values, purpose, and goals; (2) open and honest communication of information; (3) a sense of responsibility shared by all who participate; and (4) an environment of trust and commitment of all to the success of the process.

Suppose for a moment that conflict has arisen among a care-giving group. They meet together in the conference room. The problem is introduced. Two points of view are offered in the form of a thesis and an antithesis. Through open and honest dialogue the ideas for and against possible solutions are listened to and synthesized until they become integrated. The answer to the problem is one of higher quality than any one person could possibly have arrived at alone, the wisdom of the group becoming greater than that of the individual.

In the decision-making process, a constant effort exists at all levels to treat conflict and conflict situations as problems subject to the problem-solving methods. A clash of ideas is encouraged and little energy is spent in conflict over interpersonal difficulties because they will have been generally worked through as they have arisen.

Basic beliefs are necessary for integrative decision making to occur. Those in conflict must believe that (1) there is a mutually acceptable solution to the problem, (2) the mutually acceptable solution is desirable, (3) others' statements are legitimate and truthful, and (4) differences of opinion are helpful.

A constructive format for the nurse-manager to implement when conflict is present or anticipated is as follows:

1. Program a special time for meeting all persons involved in the disagreement, making sure that there will be time to discuss the issue and that there will be no interruptions.
2. Present the problem and have people give full expression to both positive and negative feelings. (As this happens more often, positive feelings will increase and negative ones will decrease.)
3. Use a paraphrasing ground rule, that is, when A says something to B, B cannot respond until A is satisfied. State what is heard and the feeling generated by the words. If done on every response, it can become very tedious, but the process forces hearing and promotes understanding. Often after two or three exchanges, B will say, "Oh, if *that* is what you are saying or feeling then we don't really have an argument."
4. Keep the focus on the problem.
5. Do not stop the meeting until a mutually satisfactory solution is reached.

CONTROLLING PROCESS

Controlling is a process designed to bring about an orderly and desired flow of activities in accordance with the requirements of plans. Controlling is like a checkup to make sure that what is done is what is intended. Purposes of control in nursing services are as follows: (1) to have sufficient quantities of staff and supplies available where they are needed, (2) to know whether the operation is economical, and (3) to determine if desired performance has been achieved. Fundamental questions as to what, when, where, how, and why are addressed in each phase of the controlling process. The basic steps in control are to (1) establish standards, (2) measure performance and compare results with standards, and (3) make corrections or adjustments in the care-giving operations to obtain results compatible with expectancies.

PREDICTIVE PRINCIPLE: Contracting for accountability of services rendered identifies the scope and limitations of the nurse-manager's span of control and provides a guide for assessment of the degree to which the nurse-manager's responsibilities are being fulfilled.

Accountability for the nurse-manager is blurred. By definition, accountability means answering to authority or becoming responsible or liable for one's actions. The accountable individual is prepared to explain and to receive credit for the results of his actions.

Multiple roles are often thrust on nurse-managers by the very nature of the organizational system. The nurse-manager may be expected to (1) set standards for quality of care and ensure their implementation; (2) manage staff through selection, staffing patterns and assignments, development, and evaluation; (3) be adept in communication and interrelational skills; (4) be an effective decision maker; (5) know how to plan, implement, coordinate, and control; (6) be involved with budgetary planning and control; and (7) serve as a role model for personnel and clients under his jurisdiction.

In accepting administrative responsibility the nurse-manager assumes accountability for management tasks and clinical outcomes. As a controller, it is his job to secure, formulate, and prepare information that makes possible effective control. He cannot be all things to all people. Before accepting the position the nurse-manager needs to know to whom he is responsible and the mutual areas of accountability. He needs to know to what degree the administration shares responsibility, because accountability depends on the authority of the position and the responsibilities inherent in the role. This function takes place between the nurse-manager and his immediate supervisor.

Unfortunately, most health care organizations are basically bureaucratic, with maintenance of the administrative hierarchy given greater importance than organizational goals. In a bureaucratic organization, authority and accountability are well defined for all employees, with rules and routine. Where decentralization is present, nurse-managers have more freedom and can become involved in developing standards and objectives more congruent with their priorities for professional practice, but with a strong feeling of accountability for hospital and medical procedures.

Independent practice is another matter. Medical personnel have made inroads within health facilities by practicing on a collegial basis with autonomy for their profession, allowing each physician to maintain control for the care of clients.

Nurses have not kept pace in developing a system in which they can function autonomously as independent nurse practitioners. Typically, nurses are employed in a department of nursing within an institutional hierarchy. The nurse-manager is delegated administrative authority and accountability but has not been granted major responsibility for the control of nursing care to the clients from the time of admission through discharge. There are some beginnings in transferring more accountability to professional nurses through the avenue of primary care, which incorporates the strong components of responsibility and accountability. There is need for the development of a nursing model that will define innovative roles for nurses within organizational conditions and that will allow for improved services to be given with greater professional nurse autonomy and accountability.

Wade* suggested a neoteric model for professional autonomy that can be adapted for hospitals, nursing homes, and similar institutions. He provides a set of conditions that, if present in an organization, are conducive to a high level of autonomy for the professional in the organization, as follows: (1) decisions made at the operational level in terms of the needs of clientele, (2) systems for services that will best meet objectives, (3) a climate that is open and receptive to new ideas and change, (4) effective interpersonal relationships among the organization's

---

*Wade, L. L.: Professionals in organizations: A neoteric model, Hum. Organization, pp. 40-66, Spring-Summer 1967.

professionals and between workers and clients, (5) equal distribution of supplies and services, (6) allowance for expressions of individuality, (7) belief that authority arises from knowledge and expertise and not hierarchy, (8) congruence among organizational professionals, and (9) goal setting and evaluation of professional behavior only by fellow professionals.

Irrespective of organizational system, contracting for accountability allows each party to see the other's perception of the role. In the process, each is helped to see the realism or unrealism in expectations. Furthermore, agreement to assume specific responsibilities provides criteria for assessment of the degree to which the nurse-manager's obligations are being accomplished.

PREDICTIVE PRINCIPLE: Setting standards serves to clarify purpose and provides a gauge for controlling quality and quantity of services.

Quality control is a foremost consideration in nursing management. The goal is maintenance of a satisfactory quality for the intended purpose. Specifically the goal sought is that which is best in terms of consistency with the standards set and satisfactory and dependable results being provided. Standards are the yardstick for gauging the quality and quantity of services. They serve to clarify purpose.

As much as possible, standards are stated clearly, objectively, and quantitatively so that they may be seen, measured, and judged and thereby become useful in the control function. There are some qualitative standards such as attitudes, morale, or relationships that are difficult to measure, but even these variables can be assessed with some degree of confidence.

It has been pointed out that there is no one set of standards used by all health care agencies for quality assurance, but that it is the task of each care giving group to develop standards and objectives to guide the actions of individual personnel into purposeful, safe, and effective client care. Standards that have been developed by many people and organizations such as joint commissions, the American Nurses' Association *Standards for Nursing Services* and *Standards for Nursing Practice,* and the National League for Nursing's *Criteria for Evaluating a Hospital Department of Nursing* are broadly stated but can be drawn on to develop appropriate standards for individual nursing care settings against which quality of care can be compared.

Standards of practice may be stated in terms of minimal or optimal activity, or any place in between. They describe the level or degree of quality considered appropriate and adequate for a single purpose.

The agency's philosophy, purpose, budget, and organizational structure influence specific standard settings. Written policies, objectives, and procedures are then formulated to assist personnel in making correct decisions in the performance of nursing care, organizational function, and personnel development. These guidelines serve as a tool for the management of nursing care and become the department or unit's official guide. They serve as evidence that standards have been set up reflective of the value system and beliefs of the organization and the individual care givers.

A committee of nursing personnel can be appointed to develop, review, and revise performance standards as necessary. Representatives from other concerned groups such as physicians and consumers may be included.

PREDICTIVE PRINCIPLE: Consideration of structural, process, and outcome standards as interrelational and interdependent serves to keep the management process balanced and in perspective.

Methods for measuring the quality of nursing care can be classified into structural approaches, focusing on the organization and management of the client care system, process approaches, emphasizing the actual delivery of care, and outcome approaches, concentrating on client welfare.

Structure of the setting in which care is given might include the scope of services, functions engaged in, education providing those services, budgetary allotment, staff development programs, and specific conditions of the environment. Structural criteria evaluate the administrative processes that arrange the flow of work. Various tools are used to make a systematic analysis of activities. Questions and checklists are typical of this style. Such audits can yield results that lead to cost control as well as general improvements in departmental operations.

Performance appraisals are a necessary part of the control process, as they provide back-up data for management decisions concerning salary, retention, promotion, transfer, or dismissal; pinpoint strengths and areas that need improvement; establish standards of job performance; and help the nurse-manager to determine if goals are being met. Methods of performance appraisal are discussed in detail in Chapter 5.

Professionals and nonprofessionals may be involved in controlling the structural aspects, for there are many facets included that could bear scrutiny from individuals who are prepared in other fields, such as business and management. The objectives of structural review are to bring into focus the activities and operations of the department and to allow a careful appraisal of the effectiveness and efficiency of work performance.

The *process* approach measures the delivery of nursing care to clients within the providing structure. In this process of quality control a comparison is made between standards set and specific nursing activities and interactions utilized to achieve them. They judge the adequacy with which the activities are performed. This is accomplished through formal and informal methods using direct observation and review of data. Whereas nonnursing personnel can engage in controlling the structural areas of nursing practice, only professional nurses should participate in determining whether or not nursing plans are adequate for the client.

The nurse-manager uses the process approach informally every day by observing work, checking on personnel, and reviewing input relating to provision of care. Comparing information obtained in these ways with existing standards is a continuous daily function of the manager as he controls his area of responsibility. This on-the-job surveillance permits the nurse-manager to remain current and accurate in his assessment and to reinforce or make necessary adjustments.

Numerous formal devices for evaluating quality of nursing care are available for use or adaptation. The most beneficial systems are set up in such a way that the evaluation can be recorded as objectively as possible. Instruments such as quality patient care scales, appraisal guides, and audits on charts and records while the client is hospitalized provide criteria that are broken down into categories and items reflecting the authors' perception of quality care. In the controlling process, data are gathered, reviewed, and acted on.

The *outcome* approach takes a retrospective look at the state or condition of the client after services have been delivered. Some define the parameters of outcome as when care is initiated and when the client is discharged. Others consider outcome as the effects of nursing care on the client after discharge. Outcome is the most difficult variable in nursing to measure, as it cannot be determined precisely how much of the outcome of client care has resulted from nursing intervention. Provision, or the lack of provision, for care through organizational design, physician control, or personal or social involvements with any number of contacts could influence the client's health outcome. One of the things that greatly increases the problems surrounding the measurement of quality nursing care is the fact that few specific nursing actions are linked to specific client outcome. This means that whichever method is selected to focus on outcome, assumptions will have to be made about its relation to the nursing process. Nursing must proceed with an attempt to develop precise definitions, criteria, and instruments that can be applied to test the quality of outcome for the client.

In using a quality control system, it is important for the staff to know how the findings will be used. There may be mixed purposes, as follows: (1) to provide information to the nurse-manager for reporting results and evaluating personnel, (2) to assist the staff in assessing their effectiveness and to guide their development, (3) to obtain feedback from the client, and (4) to increase the quality of care delivered.

A determination is made by the governing group at the centralized or decentralized level as to the format that will be used for quality control. Then the group needs to know the logistics of the plan. Stevens* suggests that the following guidelines have been found useful in some organizations for the study of process and outcome:

1. Schedule evaluation sessions at regular but unannounced intervals to reflect a more normal pattern of nursing care.
2. Use a sample of the clients.
3. Select clients at random or study those who require or required challenging nursing care.
4. Appoint only those people who are familiar with the evaluation process.
5. If nurses divide the work of evaluation, each member should grade the same portion of the evaluation tool on all clients or units evaluated.

---

*Stevens, B.: First-line patient care management, Wakefield, Mass., 1976, Contemporary Publishing, Inc., p. 121.

APPLICATION OF PREDICTIVE PRINCIPLES OF MANAGEMENT

Included in the agency's statement of philosophy is the belief in providing individualized care to each client. Primary nursing care has been selected as the delivery system. Primary nursing is defined by the agency as individualized, total client care given by the same professionally prepared person from the time of admission until discharge. In this setting the primary nurse is an autonomous practitioner with the right to make decisions with the physician, client, and significant others regarding his care. Administration recognizes that all nurses may not be prepared adequately to fulfill the role of primary care nurse and are committed to a staff development program. Because of unexpected turnover, you are the nurse-manager and have been assigned a newly employed RN. Unless help is forthcoming, he will have to be assigned to give primary care to five acutely ill clients without benefit of orientation.

Problem	Predictive principle	Prescription
How to incorporate the new RN into the system and meet client needs	A statement of the philosophy and goals of the total health institution gives direction to the number and kinds of nursing services that will be provided in performing the mission of the institution.	State to immediate supervisor that you cannot assign major responsibility for five clients to a new RN on his first day. Insist on an experienced RN until the new RN understands the system.
	Excessive turnover in nursing personnel causes the client to suffer loss of efficient and effective service and increases the cost factor.	Record the reason for the additional cost factor.
	A successful staffing process promotes job satisfaction. Standards of care, clearly defined, allow for descriptions of personnel necessary for implementation.	Have frequent, two-way communication with the new RN to be sure that he understands role.
	Establishment of policies that ensure fairness, consistency, and professional development of human resources enables recruitment and maintenance of a sufficient number of qualified nurses.	Obtain feedback from nurse orienting the new RN; make arrangements for new RN to study primary care nursing through staff development program.

BIBLIOGRAPHY
Books

DiVincenti, M.: Administering nursing service, Boston, 1972, Little, Brown & Co.

Donovan, H. M.: Nursing service administration: managing the enterprise, St. Louis, 1975, The C. V. Mosby Co.

Drucker, P. F.: Managing for results, New York, 1964, Harper & Row, Publishers, Inc.

Drucker, P. F.: Management tasks, responsibilities, practices, New York, 1974, Harper & Row, Publishers, Inc.

Filley, A.: Interpersonal conflict resolution, Palo Alto, Calif., 1975, Scott, Foresman & Co.

Ganong, J., and Ganong, W.: Nursing management, Germantown, Md., 1976, Aspen Systems Corporation.

Georgopoulos, B. S., and Mann, F. C.: The community general hospital, New York, 1962, Macmillan Publishing Co., Inc.

Longest, B., Jr.: Management practices for the health professional, Reston, Va., 1976, Reston Publishing Co.

Stevens, B.: First-line patient care management, Wakefield, Mass., 1976, Contemporary Publishing, Inc.

Stone, S., et al., editors: Management for nurses: a multidisciplinary approach, St. Louis, 1976, The C. V. Mosby Co.

Periodicals

Archer, S.: Pert: a tool for nurse administrators, J. Nurs. Admin., pp. 26-32, Sept.-Oct. 1974.

Aydelotte, M.: Staffing for quality care, J. Nurs. Admin., pp. 33-36, March-Apr. 1973.

Bloch, D.: Criteria, standards, norms—crucial terms in quality assurance, J. Nurs. Admin., pp. 20-30, Sept. 1977.

Cain, C., and Luchsinger, V.: Management by objectives: applications to nursing, J. Nurs. Admin., pp. 35-38, Jan. 1978.

Cantor, M.: Certifying competencies of personnel, J. Nurs. Admin., pp. 8-10, June 1975.

Clark, E.: A model of nurse staffing for effective patient care, J. Nurs. Admin., pp. 23-27, Feb. 1977.

Clinton, J., et al.: Developing criterion measures of nursing care: case study of a process, J. Nurs. Admin., pp. 41-45, Sept. 1977.

Donna, M.: A nursing unit as a political system, J. Nurs. Admin., pp. 28-36, Jan. 1977.

Eusanio, P.: Effective scheduling—the foundation for quality care, J. Nurs. Admin., pp. 12-17, Jan. 1978.

Everly, G., and Falcione, R.: Perceived dimensions of job satisfaction for staff registered nurses, Nurs. Res. **25**:346-348, Sept.-Oct. 1976.

Fuller, M.: The budget: standard V, J. Nurs. Admin., pp. 36-38, May 1976.

Gahan, K., and Talley, R.: A block scheduling system, J. Nurs. Admin., pp. 39-41, Nov.-Dec. 1975.

Haar, L., and Hicks, J.: Performance appraisal: derivation of effective assessment tools, J. Nurs. Admin., pp. 20-29, Sept. 1976.

Hegyvary, S., and Haussmann, D.: Monitoring nursing care quality, J. Nurs. Admin., pp. 3-9, Nov. 1976.

Hilgar, E.: Unit management systems, J. Nurs. Admin., pp. 43-49, Jan.-Feb. 1972.

Lewis, J. H.: Conflict management, J. Nurs. Admin., pp. 18-22, Dec. 1976.

Little, K., and Matthews, L.: Staffing function and management techniques, Nurs. Admin. Q., pp. 27-30, Summer 1977.

Lindeman, C.: Measuring quality of nursing care. Part I, J. Nurs. Admin., pp. 7-11, June 1976.

Longest, B., Jr.: Job satisfaction for registered nurses in the hospital setting, J. Nurs. Admin., pp. 46-52, May-June 1974.

Mayers, M., and Watson, A.: Evaluating the quality of patient care through retrospective chart review, J. Nurs. Admin., pp. 17-21, March-Apr. 1976.

McClure, M.: The long road to accountability, Nurs. Outlook **26**(1):47-50, 1978.

Moore, M.: Philosophy, purpose and objectives: why do we have them? J. Nurs. Admin., pp. 9-14, May-June 1971.

Naber, M., Seizyk, J., and Wilde, N.: Standards and nursing care needs—staffing methodology, Nurs. Admin. Q., pp. 1-12, Fall 1977.

Norby, R., and Freund, L.: A model for nurse staffing and organizational analysis, Nurs. Admin. Q., pp. 1-14, Summer 1977.

Odiorne, G.: Management by objectives: antidote to future shock, J. Nurs. Admin., pp. 27-30, Feb. 1975.

Onchken, W., and Wass, L.: Management time: who's got the monkey? J. Nurs. Admin., pp. 26-30, July-Aug. 1975.

Palmer, J.: JONA refresher: management by objectives, J. Nurs. Admin., pp. 55-60, Sept.-Oct. 1973.

Poulin, M.: Nursing service: change or managerial obsolescence, J. Nurs. Admin., pp. 40-43, July-Aug. 1974.

Ramey, I.: Setting nursing standards and evaluating care, J. Nurs. Admin., pp. 27-35, May-June 1973.

Ryan, B.: Nursing care plans: a systems approach to developing criteria for planning and evaluation, J. Nurs. Admin., pp. 50-58, May-June 1973.

Ryan, T., et al.: A system for determining appropriate nurse staffing, J. Nurs. Admin., pp. 39-38, June 1975.

Schaefer, M.: Managing complexity, J. Nurs. Admin., pp. 13-21, Nov.-Dec. 1975.

Schmied, E.: Allocation of resources: preparation of the nursing department budget, J. Nurs. Admin., pp. 31-36, Sept. 1977.

South, J.: The performance profile: a technique for using appraisals effectively, J. Nurs. Admin., pp. 27-34, Jan. 1978.

Thurkettle, M., and Jones, S.: Conflict as a systems process: theory and management, J. Nurs. Admin., pp. 39-43, Jan. 1978.

Wade, L. L.: Professionals in organizations: A neoteric model, Hum. Organization, pp. 40-66, Spring-Summer 1967.

Warstler, M.: Cyclic work schedules and a nonnurse coordinator of staffing, J. Nurs. Admin., pp. 45-51, Nov.-Dec. 1973.

3 PREDICTIVE PRINCIPLES OF TEACHING AND LEARNING

ASSESSMENT

The learner's developmental stage, personal characteristics, and prior experiences influence learning potential and dictate content.

The learner's sociocultural and religious group determines the nature, content, and acceptability of learnings.

The learner's prevalent life needs determine what he will learn.

FORMULATION OF OBJECTIVES

Participation of the learner in setting learning goals increases the number of learning activities meaningful and useful to the learner.

The more congruent and relevant that goals are to life needs of the learner-client, the more likely the goals are to be achieved.

Realistic behavioral goal setting enables selection of appropriate and meaningful content.

Setting goals that specify the precise degree of attainment required provides the learner with guidelines that can be followed.

MOTIVATION AND REINFORCEMENT

An obvious relationship between learning activities and stated goals increases the motivational value of the activity.

Accomplishment of beginning objectives reinforces belief in ability and motivates to greater effort for greater accomplishment.

Closely monitoring the level and source of anxiety and excitement in the learner enables the teacher to adapt the learning plan to learner needs.

Teaching in times of crisis about how to handle the crisis increases the opportunity for reinforcement and retention of learned behaviors.

Rewards consistent with the value system of the learner, such as recognition, praise, peer status, or valued gains, are motivating and reinforcing influences and thus facilitate learning rate, amount of retention, and degree of behavior change.

Practice of learned activities in a variety of ways reinforces learned behaviors and promotes the ability to generalize and discriminate.

ESTABLISHING THE LEARNING ENVIRONMENT

A reciprocal relationship of trust and security facilitates teacher-learner communication and allows accurate assessment, learner participation in goal setting, and better utilization of resources.

Recognition of the effect environment has on learning enables the nurse-teacher to mobilize environmental factors for the reinforcement of content.

Accountability for learning that rests with the learner enables the learner to meet his own learning needs and goals and enables the teacher to act as resource person, facilitator, validator, conferee, and consultant.

Verbal or written contracts with client-learners for attainment of specific learner needs enable the nurse-teacher to enact the teaching role more precisely.

Structure, limits, and feedback provide an environment that promotes security and trust.

LEARNING ACTIVITIES

Ability to use a varied number of learning theories increases the probability that varied strategies will be used in the nurse-teacher's teaching repertoire.

Learning episodes that contain input, operations, and feedback increase retention and utility of learning.

The more teaching strategies and operations available to and usable by the nurse-teacher, the better able the nurse-teacher will be to select a strategy based on learner and situational needs.

Utilization of problem-solving processes promotes continuity and ease of learning.

Increasing the difficulty of learning material in small increments promotes learning success.

EVALUATION

Objectives expressed as learner behaviors enable the teacher and learner to know the limits of expected outcomes and to evaluate in meaningful, specific terms.

Criteria by which to measure success, established through collaboration between teacher and learner, provide motivation, reinforcement, and guides for determining achievement.

STAFF DEVELOPMENT

In-service education programs structured to separate orientation, clinical experience, and management aspects promote clarity of content and staff growth.

All nurses function as teachers. Nurses teach patients, families, ancillary personnel, and one another. Teaching is inherent in the nurse role whether or not the nurse consciously cultivates and exhibits teacher behaviors.

The teaching role in nursing usually is the responsibility of lower and middle level management. It seldom is assumed by upper level management. Upper level management people usually delegate their teaching functions to others, for example, the staff development director, the patient education coordinator, the clinical specialist, the clinical coordinator, the supervisor, the head nurse, the team leader, or the staff nurse. Middle management and lower management people find teaching one of their major responsibilities. The formal classroom setting, where clearly delineated teacher-learner roles are established, is increasingly common in practice settings. However, more commonly, because of the nature of nursing practice, the nurse-leader serves as teacher in a wide variety of everyday activities. These activities range in scope from role modeling, to tutorial one-to-one methods for solving nursing problems, to preplanning and teaching small and large groups using a formal structure.

The nurse who assumes responsibility for assessing problems and for seeking ways to teach will be concerned with principles and methodology of the teaching-learning process. The problem facing all nurses is how to develop structures and relationships in which learning can occur.

Vaccines are helpless to prevent diseases unless people use them; heart patients live longer if they learn how to cope with their disabilities; people with diabetes live fairly normal lives if they learn how to balance their body needs, food, and insulin; cancer can be diagnosed and treated early if people learn to watch for the signs and symptoms; contagion can be stopped when people learn how to intervene in the transmission and resistance systems. The health status of any individual, family, community, or country is directly related to that individual's or group's ability to learn to prevent disease and to maintain health, to get well and to stay well. Medical science is helpless against ignorance, and information is useless without changes in behaviors that translate the information into healthful activities.

Nurses are the single largest health worker force in the world. They teach health to people and in so doing prevent disease, maintain health, facilitate coping, and enable individuals to learn to reestablish healthful living patterns. Several factors influence the teaching-learning process. These factors include the following:

1. A value need, problem, or dilemma that will motivate people to learn
2. Information that will enable people to make realistic decisions about behaviors
3. Support, structure, and direction that will enable people to alter behaviors to conform to decisions that have been made
4. Reinforcement, which will ensure the continuation of changes in behavior

Teaching is often considered to be primarily a process of giving information to others; however, information alone will not enable the learner to change his behavior. As T. S. Eliot wrote in "The Hollow Men,"

> Between the idea
> And the reality
> Between the motion
> And the act
> Falls the Shadow.

The nurse, whether leader or manager, teaches individuals and groups to ensure that applicable information is available and, additionally, helps the learner translate that information into behaviors so that no "shadow" falls between the idea and the behavior.

A teacher is a catalyst in that he can bring knowledge and learner together and stimulate a reaction. The teacher can engage in activity that either facilitates or inhibits the reaction; he can function in ways that make the reaction either transient or more stable. Teaching causes learning to take place. Learning is the acquisition of knowledge with subsequent changes in the behavior of the learner. Behavior, as used here, means anything a person does in response to an internal or external stimulus. This response can take the form of overt physical activity, emotions, or mental processes. Teaching and learning are inseparably linked in a cause-and-effect relationship and are consequently treated here as a single topic.

Teachers work with feelings just as often as with information because teaching involves human beings. It is a popular misconception that if the teacher is dealing with feelings, the activity is not teaching but psychotherapy. There is conflict and disagreement among authorities about the similarities and differences between psychotherapy and teaching. Teachers are anxious not to blunder into areas that should be handled by a skilled therapist and are eager to establish some way to discriminate between the two. Basically, both psychiatric therapy and teaching have as their purpose behavioral changes, and this is what generates much of the confusion. In both teaching and therapy the client or the learner must rearrange relationships between himself and other people, himself and a task, or himself and his environment. One of the key differences between the person needing therapy and the person needing teaching is the degree to which society has difficulty with the person. The person who needs psychotherapy is perceived either by himself or by others as behaving in a socially unacceptable manner. The person who needs teaching may not be using himself to his fullest potential, but he is not ostracized by society. The difference is essentially a matter of degree.

Nurses must exercise considerable judgment in determining the differences between teaching and psychotherapy. There are few definite rules, but there are some guidelines that will help the nurse-teacher to determine if the teaching role is appropriate. Following are some of these guidelines:

1. Does the learner have the mental and physical potential to learn (can he alter his present behavior to the desired behavior)?
2. Does the learner have a behavioral or thought disorder?
3. Can changes in behavior be brought about by:
   a. increased self-awareness and sensitivity to others?
   b. additional information?

c. additional physical or cognitive skills?

d. additional choices or alternatives?

e. change in habit patterns?

f. encouragement, reinforcement, or evaluative feedback?

The following example illustrates the use of the foregoing criteria:

Mr. Nesbit, a 38-year-old man, was suffering his first episode of duodenal ulcers. The nurse making the initial hospital admission contact with Mr. Nesbit asked him if he had any idea why he had ulcers. Mr. Nesbit replied that he thought he knew. He stated that there were times when he could feel his "stomach tighten up and the acid just pour in." When the nurse reported this to the team, the group asked, "Why not teach this man a different way to handle his feelings so that he need not jeopardize his health?" The nurse-leader replied, "I can't do that, I'm not a psychiatrist!"

The group decided to apply the criteria to determine if they could teach Mr. Nesbit and thus change his behavior response to feelings.

The following is the use of the criteria and the group's findings. No effort is made to discuss clinical content. The focus of the discussion is on the methodology of using the criteria given for the preparation of patient teaching plans.

Criteria	Group conclusions
1. Has the mental and physical potential to learn	Mr. Nesbit is of normal intelligence, has no physical handicaps, and has held a stable job for many years.
2. Does not have a behavior or thought disorder	The patient has socially acceptable behavior, can carry through in ordinary conversation, and makes appropriate responses to interview questions.
3. Changes in behavior can be brought about by	
a. increased self-awareness and sensitivity to others	Mr. Nesbit indicated an honest and well-developed sense of self-awareness as early as the first contact.
b. additional information	Additional information about stress, ulcers, and his behavior was available that would provide further data on which the patient could base changes of behavior.
c. additional physical or mental skills	Earlier awareness of rising stress would enable him to perceive impending situations that would elicit gastric responses.
d. additional choices or alternatives	Mr. Nesbit could participate with the nurse-teacher in exploring helpful ways to deal with stressful situations.
e. a change in habit patterns	Once new ways of handling stress are identified and tried, successful ones can be developed into new habits.
f. encouragement, reinforcement, or evaluative feedback	Close and honest working relationships with Mr. Nesbit can provide the nursing staff with opportunities to participate in identifying and reinforcing successful ways of handling stress. Reduced acid flow will be reinforcing.

When the discussion was completed, the team decided to work with Mr. Nesbit and teach him a more healthful way to handle stress. The nurse talked extensively with the patient and discovered that with some help he could identify some recent, very consistent sources of stress. The nurse supplied information about the physiology of duodenal ulcers and the stress–acid–intestinal motility relationship, and together Mr. Nesbit and the nurse worked out several alternative ways of dealing with the stress at the time it occurred. His hospital stay was of sufficient length to allow him several opportunities to cope with stressful situations successfully. The nursing team collaborated to reinforce his changing behavior.

ASSESSMENT

Assessment is determining the present status of the individual; goal setting is establishing the changes that are necessary; teaching is facilitating changes; and evaluation is assessing what changes occurred and whether they were the desired changes.

Assessment is the first step in the teaching process and is necessary to establish need, content, and method. Even when incidental teaching occurs, quick assessments are made by the nurse-leader. Often these are so natural that they are engaged in without planning or conscious thought. Some of these easy and obvious assessments are the general health status of the learner, his age, general alertness, and any of his more obvious characteristics.

Planned change requires detailed and methodical assessment of the learner and those things that influence his learning. Assessment is not something that ends before teaching begins; it continues throughout the teaching process. Information gathered during all phases of teaching adds to the teacher's total knowledge of what the learner brings to the teaching-learning situation, and this knowledge contributes to better teaching.

The effective teacher gathers information from all available and appropriate sources. The patient, family members, friends, other members of the nursing and health teams, charts, observations, and other agencies contribute to the total data about the learner. The principles elaborated in this section are designed to help the nurse-leader assess the learner so that content and methodology have meaning and are useful.

PREDICTIVE PRINCIPLE: The learner's developmental stage, personal characteristics, and prior experiences influence learning potential and dictate content.

The age and central stage of development of the learner will determine how he interprets what he hears, sees, and experiences.

The age level is an indication of "normal" growth and maturation. The average child grows at a given rate and develops physical and mental skills at certain mean ages. With knowledge of normal growth and maturation the teacher will know at approximately which ages muscular coordination is developed, abstract thinking is developed, and physical decline will begin to occur.

Erikson's stages of development are briefly outlined here. Only the positive senses are listed. The negative senses, which Erikson calls the "dynamic counterpart," are omitted for brevity. The development of these "senses" is a problem or task facing each individual.*

1. Sense of trust (first year)—satisfying experiences or finding biologic and emotional needs taken care of consistently in appropriate ways without pain or harm

---

*For a full discussion of the stages of development see Erikson, E. H.: Childhood and society, ed. 2, New York, 1963, W. W. Norton & Co., Inc., pp. 247-273.

2. Sense of autonomy (12 months to 3 or 4 years)—asserting and concluding that he is an individual with a choice and responsibility
3. Sense of initiative (4 to 6 years)—finding out what he can do; period of vigorous learning and intrusion into other people's worlds by physical attack, incessant questioning, and locomotion
4. Sense of industry and accomplishment (6 to 12 years)—engagement in real, worthwhile, socially useful tasks that can be completed correctly and well
5. Sense of identity (early adolescence, 12 to 15 years)—clarification of who he is, what his role in the world will be, and to what group or groups he belongs; whether he is independent or dependent, adult or child
6. Sense of intimacy (middle to late adolescence, 15 to 20 years)—friendship and companionship; need for warm, close bonds with others, even a need for an inner feeling of fusion with others
7. Sense of generativity (adulthood)—interest in producing and caring for one's own children
8. Sense of integrity (maturity)—healthy integrated personality that accepts his life, limitations, people, group, and time period; recognition and acceptance of limitations and potentialities

These categories are presented briefly and incompletely. The ages given are approximate ages of focus for each task. No task is mutually exclusive of other tasks, and most of them overlap and are repeated at subsequent stages of development.

The nurse-leader who can recognize the developmental level and central tasks of the learner can use this knowledge effectively in teaching. For example, the child who has not developed a concept of time cannot be taught about "tomorrow," for time has no meaning or reference point. The 6- to 10-year-old child can best be taught by utilizing his sense of industry and accomplishment, and the adolescent can be taught by using his sense of identity and independence from adult domination.

The use of central tasks of development in teaching patients can be seen in the following situation:

Carolyn, a 16-year-old girl, was admitted to the orthopedic ward with a fractured femur and was placed in balanced traction. She was 30 pounds overweight and was placed on a 1000 calorie diet. Maintenance of the diet quickly became a power struggle between Carolyn and the nursing and dietary staffs. The physician ordered dietary teaching for Carolyn, which was given by the hospital dietitian using didactic methods.

High school friends participated in the power struggle by smuggling in favorite candies; parents became caught up in the cross fire between pampering a loved child and cooperating with the prescribed regimen. One day the team leader asked, "Carolyn, does food really mean that much to you?" Carolyn replied, "Not really, but I don't like to be *made* to do anything. I'm old enough to eat what I please."

The nurse assessed Carolyn's present task of development as the need for identity and independence from adult domination. This developmental task was then used by the nurse to foster personal growth. The nurse obtained the physician's cooperation, and the diet order was changed to a "regular select." The nurse then acted on the knowledge that the adolescent needs to plan her own life and course of action in collaboration with others but maintaining some degree of independence.

The teacher used Carolyn's additional need for intimacy with the concomitant adolescent preoccupation with appearance and attraction of the opposite sex to interest her in personal hygiene and grooming. Dietary facts and information were supplied in the form of booklets and pamphlets. Carolyn was soon asking for explanations about food values, calories, fats, protein, and carbohydrates. A high school friend brought her a home economics book, and Carolyn requested the dietitian to come back so questions could be answered. By the time Carolyn returned to school, she had lost the 30 pounds and was helping her mother lose weight by planning the family meals. The nurse's skilled use of the central tasks of development of the middle teens enabled the accomplishment of the desired health goal for Carolyn.

Personal characteristics, such as intelligence, curiosity, perseverance, ways of handling stress, and adaptability, help to determine the content and method of teaching. Often a learner's inability to speak English, or health problems such as blindness or deafness, mask intelligence or obscure other personal characteristics. These factors should be carefully considered when assessing the learner.

The nurse-teacher can make some personal characteristic assessments by observing the learner's ability to solve small problems and cope with minor life situations. Entering into ordinary discourse with people can give the nurse further clues about their intelligence and level of curiosity. The nurse can observe (1) the kind of questions that are asked, (2) the frequency with which the same question is repeated, (3) the rapidity with which simple instructions and routines are grasped, and (4) the difficulty or ease with which new ideas and ways are adapted. These observations help the nurse build a picture of the learner's personal characteristics and assist with the adoption of content useful to the learner.

Prior experiences influence present responses by providing the conditioning and context for understanding the meaning of educational stimuli. Concepts are learned by building ideas, facts, knowledge, and antecedent concepts, one on the other, pyramiding them into an interrelated whole.

Everyone has antecedent knowledge and concepts on which to build new knowledge. The nurse cannot assess all prior experiences of learners but can evaluate selected prior experiences. Education, family constellation, experiences with teachers and health personnel, hobbies, interest areas, and occupation provide reference points, context, and antecedent knowledge for learning. This information allows the nurse-teacher to start where the learner is and to relate new material to familiar material in meaningful ways.

PREDICTIVE PRINCIPLE: The learner's sociocultural and religious group determines the nature, content, and acceptability of learnings.

The learner's sociocultural and religious group usually determines his value system. The value system dictates what is right and wrong, moral and immoral, fair or unfair, honest or dishonest, desirable or detestable. A value system influences ideas and feelings about others and provides guidelines to behaviors.

Teaching and learning objectives consistent with the learner's value system are realistic and achievable; the value system itself can be used as a motivation factor. Objectives in conflict with the learner's values are unrealistic and almost impossible to achieve without first changing the values.

An example of the influence of values derived from cultural groups can be seen in the following:

Alfonso is a 22-year-old Mexican-American with diabetes. Alfonso resisted all health teaching, regardless of methodology, until he saw another diabetic, aged 40, with a below-the-knee amputation as a result of gangrene. The knowledge that a loss of limb could be a consequence of uncontrolled diabetes and inattention to special foot care shocked Alfonso and threatened his "macho" (self-concept of manliness). He became interested in preserving his feet and legs and learned rapidly about all aspects of diabetes. He also helped the nurse to understand the importance of the "extended family" in the Mexican-American culture so that more valuable and realistic teaching could include reference to the extended family.

Knowledge of and respect for the learner's value system will be a major determinant in the teacher's success or failure and may influence the learner's future relationship with health care personnel. Values govern both the learner's and the teacher's behavior; interpretations of and judgments about other people's behavior are made within the framework of each person's value system. The nurse-teacher must not only be cognizant of the learner's sociocultural or religious values but also must have insight and self-knowledge.

PREDICTIVE PRINCIPLE: The learner's prevalent life needs determine what he will learn.

The learner, as does any other organism, responds to the strongest stimulus. A strong need is a strong stimulus, and the teacher must identify early the most urgent need, for until this need is met little else will be learned. The needs of the learner determine what he will see and hear and the interpretation he will place on sensory input. A patient who had just had an electrocardiogram and was anxious over the results was asked by the team leader, who was making patient rounds, if he had been up yet that morning. The patient replied, "Why, what's the matter, is something wrong with my ECG?" Another patient, responding to a different need, might reply, "No, not yet, I wake up slowly, and I haven't had any coffee yet."

A strong stimulus can create a need and facilitate learning or can interfere or distract the learner so that the stimulus becomes an inhibitor. A patient who is concerned about an errant husband or a sick child may not be able to learn about prenatal diets because of the more pressing worry.

Selective hearing, need, and readiness become problems to the teacher only if the teacher has not assessed the most pressing and current need of the learner collaboratively with the learner. Frequently what the learner wishes and is ready to learn is more important and achievable than what the nurse wishes and is ready to teach. Developing common goals may require a synthesis of teacher and learner goals.

FORMULATION OF OBJECTIVES

An objective is a destination, goal, or expected or desired outcome. An objective defines where one wishes to go and what one wishes to accomplish. It tells what the learner will be able to write, recite, construct, identify, differentiate, contrast, solve, compare, discriminate, judge, do, and so on. Objectives tell the teacher what is to be taught and the learner what is to be learned, and they enable both to determine the extent of accomplishment.

Objectives cannot be assumed, for such assumptions lead to conflict of purpose and misunderstandings and defy evaluation. Objectives need to be clearly and concisely stated so they can be understood, accepted, and used. Vague objectives, couched in erudite but trite jargon, are useless to most teaching-learning participants. Simple, direct, and explicit sentences that spell out in common language the desired outcomes enable the teacher and learner to select content, methods, materials, and activities that are appropriate and can promote goal accomplishment.

PREDICTIVE PRINCIPLE: Participation of the learner in setting learning goals increases the number of learning activities meaningful and useful to the learner.

PREDICTIVE PRINCIPLE: The more congruent and relevant that goals are to life needs of the learner-client, the more likely the goals are to be achieved.

Setting goals with the learner helps to keep them realistic and meaningful. Participation of the learner in goal setting enables goals to be set that are within the framework and context of his life and needs and ensures that established objectives are goals to which he is committed.

Learners have information, insights, awareness, and cognizance of problems pertaining to their own lives and needs; the teacher has specialized knowledge, skills, experiences, insights, perspectives, and often an objectivity that the learner does not possess. Working together, teacher and learner can set goals best suited for specific needs.

PREDICTIVE PRINCIPLE: Realistic behavioral goal setting enables selection of appropriate and meaningful content.

PREDICTIVE PRINCIPLE: Setting goals that specify the precise degree of attainment required provides the learner with guidelines that can be followed.

Inevitably, content is dictated by goals. Specific behavioral objectives enable the teacher to determine what content is realistic and relative to the attainment of each goal. The teacher need only answer the question "What does the student need to learn in order to behave in the described manner?" to select the specific content necessary to goal achievement. This is seen in the following example:

Goal: To be able prior to discharge to change the dressing on your leg using aseptic technique.

Attainment of this goal requires a knowledge of the concepts of asepsis from which theories of asepsis are derived, a knowledge of selected bacteriologic facts, and a knowledge of principles formulated on the basis of those facts. Achievement of the goal requires a knowledge of the dangers or risks involved and an ability to make valid judgments and discriminations when applying a sterile dressing in a variety of circumstances. Finally, attainment of that goal requires the enactment of specific behaviors.

The actual content selected to be taught or included is influenced by the assessment of the learner—his previous experience, his basic bacteriologic knowledge, and his particular needs. When the goal is *the ability to change a dressing using aseptic technique,* two hours are not spent discussing the pharmacologic properties and physiologic action of penicillin, even though there is a tenuous relationship of topics. In other words, specific goals help to decrease tangential and noncontributory activities.

Without specific, realistic goals, content selection becomes arbitrary and is frequently motivated more by what the nurse-teacher is comfortable in teaching than by what the learner needs to know. Therefore realistic, specific behavioral goal setting gives structure to learning situations, which decreases the frustration and lowers the anxiety of both teacher and learner by enabling the learner to understand how content will be useful to him.

MOTIVATION AND REINFORCEMENT

Theorists differ in basic assumptions about the role of motivation and reinforcement in learning. In this discussion, no attempt is made to explain or reconcile differences among learning theorists, but an attempt is made to choose those theories or aspects of theories that will be most helpful to the staff nurse during his everyday teaching responsibilities.

Motivation can be intrinsic or extrinsic. Intrinsic motivation is the impetus, incentive, or driving power within an individual that propels him into action. The teacher who can capitalize on an individual's motivation can concentrate on the activities of being mentor, guide, validator, supervisor, enabler, supporter, reinforcer, and evaluator. Extrinsic motivation is provided by the teacher or other external factors that influence the learner's desire to learn. These factors can be identified and manipulated to develop maximally and influence directionally learner motivation.

The nurse-teacher will discover that motivation may be influenced by personal and individual circumstances but that intrinsic motivation is the more important of the two types of motivation. Some motivating factors are common to most individuals and groups. This section relates to the common principles of motivation and learning and is primarily concerned with intrinsic motivation.

PREDICTIVE PRINCIPLE: An obvious relationship between learning activities and stated goals increases the motivational value of the activity.

The more reasonable and meaningful the activities appear to be to the learner, the more effort he will invest in their accomplishment. For example, the patient or aide learning about changing dressings using aseptic techniques may balk at learning the physical principles governing the capillary action of fluids until he sees the influence of those principles on the transportation of microorganisms by moisture.

The nurse-teacher can demonstrate relationships between necessary knowledge antecedents, content, and objectives by planning overall teaching content with the learner in a graphic way. To the uninitiated learner, knowledge basic or preliminary to goal accomplishment may appear to have little relevance to the goal. Content and activity plans, either written or carefully described so that relationships between necessary learning activities and accomplishment of goals will be conspicuous to the learner, can stimulate motivation.

PREDICTIVE PRINCIPLE: Accomplishment of beginning objectives reinforces belief in ability and motivates to greater effort for greater accomplishment.

Probably nothing is quite so motivating as success. Success is a lessening of anxiety or tension, because a goal has been achieved. It is a moment of accomplishment when confidence grins a little and takes a deep breath. The next task is then begun with confidence reaffirmed and reinforced. Anxiety about failure is somewhat relieved, and fear of falling short of an established goal is decreased.

Success early in the learning process is necessary even to those who appear most confident. The nurse-teacher who sets a few small but challenging goals that can be met early in the learning process ensures greater motivation and effort for the larger learning tasks. Success can be planned by structuring learning situations with a high probability of success. The reinforcement of having succeeded, even in a small learning task, can be highly stimulating to the student and can motivate him to greater effort. Success early in learning will promote greater tolerance of failure.

PREDICTIVE PRINCIPLE: Closely monitoring the level and source of anxiety and excitement in the learner enables the teacher to adapt the learning plan to learner needs.

PREDICTIVE PRINCIPLE: Teaching in times of crisis about how to handle the crisis increases the opportunity for reinforcement and retention of learned behaviors.

People learn best when they have a value, need, obstacle, obstruction, puzzle, dilemma, or interruption of some kind. Under ordinary circumstances, this interruption creates a state of mild anxiety, an excitement, and/or anticipation. Resources are mobilized to overcome, solve, or bridge the problem. At this stage the learner is highly motivated to learn things that will contribute to his ability to solve the problem or achieve his goal. Statements such as "I function more efficiently under pressure" or "I'm so excited I can't wait to get on this project" refer to the level of anxiety or anticipation described.

When the pressure is increased, anxiety increases and diminishing returns are realized. The learner's activities are no longer goal oriented and tend to function as a pressure release valve without actually contributing to solving the problem itself. Activities such as telling everyone how overworked one is, making elaborate preparations for work, and making several trips gathering books or equipment when one trip would suffice are all clues to the nurse-teacher that learner anxiety has increased.

Mild anxiety is the natural state of the human organism. Dynamic tension is the mechanism by which homeostatic balance is maintained. The healthy state is not a tension-free state; it is a state of tension balance. Anxiety or excitement is energy—energy is a pivotal learning force. Without an increased level of energy, no learning takes place. Anxiety or excitement results from encountering a problem. Sometimes the energy level is so low that it is not readily observable, or it may not be within the learner's level of awareness. Encountering a problem, or recognizing a goal, is always accompanied by an internal "toning up," a sharpening of wits, an increase of alertness that is called excitement or anxiety. McDonald* calls it "anxiety" and labels it "intrapersonal energy change." The energy change then becomes the precursor to motivation. McDonald characterizes motivation as a condition necessary for learning but not sufficient to make learning occur. He defines motivation as having three characteristics: (1) intrapersonal energy change, (2) affective arousal, and (3) anticipatory goal reaction. The *intrapersonal energy change* may be caused by autonomic response mechanisms (as with fear) or basic life support needs. Most of the time the exact nature of the causal sequence of the energy change is unknown. The *affective arousal* is a feeling state or emotion. This state may not be in awareness or it may be a highly charged, intense emotion and well within the level of awareness. The *anticipatory goal reaction* is the purposefulness of motivation. Motivation is goal oriented, for it is through movement toward the goal that anxiety is reduced and satisfaction or pleasure achieved. The consequence is that goal achievement returns the arousal state to normal and reduces the energy change to its prior level.

Generally speaking, the higher the anxiety, the more specific and focused the learner's attention, so that learning goals unrelated to the anxiety are not achieved. Learner attention becomes highly focused on the stimulus causing the anxiety. Teacher activities begin to center around reducing the anxiety, strengthening coping mechanisms, or teaching coping behaviors directly related to the source of the anxiety. Crisis, a state of very high anxiety and acute problems, provides a fertile field for learning. The person in crisis needs solutions so desperately that he is very receptive to cues and models, information guidance, and so on. The nurse-leader who takes the person in crisis through the activities necessary to resolve the crisis is capitalizing on prime learning time. The learner uses a real situation to learn behaviors that are immediately useful and have instant reinforcement.

Anxiety is one of the most delicately balanced factors influencing motivation. Perception of anxiety, accurate assessment of the levels of anxiety, and responses designed to control anxiety can mean the success or failure of any teaching endeavor.

PREDICTIVE PRINCIPLE: Rewards consistent with the value system of the learner, such as recognition, praise, peer status, or valued gains, are motivating and reinforcing influences and thus facilitate learning rate, amount of retention, and degree of behavior change.

Reinforcement of desired behaviors is the most influential factor contributing to the retention of learning. Reinforcement takes many forms and assumes many meanings, depending on the reinforcing stimuli and the learner's value system.

Recognition of a successful experience is a prompt reinforcement. Success is probably the greatest reinforcer. The nurse-teacher can promote the reinforc-

*McDonald, F. J.: Educational psychology, Belmont, Calif., 1966, Wadsworth Publishing Co., pp. 111-113.

ing value of success by preparing the learner to recognize the characteristics of a successful experience. Behavioral objectives that are spelled out enable the learner to identify what successful behaviors are and to recognize his own success immediately.

Reward and punishment reinforcement are helpful, depending on the form taken. Reward tends to be more successful than punishment. Rewards can be something tangible received for desired behaviors or positive feedback that causes good feelings. For instance, the relief of anxiety, as discussed previously, can be an important positive reinforcer.

Recognition by others can be highly reinforcing. Success recognized and appreciated by a meaningful individual or group and mentioned to other people important to the learner acts as a strong reinforcer in the learning experience.

For employees, rewards may take the form of statements in efficiency reports, letters to the employer or supervisor, commendations made to committees on promotions, and written memos to people in a position to give employment rewards such as salary raises, promotions, bonuses, and educational leaves. Copies of all such commendations should be sent to the employee.

Reinforcement therapy is being conducted currently for both selected psychiatric and pediatric patients. This reinforcing method uses rewards of valued objects, tokens that can be exchanged for privileges, favored foods, candy, or other desired objects as tangible rewards that can reinforce desired behaviors effectively. There must be careful selection of candidates for the controlled use of this teaching technique; if used inappropriately, it can become a way to obtain a desired object rather than a way to learn successfully.

Status rewards can be very important to learners. "Face," family pride, superior achievement, special mention, or public acclaim can fit into a value system and fulfill a need that can be more reinforcing than any tangible form of reward.

Punishment is an often-used negative reinforcer, but it has limited effectiveness in the teaching-learning process. Punishment of patients usually takes the form of reprimands, deprivation of privileges, exhibition of angry behavior by authority figures, ridicule, or sarcasm. Punitive statements such as "I'm not speaking to you today; I heard how bad you were last night" or "That was a stupid thing to do; what in the world made you do that?" do not contribute to the motivation of the learner and probably only serve some ego need of the nurse-teacher. Punitive measures may cause the learner to avoid the teacher and withdraw from learning situations. Fear of punishment or failure can cause learners not to try. This does not imply that failure should be ignored, nor can the teacher positively reinforce *nonlearning,* for that would negate *positive* reinforcement of *learning.* The teacher can make an evaluative statement about whether the objective has been accomplished and/or can help the learner learn to evaluate his own progress.

The optimal use of the reinforcements most meaningful to each individual requires the nurse-teacher to utilize the reinforcement judged effective for each person or group in each separate learning experience. The closer the reinforcement follows the successful learning experience, the more valuable the reinforcement for both motivation and retention. Continued reinforcement at later times also provides increasingly greater reinforcement and greater motivation and retention. The reinforcement that takes place at a later time can take the form of additional comments from the nurse-teacher or opportunities for repetition of the successful experience.

PREDICTIVE PRINCIPLE: Practice of learned activities in a variety of ways reinforces learned behaviors and promotes the ability to generalize and discriminate.

Repetition of the same material over and over again has little value for learning beyond habit fixation. Repetition, to be valuable, must have an improvement aspect. When repetition contains an improvement aspect, it becomes practice. Accompaniment of each repetition of the behavior by a feedback and correction cycle enables the learner to improve, if only slightly, each time he performs the behavior.

Repetition and overlearning are necessary for the purpose of achieving skill. Beyond achieving the required skill, repetition of learned behaviors in the same manner or in a similar situation is unnecessary and adds nothing to the learner's knowledge or skill.

Learning experiences spaced to allow the time lapses necessary for maturation are most effective for promoting retention. Rapid repetition of activities within a short period of time increases skill in narrow or single applications but contributes little to the learner's ability to generalize and discriminate.

Providing the learner with situations that require extraction of central principles and application of these principles to several problems or learning situations does three things: (1) it requires the learner to recognize and extract the central and uniting themes of situations (conceptualization); (2) it requires the application of principles to like situations (generalization); and (3) it requires the learner to perceive variables and make decisions and judgments about the selection of principles to apply to a given situation (evaluation and discrimination). An example of this type of reinforcement can be seen in the learner who had learned that microorganisms can move rapidly through moisture, which was an important consideration when sterile dressings were changed. Opportunities to work in other situations where sterile fields were important enabled him to extract selected central uniting concepts and principles of asepsis. The preparation of injections and emptying and changing urethral catheter drainage bags required that he select and apply the applicable aseptic commonalities discriminately.

Practice, either spaced or continuing, or application to similar situations requires periodic review, supervision, or evaluation by the learner and the teacher to ensure continued quality behaviors.

ESTABLISHING THE LEARNING ENVIRONMENT

The learning environment is not so much a matter of architecture as a matter of atmosphere. The building, patient units, classrooms, conference and office spaces, lighting, temperature, air circulation, paint color, piped-in music, and intercommunication systems affect the teaching-learning process to some degree. Physical environment can facilitate teaching and learning through technologic aids, convenience, and comfort. However, the teacher with something to teach and the imagination, enthusiasm, and will to teach and the student with the need, ability, and determination to learn will create an environment where teaching and learning can take place regardless of the surroundings.

Authority figures in the teaching-learning situation in health agencies set the tone and atmosphere for learning. However, learners are equally important contributors to the learning environment. The learner who brings negativism into the learning situation as a predominant characteristic can negate efforts of the nurse-teacher to establish an environment conducive to learning. Mutual contributions and consistent effort to create and maintain a positive learning environment are required of all participants. The nurse-teacher sets the pattern for learning interactions by implementing principles of teaching and learning that elicit positive responses from the patients, co-workers, and ancillary workers who are the learners.

PREDICTIVE PRINCIPLE: A reciprocal relationship of trust and security facilitates teacher-learner communication and allows accurate assessment, learner participation in goal setting, and better utilization of resources.

The optimal learning environment is basically one in which freedom is fostered by mutual trust. This allows the learner (1) the freedom to question without feeling foolish or stupid, (2) the freedom to participate in decisions, (3) the freedom of choice when there is a choice, (4) the freedom to learn as much as possible, and (5) the freedom to establish his own goals and obtain help in reaching them. These are important freedoms in learning, and either the teacher or learner can alter the learning climate and decrease learning potential by tampering with the trust on which the learning freedoms exist.

Accurate assessment, learner participation in goal setting, and full utilization of resources are possible only if the teacher has self-trust. If the knowledge of self as a competent, adequate nurse depends on knowing all answers and solutions to nursing problems, then the nurse-leader will not have the ability to participate freely in the teaching-learning process. Lack of self-trust can cause the nurse-teacher to guide learners only into content areas in which the teacher feels secure. This lack of self-trust places a rigid restriction on both content and method. (For a further discussion of self-trust, see Chapter 4.)

PREDICTIVE PRINCIPLE: Recognition of the effect environment has on learning enables the nurse-teacher to mobilize environmental factors for the reinforcement of content.

The physical environment and the climate in which learning takes place have a major effect on all phases of learning, and the inclusion of environmental considerations in teaching plans will help determine what is learned. Nurse-teachers often comment, "He knows better; why doesn't he do it?" The factors causing a discrepancy between what an individual "knows to do" and what he "does" are not specifically known. It is known that all behavior is meaningful, although not always understandable, and all behaviors are in response to some internal or external stimulus. The most usual approach to solving this problem is for the nurse-teacher to attack the overt behavior when some simple alteration in the forces that cause the behavior could enable real learning to take place.

Teacher behavior frequently exerts more influence on learning environment than does the material being taught. Following is an example of behavioral influence on the learning environment:

A nurse-leader was orienting two new ancillary workers. After describing their duties, the leader assigned them to care for two patients and told them, "If you have any questions or are in doubt at all, just come and ask me." Later, when they did ask for information from the leader, the nurse answered the questions, but by her behavior she communicated impatience at being interrupted, and the ancillary workers felt stupid for asking questions. The verbal response was clear and simple; it was the behavior that communicated negatively. The ancillary workers sought no more help from the nurse-leader because her behavior created an environment that taught them not to ask when in doubt.

Contradictions between content and climate and lack of congruity between words and behavior cause confusion. Learners will respond to the clearest or least threatening message.

PREDICTIVE PRINCIPLE: Accountability for learning that rests with the learner enables the learner to meet his own learning needs and goals and enables the teacher to act as resource person, facilitator, validator, conferee, and consultant.

PREDICTIVE PRINCIPLE: Verbal or written contracts with client-learners for attainment of specific learner needs enable the nurse-teacher to enact the teaching role more precisely.

The nurse is in the peculiar position of being employed (usually) by an agency, yet being the servant of the client. As in any profession, the professional loyalty of the nurse belongs to the client. Seldom do the nurse's allegiances to the client and to the employing agency conflict, because in health-related fields the objectives of all are geared to attaining and maintaining or retaining the highest possible health level. Teaching needs of clients do sometimes cause some conflicts, since hospitalization of a patient may not be timed for the best possible teaching, and teaching needs may span the involvement of several agencies. There are several ways around this problem, but none is entirely satisfactory and gets at the problem created by the nurse's being agency based rather than client based. Some of these ways are discussed here.

1. *Involvement of the learner.* The nurse-teacher involves the learner to such a great extent that he assumes the responsibility for his own learning program. Continuity then rests with him. The client collaborates with the nurse, who makes the placement of responsibility explicit and helps him establish what he needs and wants to learn to solve his health problems. Together they attempt to establish alternative ways he might go about learning and establishing checkpoints or criteria for measuring progress. The client can then call in other nurses, other resource people or agencies, his public health nurse, or his physician for help in carrying out his learning program.

2. *Use of learning contracts.* A second alternative for solving this problem is through the use of learning contracts. Once the learning program is established, the nurse and client enter into a learning contract that incorporates both content and time so that mastery of specific content is completed within certain time constraints. Mastery of content is recognized by the attainment of certain specific criteria. Mastery means the ability to perform up to some established standard

considered to be within the parameters of safety or desirability by both nurse and client.

3. *Continuity of care on a contractual basis.* Some acute agency–based nurses have a third alternative. With agency support they can incorporate, enabling them to follow patients into their homes on a fee-for-service basis to ensure continuity of nursing care. This makes them available for helping the family and the patient and makes teaching continuity possible.

4. *Continuum of care on a donated basis.* Nurses often follow patients into their homes or other agencies on their own time. Having entered into a contract with a patient whose time constraints in a given agency did not permit closure of the learning episode, the nurse uses time off to conclude the contract. Care-oriented nurses find it satisfying, yet this activity overextends them. Nurses who make a practice of this should see their tax consultant to determine deductibility of related expenses.

PREDICTIVE PRINCIPLE: Structure, limits, and feedback provide an environment that promotes security and trust.

Structure means guidelines and road maps. Structure in learning situations means the provision of directions, limits, specific goals, specific outcomes, time constraints, and other formats that enable the learner to know where he is going; it provides a means for getting there and signposts useful for determining when he has arrived. Structure does not mean control or restriction on the independence of the learner; quite the contrary, structure is often a mechanism for providing for learning independence. One can provide a little structure and therefore a lot of independence, or a lot of structure and less independence. Often all the learner wants or needs is for someone to validate his learning or his perceptions and to help detect his misconceptions. Establishing a mechanism for validation is a form of structure. The balance between structure and nonstructure is delicate and difficult to maintain. However, it is essential to the learner's independence, creativity, and own need system to provide him with some sense of the parameters of environment, for example, time constraints and the type of learning aids available, and the parameters of his learning needs, that is, the value of knowing certain things or behaviors.

Structure in the form of telling the learner what is going to happen, what is expected from him, what are the acceptable limits and specific time limitations, and what the learner may expect from the nurse-teacher in teacher-student relationships and guidance provides a secure learning environment and decreases anxiety. Terms such as "positive environment," "freedom," "trust," and "security" need not be equated with lack of limits and structure. Lack of structure promotes insecurity, fear, and inhibition—not the desired security, trust, and freedom.

Structure in the form of specific learning objectives, limits, available learning experiences, expected relationships, and requirements for success provides a secure environment that promotes learning. Comments such as "I never really knew where I was with that nurse; I did not know what I was supposed to do or what was expected of me" indicate distrust caused by a lack of the structure necessary for optimal learning.

LEARNING ACTIVITIES

All nurse-teachers utilize activities in teaching, whether by accident or by intention. Activities are all those things that will make learning take place. Activities can involve people, agencies, books, charts, or any source of content; they can be projects, audiovisual aids, or any teaching tool. Thus learning activities enable the acquisition of knowledge and recall; they reinforce, promote, transfer, and foster generalizations and discrimination. The planning of learning activities for the maximum benefit of the learner will ensure efficient accomplishment of behavioral objectives.

PREDICTIVE PRINCIPLE: Ability to use a varied number of learning theories increases the probability that varied strategies will be used in the nurse-teacher's teaching repertoire.

There are many theories of learning. This book presents only two—behaviorism and cognitivism. These two theories are at opposite ends of the learning spectrum. Behaviorism is sometimes called stimulus-response associationism. Whereas classical conditioning deals with inevitable, or reflex, responses, operant conditioning deals with voluntary behavior. Other names for operant conditioning based on behaviorist learning theory are instrumental conditioning and behavior modification. When the desired response occurs, whether accidental or guided, a reward meaningful to the learner is provided so that the probability of the desired response recurring is increased. The basic thesis of operant conditioning is that *the frequency with which any act occurs may be altered by the consequence of the act.*

Gestalt field theory or cognitive field theory has as its salient feature that *man in his environment is a unit participating in what is called a simultaneous mutual interaction.* This theory of learning conceives of perception as all the different ways one becomes familiar with his environment and not mere consciousness of his environment. Things and people are perceived differently by different individuals because perception depends on the sum total of life experiences and the way other things in life space are perceived concomitantly. (Whereas stimulus-response associationism emphasizes single units—one organism [human being], one stimulus, and one response—and an effective reinforcer, cognitive field theory deals with the concept of person [meaning the individual] within his whole field.) Cognitive field theory proposes that hypotheses that help to determine causal interrelationships and organize facts to provide direction and predictability are the heart of a science. Reality for the cognitivist is what that individual perceives and experiences it to be for himself. Nothing exists in and of itself to people; things exist in relationship to a person's total experience. The cognitivist theory has the following characteristics:

1. Insight
2. Putting things together to make a pattern
3. Seeing things in relationship to each other (For example, sickness can only

be viewed in relation to health; passive can only be viewed in relation to active; and happiness can only be viewed in relation to sadness.)

4. Always developing

Other theoretical frames of reference for learning can be derived from learning-theory source books. Several are given in the bibliography. Since the nurse-leader has a teaching role, one of the tasks essential to role development is an exploration of learning theories. From this base the nurse-leader can develop a useful eclectic approach to teaching-learning situations.

PREDICTIVE PRINCIPLE: Learning episodes that contain input, operations, and feedback increase retention and utility of learning.

Learning is a change in behavior that is acquired as a result of practice and that can be repeated when the need is aroused.

Learning has three identifiable aspects that exist regardless of the learning theory adopted:

1. An input aspect
2. An operation aspect
3. A feedback aspect

These aspects are variously called sequences or phases, but since both sequence and phase imply a serial order in time, "aspects" is used here, for aspects can occur simultaneously. Graphically, learning is like a pyramid with three sides, one each for input, operation, and feedback.

1. *Input* is the acquisition of information and the organization of the information into action hypotheses (predictive principles). These activities may be assessments, content information, instructions, recognition that a response is appropriate, or any of the *cognitive* activities associated with acquiring input.

2. *Operation* is the *activity phase;* it is directly observable behavior, responses to the input and interactions. It is practice (prescriptive theory). In memorization, it is repetition (either oral or written). In discovery learning, it is testing out ideas, either by putting them into action or interacting with another person. The operation aspect is *response*.

3. *Feedback* is the result of the operational test or the result of evaluation. The feedback becomes input that confirms, alters, changes, or refutes the cognitive phase or input.

The three aspects of a learning episode frequently occur with such speed that clear delineation between aspects is not always possible. For instance, the operational phase is in effect a test or trial or acting out of the input. The very act of doing generates immediate "fingertip" feedback that becomes input for corrections. The most useful element about familiarity with the three phases is that the presence of all three phases in any learning episode increases the likelihood of the learner actually having a change of behavior.

PREDICTIVE PRINCIPLE: The more teaching strategies and operations available to and usable by the nurse-teacher, the better able the nurse-teacher will be to select a strategy based on learner and situational needs.

Choosing a teaching strategy depends on several variables. Most of these variables are simple logical ways of looking at the factors governing the means by which the learner and the teacher can find a common learning medium. If the learner is a patient in the hospital or home, consideration must be given to his mobility, his energy level, the availability of resources (books, pamphlets, audiovisual materials), the content to be taught, the amount of anxiety surrounding the teaching subject, and the number of other stimuli being received by the patient and his family. Families and other people significant to the client have a part in choosing the learning strategies if they are going to participate in the learning episode.

Most teaching strategies are passive in nature. The learner reads, watches, and listens. These teaching strategies provide the major modality for cognitive input. They will probably continue to remain a central learning modality because early in a human's life reading, listening, and watching play prominent roles in gathering information. People seldom experiment and rediscover information each time it is needed—that method is too inefficient. Many advances in modern technology assist learning—television, super 8 millimeter film, tape cassettes, telephone dialing information systems, film strips, slides, programmed books, transparencies, and the whole gamut of audiovisual materials, which bring information to learners in a wide variety of formats. These informational packages can be put together in learning modules tailor-made for learner and situational idiosyncrasies. The bibliography for this chapter contains references to resources helpful to the nurse who wishes to make multimedia learning modules for clients or other health care givers.

The nurse-leader who teaches the same or similar content repeatedly to clients may wish to make, or work with the agency to purchase, learning modules using several media as the input mode for selected clients. Other patients, depending on their cognitive style, may wish to participate in the development of an individualized program of study, to complete a programmed text designed to meet their needs, or simply to read or listen to the nurse-teacher talk with them about the content.

The operation sequence of learning demands that the learner *do* something with the information. This activity may involve solving a simulated problem, practicing a procedure, recalling, building, creating, making, using, or any other active operationalization of the input (information). The act of *doing* provides a basis for the feedback sequence. Feedback arises not only from the formal evaluative material available on tests but also from the act itself. As learners practice or get involved in some utilization of information, the information begins to correct itself, to make further sense, to fit into patterns, and to make generalization insights possible.

Each phase of the learning process—input, operation, and feedback—needs to be devised in collaboration with the learner and chosen for its ability to meet his specific needs and the needs of the situation in which he finds himself during learning.

Simulation teaching techniques offer the nurse-teacher an opportunity to develop teaching skills with exciting dimensions. Usually health teaching involves information giving, demonstration, and return demonstration. Creative teaching strategies provide the client-learner, the co-worker–learner, and the nurse-learner the opportunity to experience behaviors that are the objectives of the learning episode. For instance, the nursing care giver who is teaching the child diabetic to give insulin often uses a syringe, a bottle of water, and a lemon or orange, or a sponge for this purpose. This technique is a form of simulation. Role playing a patient interview with a colleague provides the nurse with alternative approaches and interviewing behaviors that are difficult to learn in the real situation. Children learning balanced dietary habits are sometimes given models of food to put on a plate for a balanced meal. These forms of simulation provide practice when the "real thing" cannot be studied directly because it is too expensive, not available, or too dangerous.

Children and adults enjoy playing games, and games lend themselves well to learning. Games are contests requiring skill or luck. Skill or good memory retention can provide the nurse with the structure for a game. Bingo provides a model for a game to aid memorization, as is needed for classification of foodstuffs or vitamin content. Guessing games such as "my ship comes in sailing" and "20 questions" are models for information games. Problem games where players are given a diabetic insulin and food balance problem make good learning exercises. For good simulations, learning experience structure, for example, supplying specific behavioral objectives and directions, make the difference between success and failure. The reader is referred to the bibliography for resource materials concerning game theory and utilization.

PREDICTIVE PRINCIPLE: Utilization of problem-solving processes promotes continuity and ease of learning.

A knowledge of the problem-solving process is a learner skill that promotes a systematic use of appropriate resources. Problem solving takes place in many ways; however, the more systematic the problem-solving, the more reliable the result. The neophyte in systematic problem solving will find that a logical format or model contributes to his skill. The following is a suggested guideline for problem solving in tasks or stages.

Stage I, problem identification or establishment of objectives, is the initial task and the keystone of problem solving. Stage II is the gathering of appropriate data or the selection of appropriate principles. This stage requires (1) a survey of all the learner or problem solver knows about the problem, (2) a collection of the antecedent knowledge patterned into concepts, and (3) formulation of the concepts into predictive principles. These predictive principles enable the learner to list possible alternatives of action (stage III). Stage IV, a listing of the risks inherent in each alternative, helps the learner to make a logical choice of alternatives, choosing the one that has the greatest chance of solving the problem with the least chance of damaging the patient or the situation. An additional stage (stage V), in which all possible applications of the theories, facts, concepts, and principles used in the problem are listed, will be useful as an aid to further generalizations. The additional stage will also help the learner or problem solver to reinforce learning. Utilizing problem-solving processes in a tangible form can make content logical and sensible to the learner. Use of such methodology will provide an overview of all elements of the content.

Since much of nursing and health maintenance is applied science, health teachers frequently draw facts, concepts, and principles from the basic sciences of anatomy, physiology, chemistry, bacteriology, physics, and the social sciences. Often the learner has difficulty in seeing the relationship between these antecedents and his goal. The nurse-teacher who begins the teaching process with the basic science concepts may lose the learner because he does not see the antecedent-goal relationship. Conversely, teachers who initiate the process with the application or "nursing action" phase may lose the learner because he does not understand the antecedent information that supplies the "why."

Objectives can be realized when the teacher and learner participate together in the problem-solving process using a simple graphic model so that individual parts of knowledge can be patterned into a meaningful whole. The table on pp. 106-109 is an example of a problem-solving tool in which the hygiene activity of mouth care is the subject. The topic chosen is simply to enable emphasis to be placed on the process and not the content. The example can be used as a model and can be successfully employed for any content regardless of complexity. The goal may be stated as a behavioral objective or as a problem, depending on which is appropriate to the situation. Both a behavioral objective and a stated problem are given here for clarity and to demonstrate the flexibility of the tool.

Problem-solving sample

Both the problem and the behavioral objective require the learner to have knowledge of facts, theories, concepts, principles, and risks involved so that he may generalize, discriminate, and perform to accomplish the objective or solve the problem.

The process enables the nurse-teacher to identify all the knowledge relevant to the development of a module or small unit of teaching. Once the necessary components of the sample model are identified, the nurse-teacher can share the overall pattern with the learner and through learner participation can select knowledge that (1) does not need to be covered, (2) needs to be reviewed, and (3) needs to be learned. In this way the teacher can start where the learner is and utilize what the learner brings into the learning situation. Once the content is selected, the methods, teaching tools, and other resources to be used can be chosen or devised. Use of the tool itself as a single method rather than as an overall guide stereotypes teaching and develops rigidity, which can decrease the creative enthusiasm in teaching and learning.

PREDICTIVE PRINCIPLE: Increasing the difficulty of learning material in small increments promotes learning success.

Difficulty is measured by complexity. Complexity in learning material is a function of four things:

1. The number of variables with which the learner must deal at one time
2. The degree or amount of structure provided by the setting, the teacher, and the learning activities

Problem-solving sample*

Statement of problem and objective	Necessary facts or concepts	Principles†
Problem: How to get the licensed vocational nurse (LVN) to use appropriate mouth care with two critically ill patients who were given nothing orally (NPO) and were mouth breathers	1. Mouth is the portal of entry for food.	A. A well-cared-for mouth during critical illness increases the patient's ability to return to normal eating habits on recovery (1).
	2. Digestion is started in the mouth, where food is thoroughly chewed and mixed with saliva, which contains the digestive enzyme ptyalin.	B. A sensitive or infected mouth produces discomfort (2). (Food is often swallowed before it is thoroughly chewed and mixed with saliva or food may not be eaten at all.)
Objective: The LVN is (1) able to select the correct type of mouth care for each patient and (2) able to give adequately the correct type of mouth care to meet the individual needs of each patient	3. If the jaws are not used for mastication and if there is no acid or alkaline intake, there is little or no stimulation of parotid secretion.	C. NPO causes the parotid glands to become inactive (3). D. Meticulous mouth care prevents the massive invasion of microorganisms from the mouth through the parotid duct to the inactive gland(s) (3, 11).
	4. Salivary flow is decreased in severe illness.	E. Decreased salivary flow creates the need for frequent and special mouth care (4).
	5. Salivary flow has a constant cleansing action.	F. Local treatment of dry mouth with fluid and emollients promotes temporary relief (5).
	6. Anaerobic organisms do not ordinarily grow in the mouth.	G. The use of lemon juice for special mouth care causes an increased secretion of saliva (5, 7, 8, 9).
	7. The accumulation of dried secretions in the mouth provides an environment conducive to the growth of anaerobic organisms.	H. The use of hydrogen peroxide, an oxidizing agent, for mouth care inhibits the growth of anaerobic organisms in the mouth (7).
	8. When the mouth is dry, local treatment with fluids and emollients gives temporary relief.	I. The use of hydrogen peroxide for mouth care results in a bubbling action that facilitates the removal of undesirable excretions in the mouth (8).
	9. Application of lemon juice and glycerine to the tongue and gums is a classic treatment for dry mouth.	J. The use of concentrated glycerine alone (which is hydroscopic) for special mouth care predisposes to dehydration and irritation of mouth tissues (9, 12, 13).
	10. State of hydration of the patient does not depend on the moisture of the mucous membranes of the mouth.	K. Small amounts of glycerine promote softening and protect mucous membranes (9, 12, 13).
	11. Antiseptic rinses stimulate saliva flow and decrease microorganism population.	L. Use of an antiseptic mouth wash results in lessening of halitosis (11, 13, 14, 15).

*This problem is the work of Honor B. Dufour and is used with her permission.
†Numbers after principles refer to number of facts or concepts used to compose them.
‡Letters after statements refer to principles used to devise action.

Prescriptions‡	Possible risks involved	Generalizations
Frequent examination of the mouth to ascertain its condition. Observe for dryness, collection of undesirable excretions, redness, and odor. If patient is responsive, question him concerning subjective condition of his mouth—discomfort, pain, difficulty swallowing, foul taste (A, B, C).	Examination may be incomplete because of poor visibility. A tongue blade may be necessary to hold tongue down during examination, but care must be taken *not* to damage delicate tissues. Patient may not give dependable answers to questions.	This procedure for special mouth care would be applicable to any patient in whom the salivary flow is decreased. Some common examples would be: Patient who is comatose Patient suffering from severe dehydration Patient unable to swallow Patient receiving oxygen therapy
Use tongue blade and light when necessary to improve visualization of oral cavity (A, B, C).	Aspirating agent used for oral care.	Patient with collection of foul debris in the mouth Patient who is NPO Patient receiving chemical therapy that has drying effect on the mouth *Discrimination:* This procedure would *not* be applicable in any situation where blood clots were necessary for healing (oral surgery).
Give mouth care with lemon juice and glycerine if there is danger of the patient swallowing the substances (E, F, G. J. K).	Glycerine must not be too concentrated, since it can be dehydrating and irritating. The nurse must obtain help to position the patient if he cannot do it alone.	
Careful positioning of patient with head to one side to prevent aspiration; suction machine should be available if patient is not responsive or cooperative (O).	If suctioning is required, care must be taken *not* to damage delicate tissues.	

Continued.

Problem-solving sample—cont'd

Statement of problem and objective	Necessary facts or concepts	Principles
Objective—cont'd The LVN is (1) able to select the correct type of mouth care for each patient and (2) able to give adequately the correct type of mouth care to meet the individual needs of each patient	12. Glycerine (concentrated) is hydroscopic and is a drying agent. 13. Small amounts of glycerine can protect and soften. 14. Excretions such as dried blood, mucus, and sputum in the mouth may be removed by the use of hydrogen peroxide, which is an oxidizing agent. 15. Saliva putrefies rapidly, giving rise to objectionable odors. 16. Water is not effective in removing odors. 17. Substances such as petroleum jelly and cocoa butter applied to the lips and tongue have a protective action. 18. Mechanical action and friction remove dried and putrefied materials and stimulate salivation. 19. Cleaning patient's mouth while he is positioned on back makes it easy for patient to aspirate.	M. Petroleum jelly applied to the lips and tongue after special mouth care results in a slower drying of these tissues (17). N. Careful use of mechanics and scrubbing promotes removal of dried blood, mucus, and sputum (18). O. Positioning of patient on side during mouth care promotes drainage of secretions outward and prevents aspiration (19).

3. The level of theory with which the content deals
4. The degree of familiarity of the content to the learner

When the nurse-teacher attempts to teach material that has a high number of variables, has very little structure, has a high level of theory, and is highly unfamiliar to the learner, successful achievement is jeopardized. When approaching new subject matter, it is easier to learn one thing at a time than to try to cope with something that has several aspects. The number of aspects or variables with which the learner must deal is directly related to the complexity of the material. Simplification can be achieved by decreasing the number of aspects of the material to be presented at one time and allowing one small part of the total learning package to be dealt with before proceeding to the next part. The second problem is to select and provide the amount of structure. Sometimes the structure is provided by the setting. Nurses who are learning new procedures have access, within health agency settings, to policy and procedure manuals that provide structure. Nurses in acute care agencies are aided by and receive guidance from nurse colleagues, ancillary personnel, other health provider departments, as well as supervisory-level management. This not only provides structure but also

Prescriptions	Possible risks involved	Generalizations
If the mouth is foul with dried blood, mucus, and sputum, use hydrogen peroxide to remove crusts, followed with antiseptic mouth wash and then apply petroleum jelly to lips and the tongue (unless the patient complains of the taste) (E, H, I, L, M).	Hydrogen peroxide can injure the gums if used improperly, may cause gingival hypertrophy if used over a long period of time. Hydrogen peroxide not diluted to a strength of about 1% can injure tissues Oils, such as mineral oil, are contraindicated because of the danger of aspiration and the development of lipoid pneumonia or lung abscess. All special mouth care performed with inappropriate tools can injure tissues or be ineffective in accomplishing goals. Applicators are rarely effective.	
Special mouth care is best carried out with a toothbrush; however, in some instances a protected forceps and soft gauze sponges may be substituted (N).	If protected forceps are used, care must be taken not to injure the buccal tissues or disturb oral injury, surgery, or dental work.	

promotes the security of the learner. The teacher's role, then, is to provide structure by formulating clear, concise, attainable behavioral objectives and by giving clear directions, instruction, or other relevant information.

The level of theory involved is an important aspect of difficulty. Low-level theories (see Chapter 1) are easier to learn than high-level theories; in other words, it is easier to learn to identify, name, describe, and list things than it is to predict or develop causal connections and prescriptions. Creative, or inventive learning, that is, at level IV, is the most difficult level of theory with which to deal. Nurse-teachers must be sure before teaching level III and IV theories that the learner is well acquainted with level I and II theories that are fundamental and basic to these higher levels. For example, identifying, naming, listing, and describing the anatomy and physiology of the skin and subcutaneous and muscular tissues is prerequisite to predicting absorption time of insulin based on whether or not it is injected into the muscle or subcutaneous tissue. The last aspect of difficulty, familiarity, is a factor that enables the learner to be the nurse-teacher's greatest resource. The teacher who assesses what the learner knows, not only about the subject in question but also about other areas of interest to him, can relate this familiar knowledge to the unknown.

For example, a maintenance worker in a factory that used steam boilers suffered a heart attack. Arteriosclerotic heart disease was diagnosed. The community health nurse used the patient's knowledge of the precipitation of mineral content of water in boilers and pipes and the resultant dangers of clogging and pressure in the boiler system to teach the patient about arteriosclerosis, blood pressure, and myocardial infarcts.

It is not always possible to teach material from the "simple" to the "complex" because "simple" and "complex" are relative terms to the learner and actually depend on the related knowledge and experience the learner brings to the learning situation.

EVALUATION

Evaluation is the bugaboo of all those engaged in the teaching-learning process. Evaluation is the process through which the teacher and the learner determine progress toward the learning objective.

Evaluation for the purpose of establishing a "grade" may only tell the learner his achievement as rated on some established scale and usually compares him to other learners attempting to master the same content. Evaluation provides the learner with a guide that will enable him to determine his progress toward accomplishing a desired goal. It helps him ascertain his goal achievement. In health teaching and problem solving, evaluation means assessing behavioral changes in relationship to the goal or defined problem.

Evaluation for better learning enables the nurse-teacher and the learner to determine (1) that a desired behavior has or has not been learned and (2) how well a desired behavior has been learned.

Quantitative evaluation is of little use to the nurse-leader. Quantitative evaluations are characterized by words like *always, frequently, sometimes, rarely,* and *never. Qualitative* evaluations are characterized by descriptions of behaviors that indicate the stage the learner has reached in the theory-building or problem-solving process and how skilled he has become in that stage. Qualitative evaluations tell the character and nature of success or failure.

An example of the differences in quantitative and qualitative evaluations may be drawn from the situation in which the nurse-leader was teaching an elderly man to administer injections to his wife, who had pernicious anemia. The man had extreme difficulty in manipulating the syringe and vial without contamination. The nurse's evaluative note, which states, "Very rarely draws up solution correctly" and "Frequently contaminates the syringe," does not convey to either the teacher or the learner what has or has not been accomplished. A qualitative evaluative statement would read, "Has identified the components of aseptic technique but has difficulty with the coordination necessary to master the handling of the vial and syringe without contamination. He is aware of breaks in techniques and is developing manipulative skills slowly." This statement conveys specifically and clearly the stage of learning achieved in behavioral terms.

PREDICTIVE PRINCIPLE: Objectives expressed as learner behaviors enable the teacher and learner to know the limits of expected outcomes and to evaluate in meaningful, specific terms.

The time required to write detailed behavioral objectives is compensated for by the efficiency with which one can plan the content necessary to accomplish the objective and the ease with which behavioral objectives can be evaluated. Behavioral objectives definitely describe the precise activities necessary to demonstrate that the desired learnings have occurred. For example, the practical nurse who was learning aseptic technique would not know what was expected of her if she were trying to achieve the objective "to become increasingly knowledgeable about aseptic technique." "Knowledgeable" does not indicate what behaviors result from the knowledge. Contrastingly, "to be able to recognize when aseptic technique is required" and "to perform tasks requiring aseptic technique in any situation" are two objectives that tell the learner and teacher exactly what behaviors must be achieved to accomplish the objective. They spell out criteria for both teacher and learner to use in judging accomplishment.

The foregoing principle indicates that evaluation in meaningful and specific terms is an activity of both teacher and learner. Evaluation carried out by either, exclusive of the other, reduces the effectiveness of the evaluation by making it impossible for one half of the teaching-learning team to use the evaluation in activities designed for further goal accomplishment. For successful evaluation, both teacher and learner profit by having the data necessary to assess the present situation and to structure additional experiences for achievement of the desired behavioral changes.

USE OF PREDICTIVE PRINCIPLES OF TEACHING AND LEARNING IN IN-SERVICE EDUCATION DEPARTMENTS

In-service education programs have three distinct purposes:
1. To increase the health care giver's ability to be congruent with and supportive of the health agency's philosophy and/or statement of mission and goals as provided in its charter, organization plan, or appropriate documents
2. To meet the specific learning needs of the individual nursing care given in order to facilitate the employee's optimal development

Both of these purposes synthesize to form a third purpose:
3. To enable each employee to provide the most effective and efficient patient care possible in the setting where employed

In-service programs are organized to meet these purposes by responding to the following three basic in-service needs:
1. The need for orientation to the health care agency, its policies, procedures, physical environments, culture, goals, organization, communication flow, and people
2. The need for mastery of health care–oriented content; learning nursing behaviors necessary to:
   a. care for clients (general or specialty content)

b. use physical plant and equipment better
c. work with nursing group
d. work with health care team

3. The need for promotional mobility, which involves:
   a. expertise needed for vertical promotions and merit raises in salary
   b. expertise needed in leadership and management group work and clinical knowledge and skill for vertical promotion up the organizational ladder

Therefore all instructional designs for in-service education programs are devised to respond to one or more of these three areas of need:

1. Orientation
2. Client care improvement
3. Promotion

PREDICTIVE PRINCIPLE: In-service education programs structured to separate orientation, clinical experience, and management aspects promote clarity of content and staff growth.

In-service education is one of the biggest problems managers face. Nursing attrition (turnover) is a constant problem for nursing managers. Nurses and ancillary help tend to go from agency to agency looking for greener grass, that is, better pay, fringe benefits, better working conditions, and greater job satisfaction.

Good in-service educational programs alone will not alter attrition rates but will provide one positive factor for staff stability. "Good" in-service education is in-service education that is:

1. Planned to separate the three aspects of in-service education
2. Planned so that it is congruent with the conceptual framework of the agency
3. Slanted toward active rather than passive teaching strategies
4. A total curriculum package
5. Tied into merit raises, promotion, retention, and other concrete reinforcements
6. A mechanism for self-improvement and for increased job satisfaction

Orientation. Orientation is the simplest, most routine, and most repetitious of the three areas. It is also the area most likely to lose the interest of the learner. Orientation tends to be uninteresting to the learner because it may lack relationship to a real or felt need of the nurse. Learning in the abstract is more difficult than learning in the concrete. There are a few practical guidelines for making orientation programs more concrete, usable, attractive to the learner, and efficient. Some of these are as follows:

1. Conduct all the tours of the physical plant, grounds, offices, etc. as taped guided tours. The in-service education director can carry a mobile tape recorder with a map around the agency and conduct a guided tour as if for one individual. Some hints for this are:
   a. Speak as if speaking to one person on a tour.
   b. Make it personal, interesting, and relaxed.
   c. Speak in the first person singular.

    d. Walk the employee around the facility using a map with numerically designated spots.

    e. Instruct the employees how to use the tape recorder, ear jack, and map to tour themselves around the agency.

    f. Allow the employee to keep the map at the end of the tour.

2. Meet important people in the situation through slides and taped voices. Take several slides of each important person doing his job in the agency. Have his voice on the tape: "Hello, I'm Mr. Important. This is my office. It's marked on your map as '10.' My job is . . ." You might ask the important person to tell something about his responsibilities, lines of authority, communications, and committees. Ask him to tell something about his professional life, previous work experiences, biographic data, work history, values, hobbies, religious affiliations, or anything else of interest or use to the employee.

3. Devise active learning experiences to teach new employees about policies and procedures. This can be done by assigning problems that must be solved correctly by using the policy/procedure manuals, for example, instead of telling a nurse what to do with diet orders, give him a "mock" chart of diet orders and allow the problem to be solved using the policy/procedure manuals. (This format will also point out areas in the policy/procedure manuals that need clarifying in order to be useful.)

EXAMPLE 1: Mr. Jones has been on a regular diet. His doctor just ordered a low-fat diet. It is ten minutes before the trays are due to be served. Use your policy and procedure manual and list the steps you would take to ensure that Mr. Jones receives the proper tray. Now fill in the correct forms and state where you would send each form.

EXAMPLE 2: Mr. Jones is admitted with orders for complete isolation. Do all the appropriate things to ensure that isolation is established for him and all appropriate departments are notified.

4. Give simulated experiences (problems) to teach all routine desk work, for example, use of tickler files; all chart work; admitting and discharging patients; handling orders such as medications, x-rays, laboratory work, activities, physical therapy, and social services; and giving public health referrals.

Client care improvement. Many nurses speak of wanting to improve client care. It is often difficult to plan a curriculum that is individually tailored for each nursing care giver and yet is common enough to be practical. If one refers to the needs of the setting, the client, and the knowledge base of the conceptual framework of the agency, cues can be found that are helpful in designing a curriculum responsive to the nurse and the agency and beneficial to the client. Some helpful ideas are as follows:

1. Keep a frequency count of the types of nursing care problems that present themselves in a two- or three-month period.

2. Keep a list of admitting and discharge diagnoses.

3. Keep a running list of the incident reports.

4. Ask the pharmacy for a list of the ten drugs used in largest volume in the agency.
5. Ask the dietary department for a list of the five most common diets issued, except regular and soft.
6. Ask housekeeping what its three most commonly recurring problems are.
7. Find out from patients (through interviews) what kinds of things they find most and least helpful.
8. Ask employees what course they would enroll in if offered any course they wanted in nursing.
9. Ask each employee what his professional goals and ambitions are.
10. Ask supervisors, head nurse, and clinical specialists what recurring problems are attributable to human ignorance or carelessness.

Regardless of the content of your in-service educational programs, there are guidelines helpful to managers that will enable the in-service education program to be responsive to the needs of the agency, the nurses, the clients, and the community. Some of these guidelines are as follows:

1. Plan as few single-topic, one-shot programs as possible. Instead, plan courses consisting of five to fifteen hours, or the equivalent of a course of study, so that the learner can become involved in the course.
2. Build in some assignments and requirements for the learner that take into consideration the learner's individual problems, needs, areas of interest, and life goals.
3. Use clients of the agency as a resource for learning activities necessary for the completion of the courses.
4. Provide some rewards for work accomplished, for example, compensatory days off, letters of commendation, efficiency reports for permanent files, merit raises, and mastery certificates.
5. Allow the nurse-learners to help structure the course, its objectives, learning activities, etc.
6. Buy, make, beg, or borrow some individualized learning materials, multimedia learning materials, books, and films on the subject(s) under study.
7. Always have topics that are immediately applicable to the "real world" work situation.
8. Tailor all interactive learning (learning where nurses interact with teacher, other nurses, or patients) to the personal needs and characteristics of the learner.

Promotion. Many agencies promote nurses who have shown promise or expertise in nursing up the managerial hierarchy into positions of greater and greater responsibility as openings occur. More and more agencies are establishing requirements for skills in organizational leadership and management for these promotions. Civil service–type examinations and/or oral interviews often are used to test for skills. Sometimes it is presumed that nurses have managerial skills because they have previous work experiences. All these methods for selecting persons for promotion have assets and liabilities. Agencies are increasingly adding another dimension to the prerequisites for promotions, that is, a requirement that employees have completed an in-service course in leadership and management especially tailored for the setting of employment. Staff development directors design courses that teach the philosophy and content of leadership and management as practiced or desired at the agency. In order to qualify for promotion up the administrative line the employee must complete a specified series of courses. Each promotional slot requires additional courses of study and preparation. Sometimes several agencies in a locale combine to offer the courses for greater cost effectiveness. Completion of a course of study does not ensure promotion; it only satisfies one qualification for a promotion.

Some topical examples are as follows:

Team leadership
Primary nursing
Principles of management
Budgeting and cost accounting
Evaluating personnel and peer review
Philosophy and goals of health care
How to critique a procedure
Working with people—a communications course
Assessing patient care—a supervisional function
Patient teaching—a basic nursing leadership activity
Teaching ancillary personnel
The nursing audit

APPLICATION OF PREDICTIVE PRINCIPLES OF TEACHING AND LEARNING

Mr. Scarborough, a 34-year-old alert man, has acute thrombophlebitis of the right leg. He is on complete bed rest with his legs wrapped with Ace bandages to midthigh (rewrap every four hours) and taking anticoagulant therapy. One of the aides reported to the nurse-leader that he had seen Mr. Scarborough twisting a towel tightly around his right thigh. When the aide asked him why, Mr. Scarborough stated, "It eases the pain."

Problem	Predictive principles	Course of action
How to teach Mr. Scarborough healthful ways of alleviating the pain of thrombophlebitis	The learner's developmental stage, personal characteristics, and prior experiences influence learning potential and dictate content.	Assess prior experiences, previous knowledge, and personal characteristics.
	The learner's prevalent life needs determine what he will learn.	Use learner need to decrease pain as starting point.
	A reciprocal relationship of trust and security facilitates teacher-learner communication and allows accurate assessment, learner participation in goal setting, and better utilization of resources.	Establish open and trustful communication using appropriate activities.

Continued.

Problem	Predictive principles	Course of action
How to teach ways of alleviating pain—cont'd	Participation of the learner in setting learning goals increases the number of learning activities meaningful and useful to the learner.	Collaborate (his need and nurse's specialized knowledge and skill) in establishing learning goals in behavioral terms, that is, identify a variety of methods for reducing the pain without jeopardizing his health; choose the appropriate method for each situation; perform the activities necessary to the implementation of the chosen alternative.
	An obvious relationship between learning activities and stated goals increases the motivational value of the activity.	Develop a brief overview of necessary content in collaboration with patient.
	Rewards consistent with the value system of the learner, such as recognition, praise, peer status, or valued gains, are motivating and reinforcing influences and thus facilitate learning rate, amount of retention, and degree of behavior change.	Determine appropriate rewards and use as reinforcers.
	Utilization of problem-solving processes promotes continuity and ease of learning.	Use flexible approach building toward a useful body of predictive principles based on valid antecedents.
	Increasing the difficulty of learning material in small increments promotes learning success.	Use meaningful similes (based on prior experiences), such as that a clogged drain causes drainage backup and overflow and collection of solids at point of obstruction, causing further clogging.
	Objectives expressed as learner behaviors enable the teacher and learner to know the limits of expected outcomes and to evaluate in meaningful, specific terms.	Evaluate patient's ability to behave in the manner specified and thereby gain relief from the pain. If possible, reinforce behavior. If not possible, determine with patient what would be necessary steps for achievement of success.

BIBLIOGRAPHY

Babcock, S. S., and Schild, E. O.: Simulation games in learning, Beverly Hills, Calif., 1968, Sage Publications, Inc.

Barton, R. E.: A primer on simulation and gaming, Engelwood Cliffs, N.J., 1970, Prentice-Hall, Inc.

Begge, M.: Learning theories for teachers, ed. 3, New York, 1976, Harper & Row, Publishers, Inc.

Biehler, R. F.: Psychology applied to teaching, New York, 1971, Houghton Mifflin Co.

Biehler, R. F.: Psychology applied to teaching: selected readings, New York, 1971, Houghton Mifflin Co.

Bower, F. L.: The process of planning nursing care, a model for practice, ed. 2, St. Louis, 1979, The C. V. Mosby Co.

Carlson, E.: Learning through games, Washington, D.C., 1968, Public Affairs Press.

De Tornyay, R.: Strategies for teaching nursing, New York, 1971, John Wiley & Sons, Inc.

Erikson, E. H.: Childhood and society, ed. 2, New York, 1963, W. W. Norton & Co., Inc.

Glasser, W.: Schools without failure, New York, 1969, Harper & Row, Publishers, Inc.

Havelock, R. G.: A guide to innovation in education, Ann Arbor, Mich., 1970, Institute for Social Research, The University of Michigan.

Interaction Associates: Strategy notebook, San Francisco, 1971, Interaction Associates, Inc.

Lefrancois, G. R.: Psychology for teaching, a bear always faces the front, Belmont, Calif., 1972, Wadsworth Publishing Co., Inc.

McDonald, F. J.: Educational psychology, Belmont, Calif., 1966, Wadsworth Publishing Co., Inc.

Mosston, M.: Teaching: from command to discovery, Belmont, Calif., 1972, Wadsworth Publishing Co., Inc.

Rogers, C.: Freedom to learn, Columbus, Ohio, 1969, Charles E. Merrill Publishing Co.

Schrank, J.: Teaching human beings: 101 subversive activities for the classroom, Boston, 1972, Beacon Press.

Shaffer, S. M., Indorato, K. L., and Deneselya, J. A.: Teaching in schools of nursing, St. Louis, 1972, The C. V. Mosby Co.

Wilson, S. F., and Tosti, D. T.: Learning is getting easier, 1972, Individual Learning Systems, Inc.

4

PREDICTIVE PRINCIPLES OF EFFECTIVE COMMUNICATION: INTERPERSONAL AND GROUP

PERCEPTION OF SELF AND OTHERS

The leader/manager's self-perception directly influences the development of positive perceptions in each group member.

The value systems of the leader and the group influence the establishment of goals and the setting of priorities and govern the amount of effort given to goal attainment.

Continuity of competent leadership and management facilitates the efficiency of the communication process.

Characteristics of client and nurse-leader/manager determine the type of communications that will evolve.

REINFORCEMENT AND FEEDBACK

Integrative positive reinforcement increases individual identification with group goals and the participation level of the individual.

Perceiving negative feedback enables group members to become aware of others' responses to them and their effects on the group and to modify behavior accordingly.

The dependent, interdependent, and/or independent natures of relationships affect the structure of the communication process.

The interdependent collaborating group facilitates group goal accomplishment.

Continuing reference to and clarification of goals enhance the ability to attain those goals.

COMMUNICATION STRATEGIES

The type of communication at work in a group dictates member perception and consequent action.

Congruent behavioral and verbal messages promote clear communication.

Threat and resulting anxiety, unless resolved, can inhibit individual and group communication.

Questions and discussion geared to second- and third-level theories promote cognition that is more useful in nursing activities than questions and discussion geared to first- and second-level theories.

Use of simulation facilitates decision making and provides efficient means for learning problem-solving methods in a nonthreatening and safe environment:

GOAL SETTING, ACHIEVEMENT, AND EVALUATION

Preassessment of individual and group knowledges, skills, and expectations establishes baseline data for measurement of progress or change.

Mutual understanding and agreement on goals appropriate to the client or agency ensure support for goal achievement.

Circumstance and member capability determine the type of directions to be communicated.

Opportunity to express expectations of the individual or group, when translated into meaningful terms to members, determines individual identification and invites commitment of members to goal achievement.

Realistic and valid goals promote achievement.

The extent of involvement of each group member determines the proficiency of the group.

Group involvement in goal setting requires the endorsement of the agency and commitment of membership to participate in the outcome.

EFFECTIVE CONFERENCES

Adequate preparation by the leader for all conferences expedites fulfillment of expectations for the conference.

Relieving care givers of responsibility while the conference is in session allows members to proceed without interruption.

Prior announcement of time, place, purpose, and duration of conferences to all concerned promotes assembly of a group well prepared and ready to focus attention on the purpose of the conference.

DIRECTION-GIVING CONFERENCES

Obtaining the most recent data available prior to conference ensures the leader that imparted information is pertinent, inclusive, and accurate.

Information to care givers and/or clients that is paced, systematic, and inclusive allows participants time to assimilate the content and provide them with information necessary to function.

PATIENT-CENTERED CONFERENCES

Interaction of conference members on an equal basis encourages active participation and leads to usable solutions to the problem.

Identification of the nursing problem to be considered expedites the formulation of nursing intervention.

Analyzing nursing care given in the light of established goals enables members to validate their behavior and to devise ways to improve nursing care.

Formation of written nursing orders or care plans from patient-centered conferences provides a central, continuous source of information.

CONTENT CONFERENCES

Member participation in problem-solving processes during content conference results in more meaningful learning.

Conferences held between nurse and client and/or significant others contribute to reciprocal development of care plans and lead to optimal health service for the client and satisfaction for the nurse.

Periodic care review conferences held with colleagues provide a mechanism for the nurse to validate care plans and maintain quality control.

REPORTING CONFERENCES

Directions given to conferees before report reveal expectations the leader has for the members.

GENERAL PROBLEMS CONFERENCES

Sharing feelings through conferences unifies and integrates the membership and allows work to progress.

Understanding and management of group behavior require ability to predict the processes through which feelings and meanings are transmitted among group members.

Involvement in group process results in specific gains or losses for the individual member.

Nurses function in high-stimulus environments, and communication is a major source of this stimulation. Leadership, as defined in the conceptual framework, is a set of actions that influence members of a group to move toward the setting and attainment of common goals; management is the manipulation of people, resources, budgets, and time to achieve organizational goals.

Communication can be defined as sending, receiving, and validating information. According to rueschian theory, communication is the ability of one mind to affect another and includes all methods for transmitting and receiving messages—pictures, paintings, sculpture, music, dance, signs, and signals, as well as written, vocal, or extrasensory transmissions. However, for the process to be communication, a connection must be made. One mind must indeed affect another and that impact must be sent, received, and validated. Therefore communication is circular, that is, it has a built-in feedback system. This chapter will deal with two basic types of communication—interpersonal and group. The same factors influence communications in these two contexts, with only minor differences.

Interpersonal communication follows the definition just given. A statement need not be verbalized, but can be conveyed through a series of signals such as posture or body langauge. It can be any expression of what is being thought or experienced. It might be an article offering an opinion or viewpoint or instructions for specific results. But it remains a statement and does not qualify as communication until it is perceived and interpreted by someone else. Reception and acknowledgment by another signifies that interpersonal communication has been established. To be perfected the message must be clarified or corrected if it has not been properly interpreted, and only through feedback, or some demonstrated response, can it be learned whether or not modification is needed for complete understanding of what the statement was intended to express.

Feedback is useful only if it is properly timed—again, contact must be made and there must be reception by another. It must also be appropriate to the situation and relayed in a clear, easily understood way. Vital to this process is an "open channel" to allow and ensure reception and response. Feedback, whether positive or negative, is thus an integral factor in communication, which cannot continue without it.

Group communication can refer to an individual and a group of people communicating with one another or to one group of people communicating with another group. Usually in group communication, feedback and correction are slow and change is more ponderous. Generally speaking, the more bureaucratic the system and the larger the group, the more slowly perception, response, and correction occur.

The purpose of group communication, like individual communication, is to enable collaboration in finding solutions to problems and meeting needs. This differs markedly from making statements and giving directions or providing information. These are one-way messages not geared to collaboration.

Communication breaks down for several reasons:

1. *Overloading the system.* Human communication shares a characteristic with animal and machine communication, that is, overloading causes them to break down. A computer will click out on overload; an animal under excessive stress will show signs of purposeless or erratic behavior, motor neuron synaptic failure, or other signs of "nervous breakdown." A human being will replace normal modes of communication with private modes or will restrict communication to the intrapersonal system (talk to himself) or use some other protective device. Reduction of the communication load and of other stimuli is necessary for intervention and reestablishment of successful communicating patterns.

2. *Malfunction of the communication apparatus.* This can be from disease or from poor or insufficient mastery of the use of the communication apparatus (eyes, ears, touch, smell, and vocal ability).

3. *Incorrect information.* This is erroneous perception or interpretation of data or faulty data. Anytime the input is faulty, the response will probably be inappropriate.

4. *Misuse of or use of too few communication strategies and tactics.* Strategies and tactics provide for the sending of messages and the obtaining and utilization of feedback. In addition to the clarifying and validating tactics discussed earlier, communication modalities are included here.

5. *Crossed ego states.* According to Berne,* each person has three ego states: Parent, Adult, and Child. Communication proceeds from one of these states. When the person with whom communication is occurring responds from a parallel ego state, breakdown does not occur. However, when communication lines cross, breakdown occurs (Fig. 9). Further discussion of the ego states and their impact on communication can be found on p. 125.

6. *Perceptual differences.* Perceptual differences exist among people because of different life experiences, different expectations, different levels of education, and different ethnic, cultural, and religious backgrounds. Two people perceiving the same message will interpret that message differently, based on perceptual "programming." These perceptual differences often cause breakdown in communication.

7. *Cognitive style differences.* Several types of cognitive style have been mapped, and differences in cognitive style account for communication problems. Some people's cognitive modes are comparative. They reason by

---

*Berne, E.: The structure and dynamics of organizations and groups, New York, 1966, Grove Press, Inc., pp. 130-138, 141-142.

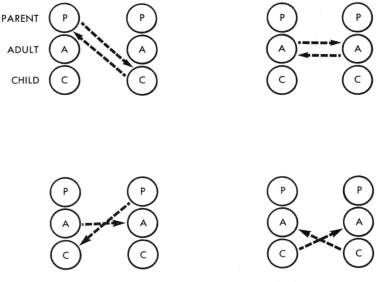

Fig. 9. Parallel and crossed communication.

comparing and contrasting. Others synthesize what they hear into categories meaningful to them and responsive to individual needs. Some people are highly theoretical and/or esoteric in their cognitive styles, whereas others are quite concrete and like examples and explanatory material. Differences in cognitive styles can lead to communication breakdown.

8. _Private fantasies_. Private fantasies occur because people's imaginations provide them with the structure they deem necessary to operate in ordinary life. When private fantasies become very real, people operate on their fantasies rather than checking out the landmarks of reality. For instance, an employee may imagine that the manager will not like a particular event in the day's work. Operating on that fantasy the employee may begin to defend himself or to dissemble. The manager in such an instance may not know from whence the defenses are coming or how to respond. Communication breaks down.

Since practice in nursing is basically group and interpersonally oriented, people do not tend to work in a vacuum or alone. All types of nursing require collaboration with other health care givers or clients. Therefore much of this chapter will deal with group work. Leadership and management communications with groups are designed primarily to facilitate groups in setting goals and carrying out the activities necessary to attain those goals.

Group work extends throughout all health services. Nurses are called on routinely to work with groups of personnel who have a diversity of experience and preparation. The nurse-leader/manager learns to use effective communication in any structural care pattern (for example, case, functional, team, or primary) or within varied organizational systems established for provision of care.

In this context, *group* refers to a number of people, small or large, who, under a leader, work for a common purpose: that of providing quality nursing care to a specific client or a number of clients in any setting. *Process* refers to the goal-oriented operations of the group and to the forces at work within the operational procedures. For many years the dynamics of group behavior have been studied intensely by psychologists, sociologists, and educators. The scientific study of group process is relatively new; hence there are no absolutes, but there are sufficient data to indicate the processes most useful to leaders and managers. Efforts to classify groups and to identify internal processes reveal that the general laws concerning group life apply to all groups, large or small.

The following section is addressed to leaders and managers who use communication in all phases of nursing. No attempt has been made to deal specifically with therapeutic communication; however, the predictive principles discussed have relevance to all phases of nursing.

PERCEPTION OF SELF AND OTHERS

Perceptions, like beauty, are in the eye of the beholder. The nurse's total self-system affects his perceptions. Value systems, ideals, life goals, experiences, presets, expectations of self and others, context—all affect perception. What a person sees and hears and how he interprets this information are regulated by the self-system. Perception is more than seeing and hearing; it also includes interpreting these data. Interpretations are functions of values, social conditioning, and life experiences and expectations. The leader's perception of himself affects his view of others. If the leader sees others with a positive preset, that will affect other's responses to him and reaffirm his predeterminations. In other words, individuals who believe they will receive affirmative responses from people condition themselves to elicit positive responses because their approach to others is with this type of expectation. The converse is also true. People who expect negative reactions usually communicate behaviorally such expectations and elicit similar negative responses from the communicant.

Perceptions of others also affect communications. Leader perceptions of an individual or group are usually only parts of the true picture. The same is true of the group's or individual's perception of the leader. The invalidity or lack of authenticity in perception greatly influences interpretation of behavior and communication. Sharing insight about perceptions and self within the group will aid the efficiency of communication.

PREDICTIVE PRINCIPLE: The leader/manager's self-perception directly influences the development of positive perceptions in each group member.

Since much of the leadership and management roles is individual and personal, these roles demand employment of self as an instrument and involvement as a person. It is essential that the leader have both the ability to share himself and the capacity for self-discipline. Perceptual psychologists have indicated that the deeply deprived self cannot afford to give itself away. The self must possess a satisfactory degree of adequacy before it can venture commitment to and provide encounter with individuals or groups. Leadership depends on entering into an interaction relationship with others, and effective leaders possess sufficient self-esteem to make sharing and supporting relationships possible. The nurse-leader needs to feel personally adequate to deal effectively with others.

The effective leader believes himself fundamentally adequate, which enables him to give adequate attention to client and care giver's needs. Those who feel inadequate and deprived cannot afford the time and effort required to lead and assist others. In the University of Florida studies of the helping professions a number of perceptual psychologists studied the nature of self-fulfillment and personal adequacy in professional leaders and directors. It was found that effective leaders felt themselves being (1) identified with rather than apart from others, (2) basically adequate rather than inadequate, (3) trustworthy rather than untrustworthy, (4) wanted rather than unwanted or ignored, and (5) worthy rather than overlooked or discounted.

The nurse-leader/manager who has a positive self-perception is able to provide the necessary positive support and reinforcement to clients and members of the health team. The nurse-leader/manager with positive perceptions of self communicates positive perception to others, thereby increasing the self-esteem of individuals and group members. With the self-concept strengthened, participants can in turn often develop into support agents for other relationships, as, for example, with clients.

Another element in positive supportive relationships is the ability to care. People who have successful caring experiences find it easier to care about others successfully. Caring managers and leaders learn names, obtain vital statistics and personal and professional information, and use these data in positive, supportive, and growth-provoking ways.

PREDICTIVE PRINCIPLE: The value systems of the leader and the group influence the establishment of goals and the setting of priorities and govern the amount of effort given to goal attainment.

Value systems are those ethics, ideas, objects, behaviors, or philosophies important to an individual. Value systems are outgrowths of life experiences, life goals, ambitions, and ethnic background. Values dictate the moral, ethical, material, and religious "set" of individuals. The leader/manager and every member bring to their group a value system. This pooling of values creates an amorphous group personality. Because of the makeup of a group and its climate, leadership, and task, the group's value system becomes evident in what is important to it, that is, in what receives its attention and efforts. Changes perceived by the leader/manager and the group as having great worth will receive high priorities and much effort, whereas changes or goals viewed by the group as unimportant or of little value will receive slight effort and be of low priority. Priority setting is a direct function of individual and group values.

If goals are established that the group does not value, usually the personnel will not work toward them. However, other extraneous factors may enter in. If rewards for goal achievement become important enough, receiving the valued reward is the group's target and the group will attain the established goal to achieve the reward.

PREDICTIVE PRINCIPLE: Continuity of competent leadership and management facilitates the efficiency of the communication process.

Continuity, with reference to nursing care, means provision for daily, uninterrupted service for a prescribed period of time. To ensure continuity there is an unbroken chain of related communications, events, and responsibilities. When a link in this chain becomes weak or is severed, discontinuity probability increases in proportion to the number of persons involved. Hence there is a return to the concept of primary care where those persons who are most concerned and involved in health care services are in communicative contact.

Continuity necessitates adequate coverage for days off, illness, vacations, and leaves if communication is to be maintained at the desired level of operation. The manager attempts to select replacements who are skilled in nursing, are familiar with client or agency policies and procedures, have the ability to work well with others, and have the potential to guide the client or group members in the achievement of their purposes.

The opportunity to experience group process in operation helps the alternate or associate leader to carry on the pattern of activity established by the primary leader and also provides a basis for joint evaluation of the process by both leaders.

Staffing formula can become inadequate when prolonged absences occur. Provision for vacations, illnesses, attendance at workshops, and leaves for other purposes requires that additional personnel be added. It is well for new nurses to become familiar with the overall plan of nursing care, to assess potential client needs, and then to be assigned for individual orientation into group processes within the work setting.

The importance of having a second person qualified to assume a managerial role is determined by the length of absence of the regular manager and the role the manager plays in the agency. Leadership does not always depend on the physical presence of the leader. If the individual or group understands its direction and its behaviors are established, basic functions can take place under minimal direction. If the absent time is extensive, it is important that a prepared person be available.

Having someone ready to take over during absences is important, but there are other benefits of having an associate manager. The process of teaching and preparing others for leadership helps the manager to learn. The manager may gain a clearer picture of the job in the process of explaining it, will learn more about the abilities of the client or care givers, and will gain increased insight into the group processes involved.

The sense of cohesiveness built up in the members when management is shared results in a much more reliable process. Each person clarifies his role and his relationship to others. There is a reinforcement of the knowledge and a sense of accomplishment in seeing that plans run smoothly.

PREDICTIVE PRINCIPLE: Characteristics of client and nurse-leader/manager determine the type of communications that will evolve.

The practice of nursing is gradually shifting its focus from that which is essentially curative and restorative, generally acute and chronic in nature, and practiced in hospitals or in patient facilities to the promotion of health and prevention of disease. This latter practice is normally a continuum process and is increasingly becoming a part of community or emergent institutional programs. Hence the consumer of nursing services is being looked on not as a "patient" but as a "client" who may initiate and participate in his own health care. This procedural shift from the client's passive to active role influences attitudes and behaviors concerned with communication.

The average consumer has increasing geographic and economic access to health care. Hospitals and similar agencies are often overcrowded and unable to provide for all the clients seeking admission. There is also the economic problem faced by those seeking health care who are unable to finance the higher cost of institutionalized service. Subsequently, there is a shift in the role of the nurse-leader from hospitals and other institutions to outpatient health care. This requires a varied technique of communications, for the nurse-leader must be acquainted with many types of facilities that offer health treatment in various locales. These range from national, state, and regional facilities to those provided by local communities, churches, and other groups interested in fostering health improvement among all strata of society. These health programs incorporate maintenance, curative, restorative, and rehabilitative services for the various types of health needs such as physical health, mental health, family planning, mother-child relationships, health supervision, teaching, and counseling.

Despite how or where client and nurse begin their relationship or contractual agreement, the nursing process involves partnership between nurse and client in planning and implementing problem-oriented care. As mentioned earlier, Berne states that every individual has three basic ego states—parent, adult, and child. The parent ego state governs an individual's values, conscience, and moral and ethical behaviors. Parent messages given to self and others contain words like "should," "ought," and "must." Parent ego states are derived from early injunctions learned in the primary family and are part of the "scripting" of early childhood. They are necessary in the socialization of an individual and enable people to conform to the mores and folkways of their cultural environments. Parent ego states can be nurturing (loving, protective, supporting, caring) or critical (cross, criticizing, discounting).

The adult ego state is the logical state that looks at consequences, weighs risks, and makes decisions on a strictly rational level. It is mathematical in its precision, objectivity, and freedom from emotional overlay.

The child ego state is an emotional, "little kid" state. It has two facets:

1. Adaptive, which can be sweet, loving, dependent, seductive, and eager to please, or rebellious, which can be easily angered, contrary, negative, and not wanting to be bossed or managed
2. Free child, which can be playful, mischievous, enthusiastic, caring, and insightful, or a "little professor," who figures out how to get what he wants

Nursing, because of social set and traditional role enaction, proceeds primarily from the parent and child ego states. Communication patterns with clients usually place the nurse in the "parent" position, "telling" the patient (child) what

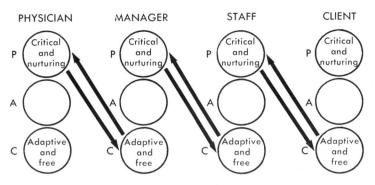

Fig. 10. Traditional ego state communication patterns in health agencies.

he should or should not do. Patients get "hooked" into playing the child ego state, whether adaptive, rebellious, free child, or little professor.

Nurse's relationships with physicians are also child-parent oriented, with the physician playing the parent role and the nurse playing the child role. The physician is nurturing and critical by turns, and the nurse adaptive, rebellious, free child, or little professor in response.

Communication flows well as long as each participant plays out prescribed roles, but when any participant attempts to establish another ego state whence to communicate, communication can break down.

Nurse-managers usually set the stage for communication. Managers who communicate with staff as "the boss" are in the parent ego state and, through role modeling, set a climate of "parenting" for their subordinates. Clients, last in the chain of command, are then treated like children and are placed in the "one-down" position. This decreases the decision-making powers of patients and strips them of individuality, rights, and responsibility for their own care and destiny.

Fig. 10 illustrates the traditional communication flow in nursing just discussed. Fig. 11 illustrates the communication pattern adult-to-adult, that is, the desirable flow of communications among physician, manager, staff, and client. This is not to say that participants in the health care setting need never proceed from any but the adult ego state. This would indeed be a coolly logical, and not necessarily desirable, communication flow. There are times when every individual needs and requests nurturing, and it is productive for a manager to play that role when requested. It is also helpful when one gets into the child ego state to have another willing to enter that state with him and "play." Indeed, this section is not intended to convey that because the adult ego state is the most reality oriented the other ego states are undesirable and should never be used. What is desirable is that each individual recognize the ego state from which his communications are derived at any given time and be aware of the ego states of those with whom he is communicating, so that adjustments can be made that keep communication flowing.

Managers who are willing to relate to staff on an adult level and reinforce

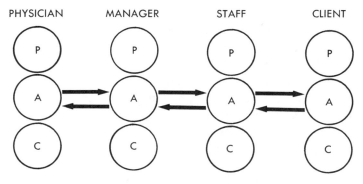

Fig. 11. Desirable ego state communication patterns in health agencies.

adult communication among staff succeed in raising the level of productivity, accountability, and shared responsiveness to clients' rights and privileges. When communication is (1) uncrossed, (2) clear, and (3) proceeding from the adult ego state, the client is the beneficiary. As a result, clients make verbal contracts and agreements about the care they want and need and participate in their own care; families can make choices about their own involvement in the family member's health problems. In general, when communications proceed from managers on adult-to-adult levels, there is a better climate for healing.

The successful leader will work to keep interpersonal relationships at a level where group efforts will be productive and will encourage members to be cooperatively interdependent. With this type of leadership and management, it is probable that a process will evolve in which there is increased member participation, increased client participation, more rapid decision making, more achievement within the group, and more progress toward accomplishing purposes and goals. Effective communication increases productivity, group cohesion, and quality of client care.

REINFORCEMENT AND FEEDBACK

In human relationships, some form of reinforcement, positive or negative, is communicated. The effective leader will use reinforcement as a means to increase each participant's identification with and effort toward individual or group goals. According to Professor B. F. Skinner of Harvard, reward, not punishment, is the most effective force for shaping human behavior. Positive reinforcement may be food, money, praise, a kiss, a smile, a nod of approval. More significant, however, is that positive feedback may consist of eliciting a right answer and knowing it is correct, working out a problem to one's satisfaction, mastering a skill, or finding new beauty and order in words, music, and art. Every culture and subculture, all institutions such as hospitals and health agencies, and every home has its own methodology, acknowledged or unacknowledged, of employing rewards and punishments. Studies have shown, however, that in many cases the direction of various group processes has relied on punishment or the threat of punishment to control subordinates and other members of the group. Ineffective forms of positive reinforcement are used, forms that are not in keeping with the value system for participating. These practices ignore the most effective forms of positive reinforcement.

Steiner* has done much work in stroking patterns. Steiner defines strokes as reinforcements. They can be (1) positive conditional, (2) negative-conditional, (3) positive-unconditional, or (4) negative-unconditional.

Positive-conditional strokes are strokes given for things well done—pleasing and acceptable behaviors. An example is "You certainly took good care of Mrs. Jones while she was in such a panic state during that procedure."

Negative-conditional strokes are those that are critical, providing negative feedback. They are given for things incorrectly and poorly done or things omitted that were displeasing to someone. An example is "You really blew that! Now we'll never get Dr. Morris to cooperate in our new drug plan."

The best strokes are *positive-unconditional* strokes. These are positive compliments and valuing a person for just being—just existing. Comments like "I really do like you," "I really like being around you," and "You're such a fine person" are positive-unconditional strokes.

The worst strokes are the *negative-unconditional* strokes. These strokes punish one for just being—not for anything that has been done or not done—but for just existing. Battered children and battered managers and staff are often the products of negative-unconditional stroking. For example, "I just don't like you" is a negative-unconditional stroke. Character assassinations that evolve during arguments or reprimands are common negative-unconditional strokes. These are such remarks as "You are such a turkey!" or "You dumb broad!"

According to Steiner,* there are five stroke injunctions. These injunctions have been taught to people in the United States as a part of their socialization process. Much of our inability to provide reinforcements can be attributed to these injunctions:

1. Don't ask for strokes—even if you want them.
2. Don't give strokes—even if they are deserved.
3. Don't reject strokes—even if they are given for something you don't want them for.
4. Don't stroke yourself—even if you think you deserve it.
5. Don't accept strokes given to you—even if you want to.

One can see by looking at these stroke injunctions why strokes are so difficult to give and receive, for the messages are mixed. A person who asks for strokes is often perceived as conceited or having excessive ego needs. A person who gives strokes often perceives himself as giving away too much or somehow detracting from his own worth and value. People are taught that if someone gives a stroke, positive or negative, one must accept it whether or not it is wanted. It somehow is not legitimate to say "Please don't compliment me on that thing— I'm not very proud of it," or "Don't criticize me for that—I'm very pleased with myself about that," or simply "No, thank you, I don't think I'll take that compliment." People who stroke themselves say "Gee, didn't I do a great job!" or "I

---

*Steiner, C.: Scripts people live, New York: 1974, Grove Press, Inc., pp. 106-107.

really like the way I handled that situation," or "I wish I had done such and such. It would have produced a better job" and may be seen as either too prideful or too critical of themselves. As a result of the injunctions listed, it is extremely difficult to enter into a healthy, even-keeled, balanced stroking system that reinforces positive growth, promotes feelings of self-worth, provides adequate feedback, and enables continued clear communications. Leaders and managers who are conscious of stroke injunctions and individual worker's stroking needs and patterns can help workers ask for and receive the strokes they need to alter behaviors, grow, and be more productive.

Positive and negative stroking patterns (or positive and negative reinforcements) form the basis for all growth patterns and communication patterns and affect the goals that are set; how one manages time, energy, resources, and materials to achieve those goals; and how one evaluates whether or not the goals have been reached.

PREDICTIVE PRINCIPLE: Integrative positive reinforcement increases individual identification with group goals and the participation level of the individual.

Since the mid-1950s Ned Flanders, Edmund Amidon, John Hough, and others have been experimenting with a system to measure verbal and nonverbal group interaction styles called *interaction analysis*. A significant aspect of this analysis scheme is to measure the group leader's or instructor's ability to reinforce verbally the participants' behavior to get the members to initiate positive action toward group goals and increase retention level of the participants. *Integrative behavior influences* of the instructor or group leader are (1) accepting feelings of participants, (2) praising or encouraging participation, (3) accepting or using ideas of participants, and (4) asking questions of participants. These are positive-conditional and positive-unconditional strokes from the adult ego state. *Directive behavior influences* are (1) lecturing to the group, (2) giving directions to individuals or the group, (3) criticizing, and (4) justifying authority. These are communications from the parent ego state and include negative-conditional and negative-unconditional strokes.

The integrative leader is one who accepts, clarifies, and supports participants' ideas and feelings and who praises, encourages, and stimulates participation in the decision-making process. Directive or dominative leaders, on the other hand, tend to focus on introspective ideas and knowledge, give many directions and orders, criticize participants, and are concerned with justifying their own position and authority. Other studies have replicated the described analysis system, indicating that the more integrative the leader (or the more he uses positive reinforcement), the higher the identification by group participants in achieving group goals. Instruments have been devised to measure group participants' retention of substance in group sessions, and again it was discovered that the greater the positive reinforcement, the greater the retention.

A direct positive relationship exists between the group leader's ability to reinforce the group members' supportive interaction and individual initiative in achieving group goals. There is a statistically significant positive relationship between a group leader's ability to reinforce group participants and the frequency of group members' support and reinforcement of each other. This is especially true in cases where the group leader uses more integrative positive reinforcement of group participants. The more a nurse-leader accepts, clarifies, or uses the ideas of a member, the more that member will tend to participate in the group process and positively support other members by recognizing, clarifying, and accepting their ideas and input. The behavior of nonparticipating members and isolates in a group may be changed from passive to active if the nurse-leader provides sufficient positive reinforcement to the group, since the more active participants will then in turn desire to support these less active group members through questions, encouragement, or praise or, in general, communicate a feeling of acceptance.

PREDICTIVE PRINCIPLE: Perceiving negative feedback enables group members to become aware of others' responses to them and of their effects on the group and to modify behavior accordingly.

Negative feedback or strokes are reinforcing in that they provide individuals with important information about what is not occurring that should be or what is happening that should not be. It enables individuals to know how they affect others in displeasing or unacceptable ways. Negative feedback is the counterpart of positive feedback, and both are important reinforcing factors. If a care provider is not contributing to group goals, not participating in collaborative efforts, or exhibiting undesirable behaviors, it is more important for that individual to know what those noncontributory behaviors are than to proceed in ignorance.

Negative feedback is difficult for most people to give or receive. People like to be liked; therefore criticism is hard to give. People want to behave appropriately, to contribute to group effort, and to be working interdependent members. Negative feedback is often interpreted as not fulfilling to a positive self-image. The pain of receiving negative input is partially offset by the knowledge of the "caring" behind the critique. Negative feedback is uncomfortable for most people and is therefore avoided. Inherent in any feedback, negative or positive, is the message of "I care about you and your contribution to this group." Negative strokes can be very effective if they begin with some positive strokes and are given in supportive ways. Brutal negative-unconditional strokes are counterproductive.

PREDICTIVE PRINCIPLE: The dependent, interdependent, and/or independent natures of relationships affect the structure of the communication process.

Dependence in relationships takes three forms: (1) dependence of one member on another for guidelines and support; (2) interdependence, where members share decision making and responsibility; and (3) independence, where a member engages in an activity on his own.

Group members seek to achieve some balance of dependence, interdependence, and independence within group structure according to group climate. Successful exercise of authority requires not only a recognized dependence on the part of the members or the leader, but also a reciprocal and acknowledged recognition of the leader's dependence on the members. This interdependence results in greater mutual confidence between leader and members.

Some people find comfort in maintaining close dependent relationships. These individuals usually seek constant direction and reassurance from others and may become attached to another person or persons. They operate primarily from the adaptive child ego state and "hook" others into communicating with them from the parent ego state. Often dependency is shown by what people do not do; it makes them unwilling to take chances, to exert extra effort, to use their imagination, or to display initiative. They achieve a degree of security without risk by getting others to "take care" of them. It is unwise to attempt to move the insecure individual beyond that which he is capable of accomplishing without a clear agreement or contract concerning goals and growth.

Interdependence is a reciprocal reliance between group leader and participants. In a cooperative environment, whenever one member performs a beneficial act, he simultaneously benefits all others.

An example of interdependence in action can be illustrated by the following:

A vocational nurse observed that Mr. Cable, a 68-year-old man hospitalized for treatment of a fractured femur, was developing a reddened area on his coccyx. He resisted lying on his side and disliked massage. In checking his record the licensed vocational nurse (LVN) noted that no reference was made to this problem. After discussing the matter with the nurse-manager and Mr. Cable and involving them in the decision-making process, the LVN obtained an air mattress for Mr. Cable and then began to make plans with him for exercises he could do to increase his circulation. She followed through by recording the care plan on the nurse's notes.

This worker initiated preventive measures that would prove beneficial to the patient (possibly saving him a long hospitalization) and would help other care givers by affording them the satisfaction of knowing they had participated in problem-oriented care and had possibly avoided many hours of unnecessary nursing care. This communication pattern proceeded from the adult ego state, avoided "preaching" parent messages (of what Mr. Cable should or ought to do), and involved all concerned persons in making the decision.

A state of dependence among members can foster characteristics detrimental to group goals. The nurse who asks the leader or manager for directions or specific instructions for every move, refuses to make decisions, blames others when things go wrong, and gets others to "rescue" her or do her work is dependent and operates from the child ego state. Each person in this relationship expects the others to keep the "status quo," and there is resentment if moves are made to alter the nature of procedures designed to keep the dependency going. The alert group membership will know when conditions warrant group decision to solve the problem. The nurse leader manager who can create conditions of interdependence and adult communication patterns will have facilitated productive communication processes.

PREDICTIVE PRINCIPLE: The interdependent collaborating group facilitates group goal accomplishment.

Group participation in coordinating activities is a natural by-product of a democratic managerial philosophy. If nursing membership can facilitate coordination at the operative level, the entire organization is benefited.

Ingredients for group success in devising plans for cooperative effort include

(1) a willingness on the part of all members to participate in the planning, (2) a sharing of common purposes, (3) careful communication, and (4) adherence to the authority of the employing person or organization. Responsibility for group action is often invested in the leader by bureaucracies, but this does not imply that authority must be given to a single individual. In an interdependent group, each member shares equally in the responsibility for group decisions and actions. Within guidelines, members are free to explore processes through which care can be administered to a number of patients.

Interdependent activity operates on the basic premise that groups have the power to produce changes in individual behavior so that more work will be accomplished collectively than would be individually.

Cooperation depends on routine relationships developed and practiced over a long period of time. It relies on codes of behavior whereby people work together in a group without conscious choice of whether or not they will cooperate. Cooperation demands a certain stability in the ways of the group. In nursing, this stability is often in jeopardy because of fluctuating staffing patterns. In agencies where round-the-clock coverage is necessary, membership is relatively unstable and ways must be found to overcome this problem.

Group consensus presents an element of danger. The presssure of conformity, the urge to become like every other member, and the fear of the consequences if group norms are not adhered to may make a member function in a manner contrary to his group expectations:

> The new nurse's aide is told by her peer, "I know they told you in in-service to bathe everybody everyday, but let's face it!—we don't have that kind of time. You do up the worst ones and take care of the rest the best way you can. I give patients assigned to me a bath about two times a week. I do the best I can and report 'bath given' when we sign off."

The new aide is in a dilemma. He needs the job and wants to give good nursing care but feels pressure from all sides. He is caught in a power struggle between the stated authority figures who set the standards and one member who digresses from the rules. The solution rests in the leader's and individual's ability to recognize that a power struggle exists and to deal with the situation openly. The leader can help the members face the problem by stating directly, "I notice there is a conflict between policy and practice. I need to know more about the situation. What is really going on? What caused this to happen? How do you feel about the situation?"

In all probability, group process will lead to the formation of a work structure that will resolve the conflict. The leader can ask the group how they believe priorities can best be established to ensure the administration of good care without rigidity. Possible alternatives are as follows:

1. Provide personal hygiene for every patient daily.
2. Every day bathe those patients having fevers, diaphoresis, or incontinence.
3. Bathe geriatric patients every other day (unless in category 2).
4. Establish round-the-clock activities (bathe some patients in the evening, unresponsive patients at night).

Through interdependent action the leader has helped turn a negative situation into one that can prove highly beneficial to all concerned.

Positive relationships facilitate cohesiveness and achievement of goals with speed and efficiency. Independent activity has a definite place in group activities. When a member experiences a feeling of security in his ability and in his relationships with others, he will begin to seek ways of utilizing his capacities and skills more fully. This active search is constructive and should be nurtured. The process of allowing independence among membership is a delicate one. A willingness to assume authority for special tasks does not ensure success. Self-development must have reached a level where the individual can move into the desired role with ability to achieve. Independence can be fostered by giving additional tasks gradually, so the worker is not suddenly made insecure by too great a load but can exercise his authority with discretion.

Independent action within nursing takes several routes, ranging from physical activity to mental exercise. The nurse might have sanction to manage and complete a complex assignment (for example, primary care), to take a responsibility for reorganizing the medicine or treatment room, or to devise a new way to administer a treatment. The individual expresses his ideas and contributes his suggestions on matters that involve the client, himself, and group operation. Participation of this kind leads to member satisfaction in knowing that individual efforts have been recognized and that opinions and ideas are given consideration in a search for increased effectiveness and efficiency and solutions to problem-oriented nursing care.

PREDICTIVE PRINCIPLE: Continuing reference to and clarification of goals enhance the ability to attain those goals.

Goals will seem more attainable to the participant if the nurse-leader provides opportunity for membership input. Often the group leader will assume that the preestablished goals are clear, relevant, adequate, and interesting to the extent that mere exposure will motivate the participant to achieve the goals. Empirical data suggest that increased group participation in clarifying individual and group goals is important to continued goal-directed effort; tangential activities are fewer and group effort more consistent.

Management by objectives (MBO) is a system in which management and labor at all levels participate through organizational strategies in the identification of worthy goals for the whole division as well as individual units and individual workers. Joint participation in goal-setting enables common or agreed on goals to be established. Once this is done, each person within the structure has a responsibility for meeting the goals defined. Each person knows what is expected in the effort to achieve the goals. These goals are then used to generate criteria by which individual, unit, and division efforts can be evaluated. MBO is a science in itself, with strategies for implementing, working with, and evaluating the system. Much research has been done on the effectiveness of MBO, and findings generally indicate it is highly effective.*

---

*From McLemore, M., and Bevis, E. O.: Planned change. In Marriner, A., editor: Current perspectives in nursing management, St. Louis, 1979, The C. V. Mosby Co. chap. 9.

Goal-setting is the key to any successful management program, whether that management is the care of one client, a team, a nursing unit, several nursing units, or a whole nursing division. Goal-setting may or may not lead to MBO, but it always leads to more effective and efficient coordination and collaboration. The goals are clear and accomplishment easily evaluated. MBO is not designed for major changes in organization but rather for the smooth, daily operation of an organization.

There are several methods the nurse-leader may use to determine whether the participant has perceived the relevancy of a purpose and accepts its value. The group leader can provide various types of incentives or positive reinforcement to encourage discussion of goals, values, and motivation. For example, when a client is motivated to learn or participate in the administration of isolation technique, his rewards may be in achieving self-protection and in demonstrating to himself and his nurse-teacher that a complex skill has been mastered. At times the reward may be so far removed from the goal that the participant does not see the relationship. For instance, the client may see no relationship between hand washing and contamination and thus may fail to become interested in the subject.

COMMUNICATION STRATEGIES

Strategies are heuristic devices or tools useful for accomplishing goals. A mechanic is equipped with a huge number of tools, and each is designed to achieve a specific purpose and has a definite use. Some of his tools are helpful for a wider number of "jobs" than others. For instance, a spark plug wrench is singularly designed for removing and replacing spark plugs and is not applicable to many other functions, whereas screwdrivers, pliers, crescent wrenches, and other more nonspecific tools can be used for a variety of mechanical problems. Strategies are similar. The direct question, as a strategy, is useful for eliciting specific answers and definite information but may not be helpful in eliciting discussions about problems important to the group but not included in the question. Nondirective techniques may enable the client to follow his own needs and line of thought but may not provide the nurse with information that is vital to a nursing diagnosis and prescription.

There are literally thousands of communication heuristics—communication group laboratory experiences, books, and courses—each filled with devices that enable individuals and groups to communicate more advantageously. This discussion does not attempt to cover even a representative number. A few devices are chosen as examples.

PREDICTIVE PRINCIPLE: The type of communication at work in a group dictates member perception and consequent action.

PREDICTIVE PRINCIPLE: Congruent behavioral and verbal messages promote clear communication.

Methods of communication employed by participants are important, for receiving and sending ideas clearly are essential to accomplishing purposes. Improvement in communcation depends on daily work among all participants.

People who know what is expected of them, who learn about changes before they take place, who feel free to clarify vague messages, and who check out unknown factors will perceive their roles in the best light and will work with heightened interest and enthusiasm.

Careful use of physical behavior and verbal delivery is an effective means of increasing communication with others. Effective communication depends on all participants understanding the meaning of the encounter. Without effective communication a group becomes merely a collection of individuals working in close proximity and engaged in ill-defined tasks.

Communication takes many forms and is expressed either verbally or nonverbally. *Verbal communication* consists of words written or spoken to convey a message. When information or instructions are being given, it is important that the message be delivered clearly, explicitly, and to the point. When the meaning of a directive is clear, it can be carried out with ease. For example, instructions to "rotate the patient's position every 2 hours in this sequence, from back to right side to face to left side" are far more likely to be carried out than instructions to "see that the patient is turned frequently today." Nursing jargon is another aspect of communication that can confuse unless the listener understands the terminology. Experienced care givers and clients might be quite comfortable hearing about "b.i.d.," "s.p.e.c.s.," "p.o.," and "s.o.b.," but the novice may be filled with consternation at hearing even a single term, especially the last.

On the other hand, much nursing communication is not instruction giving but collaborating for problem solving. This requires techniques that will elicit remarks and responses, provide feedback, clarify, generate ideas, help evaluate alternatives, and ultimately make goal-fulfilling choices.

Feedback is essential in determining progress toward goals and enables corrective action to put individuals and groups more on target. Without feedback, individuals and groups flounder.

Listening is another important behavior in the communication process, for it can convey various patterns to the speaker and other group members. The manner in which a person listens often indicates attitudes ranging from rejection or indifference to keen interest. When one listens, he makes a conscious effort to hear. The degree of attention given to the words spoken determines, to a large degree, the responses made and satisfactory performance in the work scene. Listening is a skill to be cultivated.

Clarifying purposes or information may be necessary before a participant can continue to follow the messages and is an element of listening—an element vital to the communication process. Clarification is necessary to determine whether or not there is comprehension. Such remarks as "Please say that another way" or "Let me see if this is what you mean . . ." are ways to ensure that the intent of the message has been understood.

Congruence between actions and words is essential to clear interpretations. If an individual says he understands but continues to look puzzled, the communicant has a conflict in verbal and behavioral messages that must then be validated to determine which message is correct. The strategy for this is clarification, which may be made operational in several ways:

1. *Check out:* Do you really understand?

2. *Playback:* Tell me what you heard me say.
3. *Feedback:* You look puzzled. Are you?
4. *Repeat:* May I go through that in a different way? I may not have been very clear that time.

A strategy is a plan for action; an operation is how that plan is put into effect. The list illustrates how the plan for clarification might be made operational in four ways.

PREDICTIVE PRINCIPLE: Threat and resulting anxiety, unless resolved, can inhibit individual and group communication.

Threat is a device that usually results in anxiety and can have detrimental effects on individuals and groups. Anxiety can appear when there is uncertainty regarding some event or series of happenings. The tension may be expressed internally, or the feeling may be communicated to all those who have contact with the disturbed person. Anxiety can be relieved constructively through exploration of the cause, with appropriate follow-up by the nurse-leader/manager.

The effect that anxiety can have on a staff member is illustrated through the following incident:

John, an aide, was evidencing anxiety that was affecting his ability to function adequately. It was nearly time for his six-month evaluation, when he would be informed whether he would be placed on permanent status or asked to leave. He was a medical student and depended on the job for his income. Besides, he liked the work and all the members of the group. When the nurse-manager had given him his three-month evaluation, he had been told that his work was "OK," but that he needed to improve. Nothing specific was mentioned. Since that time, he found himself increasingly anxious.

The nurse-leader talked with John. Through discussion it was revealed that he was "worried sick," and because he had not heard any positive feedback except for an occasional noncommital remark from his group leader, he knew no positive ways to improve. Together they devised a plan of improvement, established evaluation and feedback schedules, and planned a program for John to ask for and receive positive strokes. He was soon clearly asking for feedback by such things as "Mr. Cox sure looked better today after I finished with him, don't you think?" "I categorized all the traction equipment this afternoon. It should be easier for everybody to find what they need from now on, right?"

The two members worked through the problem by analyzing the specific incidents and recognizing when feelings of anxiety were generated. The leader recognized the lack of specificity in the three-month evaluation and failure to provide structure for follow-up. John sought more direct ways for ascertaining his progress from the leader.

Another manifestation of problems with the communication process is the introduction of threatening stimuli. Threat occurs when impending danger is made known by word or action. The term is applied to both important and trivial matters. When the member becomes aware of the threat, he concentrates on ways to handle the problem. In interrelationships, threats are conveyed both through conscious and subconscious means. If, for example, two members of a group distrust each other, threatening actions expressive of their feelings may be manifested in both overt and covert ways. Innuendos, verbal exchanges, and failure to assist one another are examples. These actions have a deleterious impact on efforts. Threats can also exert a positive influence by serving as strong motivators to action. The group, for example, that is presented with a challenge for which it feels ill-prepared can offset the threat of failure by mobilizing forces to obtain the tools that will enable its members to accomplish the charge. Overt threats are usually more counterproductive than productive.

Resistive behavior is another negative force that can deter the communication process. The apprehension of not wanting certain things to take place can evoke resistive responses in clients or group members. The inspection process may create feelings of resentment. The client or care giver may ask "Why should I be checked on? I'm capable of completing an assignment." Opposition may also take the form of reluctance or failure to accept assignment, hostility, rigidity of action, regression, absence, or nonresponsiveness.

PREDICTIVE PRINCIPLE: Questions and discussion geared to second- and third-level theories promote cognition that is more useful in nursing activities than questions and discussion geared to first- and second-level theories.

Alert observers will show that more than 80% of the verbal exchanges in group process are initiated with a question. Traditionally, questions are used to determine what has been learned or the status of one's thinking. Most questions posed by group leaders or instructors are asked so that the response and thinking of the respondent are at the first two levels of theory and require only memory or recall. There is, then, a wide range in the quality of questions. The effective leader will use questions geared to levels III and IV of theory (discussed in Chapter 1), which call for prediction or prescription. Responses to these levels of inquiry require synthesis, imagination, and creativity and encourage varying forms of problem-oriented thinking.

In developing a questioning strategy the leader will realize that (1) raising questions and issues helps to increase group interaction and establish feedback, (2) questions are used to assist participants in sharing, (3) questions are employed to lead the participant step by step to think about experiences, and (4) questions are a means of sampling respondents' understanding of or ability to make application of concepts.

The skilled leader tends to have other techniques at his disposal to accomplish the goals itemized. Statements that elicit remarks are one way; examples of these "eliciting remarks" are "Please tell me about . . ." or "Help me to understand. . . ."

John Gallagher and Mary Aschner* developed a system that classifies questions into four categories:

1. *Recall-descriptive*—narrow questions calling for specific facts, information, or descriptions to be presented by rote. Participants are asked only to give a response, not to do anything with it. Answers to these questions require only the lowest intellectual level (first- and second-level theories).
2. *Convergent-explanation*—calling for the analysis and integration of given or remembered data. Problem solving and reasoning are often involved in

*Gallagher, J., and Aschner, M.: A preliminary report on an analysis of classroom interaction, The Merrill Palmer Quarterly of Behavior and Development **9**:3, 1963.

this category. The answers may be predictable, but the task requires application of two or more recall items (second-level theories).

3. *Divergent-expansion*—calling for answers that are creative and imaginative and not empirically provable. Many different answers may be correct and acceptable (third-level theory).

4. *Value-evaluative*—dealing with judgment, value, and choice. The participant states his preference based on individual values and standards (third- and fourth-level theories).

Productive groups soon learn the value of third- and fourth-level discussions and concentrate remarks on those two levels. The payoff for the group is more efficient and valid problem solving.

PREDICTIVE PRINCIPLE: Use of simulation facilitates decision making and provides efficient means for learning problem-solving methods in a nonthreatening and safe environment.

Simulation, as used in this discussion, affords the participant opportunity to elicit various response patterns to a set of circumstances, the content of which is comparable to that found in a real-life situation. Thus the member attains particular knowledge, understandings, or skills while being confronted with lifelike situations; also he is required to apply these learnings in constructing a response. The manner in which he responds becomes a measure of the participant's grasp of the original learnings and an indicator of his abilities in reality situations.

Simulation is useful to develop decision-making skills (see Chapter 1). Since it is a structured method, feedback can be built into the format, which enables the participant to benefit from the experience in one of two ways: (1) He may observe if the course of action embarked on resulted in a desired payoff, which improved understanding of the problem-solving process. If this is so, then wise action is reinforced by the simulation. (2) Conversely, if the feedback shows the procedure resulted in ineffective decision making, he will then resort to alternative steps that lead to desirable results. One advantage of simulation is that an individual can alternately be participant and observer and can see the whole situation in a nonthreatening and safe environment.

Participation builds a high degree of motivation and gives purpose to activity. A major benefit of using the simulation process is that more members of a group are immediately and actively involved in problem solving or decision making. Because of increased insight, changes in behavior are more rapidly facilitated. Simulation also supplies a number of contingencies that may often be encountered in the nursing arena and may not be experienced in the clinical work setting.

A further advantage of the simulation strategy is the acquisition of particular skills and knowledge. In life, normally a time lag occurs between making a decision and receiving information about the effects of the decision; there is also the possibility of making costly mistakes. Simulation provides a laboratory where experience can be gained and mistakes made. It also accelerates training and shows the effects of decisions quickly.

If properly structured, simulation will make it necessary for the participants to envision the whole of the problem: to be certain of their observations and facts;

to collect, evaluate, and analyze the available information; and to develop prescriptions for nursing action. Another advantage is that alternative actions for a given circumstance can be identified and explored. During the postsimulation stage, reflection, interpretation, and discussion are often needed for final synthesizing and evaluating.

GOAL SETTING, ACHIEVEMENT, AND EVALUATION

Goal setting, prescribing nursing actions, and evaluating progress are key nursing responsibilities requiring a network of communication. Determining goals for effective nursing leadership and management depends on an accurate assessment of what comprises effectual management for the work situation. The goal-setting individual or group must know professional standards for nursing care, be cognizant of policies and expectations for the nurse-leader set by the client or employer, be familiar with the work environment (physical setting, design for administration of nursing services, personnel, lines of authority), and be aware of needs and wishes of the clients who are served. Since democratic groups are facilitated by leaders to set their own goals, this task is a shared one.

Furthermore, the nurse-leader helps goals to be communicated in meaningful terms, recognizing that (1) behavior implies active participation, (2) the learning procedure consists of acts that require a change in behavior, (3) people respond more quickly if they assist in establishing their own goals for learning, and (4) the committed individual is motivated to achieve optimal levels of performance.

The effective leader/manager develops skills in awareness of problems, formulation of goals, appropriate activities, methods of evaluation, and sharing this process with involved participants in establishing aims and devising activities for their accomplishment. With this leadership, efforts are more effective, quality of care is improved, job satisfaction is increased, and costs are reduced.

PREDICTIVE PRINCIPLE: Preassessment of individual and group knowledges, skills, and expectations establishes baseline data for measurement of progress or change.

The primary purpose of the preassessment process is to determine what the individual or group brings to the nursing arena in terms of prerequisite knowledge for nursing activity. Planning nursing prescriptions without first making an assessment of participant characteristics is akin to prescribing medicine without first diagnosing the patient. If individuals from the least to the most skilled are to be given adequate opportunity to progress and achieve, the nurse-leader/manager needs to assist members in determining their status and the procedural methods. As the nurse-leader/manager gains information regarding each care giver or related person, strategies can be developed and plans made for reducing the discrepancy between what the participant is able to achieve now (at the point of preassessment) and what he can be expected to accomplish within a prescribed period of time.

It is vital to ascertain what the participants have learned, what skill levels they have achieved, and what characteristics they possess in order to avoid problems and facilitate growth. Through the preassessment process the nurse-leader/manager can develop baseline data for the measurement of progress or change that results from the members' experiences and instruction in nursing practice. For example, the leader determines from preassessment that a nurse is unable to take a maternal-child health history at the beginning of the work experience. If at the end of the designated learning period the member is able to make a complete nursing assessment, success has been attained. Without preassessment it would be difficult, if not impossible, for the leader to ascertain how or when learning and change in behavior occurred.

Although it would seem impossible for the nurse-leader/manager to be totally aware of the interests, concerns, and expectations of each entering nurse-participant, goals are achieved with greater efficiency when the leader communicates closely with the members by preassessing, accepting, and clarifying the expectations, interests, and concerns of each member. Often a client or worker enters the nursing scene expecting a certain experience only to be disappointed, confused, and frustrated because the direction and focus are not what he expected or perceived himself as needing. The effective leader will preassess individual participant expectations and align these expectations with related activities to the extent that the care plan and environment permit.

PREDICTIVE PRINCIPLE: Mutual understanding and agreement on goals appropriate to the client or agency ensure support for goal achievement.

Agencies are established for specific and defined purposes. These purposes are dictated by social and community health needs and are written into charters and agency objectives. When an individual becomes an employee of an agency, he commits himself to the agency's established purposes. Agencies support activities designed to accomplish goals in keeping with the defined purposes of the agency. Support for activities outside the defined purposes is not economically feasible and dissipates the manpower necessary for the accomplishment of established agency purposes. Such purposes change when social, health, or community needs dictate alteration, either by evolution or through responses to emergency situations (civil, natural, or national disasters). Agency purposes seldom change simply because nursing care groups adopt goals not in keeping with established ends. Therefore it behooves nursing groups to select goals appropriate to the institution to ensure its support. The following example is illustrative of the principle under discussion:

Jimmie Bigalow, an 8-year-old boy, had been in Sundown Children's Convalescent Hospital for 18 months for convalescence from rheumatic fever with several complications when he became acutely ill with pneumonia, laryngeal edema, high fever, and severely compromised respiration. The hospital management wanted Jimmie transferred to an acute care hospital immediately. The nurses had become extremely attached to Jimmie and were very concerned about his care. The nursing group volunteered to "special" Jimmie and to devote their days off to his care. They requested that the hospital secure the necessary equipment through rental or purchase and give permission to the unit to keep and care for Jimmie. The request was denied for the following reasons:
1. The hospital plant and equipment were designed for convalescing children.
2. Other patients on the unit would feel the impact of a critically ill patient through the nurses' preoccupation with Jimmie and the necessity of maintaining a quiet atmosphere.
3. Time off should be spent away from the job to enable full devotion to the job during scheduled work time.

An astute nurse-leader/manager would have determined if group purposes were consistent with the agency goals and attempted to lead the membership to adoption of objectives compatible with the agency. Examples of appropriate objectives for the nursing group and goals that would have secured the support of the agency would have been (1) to prepare Jimmie for smooth transfer to another hospital and (2) to adopt measures that would decrease the separation anxiety of both patient and nursing staff.

To ensure successful cooperation of and support from the client in primary nursing or independent care systems, it is of vital import that communication lines exist in the operation. Goals, implementation, and evaluative measures must be defined by the nurse-leader in conjunction with the client or his representative, the group or agency, where appropriate. Of equal significance in establishing a procedural health measure is the nurse-leader and the client. In all independent negotiations, care will be exercised that the legal rights of both the consumer of health care services and the rendering person or agency be protected.

PREDICTIVE PRINCIPLE: Circumstance and member capability determine the type of directions to be communicated.

The types of directions most nurse-leaders are likely to give are (1) the command, (2) the request, (3) the suggestion, and (4) the call for volunteers.

A *command* is an authoritative direction or order; it is an exercise of direct authority. Commands imply set directives and structure and require little discussion. Some directions are communicated as commands because the implementation of the directives is important to safety, subsequent activities, cooperation with other departments, or the implementation of physicians' orders.

There are times when the *request* can be used to better advantage and, as far as the worker is concerned, carries almost the same weight as a direct command. Usually the request is given in situations where the time schedule is flexible and the worker is capable of exercising judgment. An example would be "Mrs. Blanton, when you have a chance would you investigate other ways of arranging Mrs. Sampson's personal effects so she can use them more easily? Her right arm is becoming less useful to her each day. She has indicated a desire to use her left arm more." Another form of request could be "Would you be willing to spend some time with Mr. Berra? He feels lonely because his son and family have moved from this area." The request indicates that compliance is expected but that freedom of choice exists. In a request the requestee has the right to refuse the requester without any negative consequences.

In the *suggestion* category, decisions are left to the worker as to whether or not something will be done. Suggestions offer alternatives or choices. "If Mrs. Hill is having difficulty swallowing liquids, you might try semisolids," and "You could call the welfare department and find out what they think" are examples of suggestions. Suggestions are offered only when requested; those offered when not requested are usually not used. Suggestions can do much to stimulate initiative and cooperation in the members, because they provide opportunities for the use of independent judgment.

The *call for volunteers* is a form used occasionally in soliciting people for assignments that are beyond usual duties, difficult, or unpleasant. Assisting in another area, serving on a special committee, or assuming responsibility for reorganizing the utility room are examples of situations for which all members have a choice. Again, the leader must exercise caution not to place himself in the awkward position of having to refuse a volunteer for a job for which he feels the worker is not qualified or of having no one volunteer for a job that must be done. If the possible candidates are limited, the call should go out only to those who are qualified to accept. For example, "I would like John, June, or Mary to take care of this; will one of you volunteer?"

There is dual responsibility (leader and member) for preventing continuous delegation of extra tasks to the same few individuals. In every group, certain workers are more cooperative than others and, unless protected, may be exploited.

Conversely, there is a reciprocal relationship in which the client may at times be the communicator of directions. He may determine in collaboration with the care giver the manner in which he desires his care or health plan to be implemented. The client may outline specific times, places, procedures, resources, and persons to fulfill his care plan.

Several rules of thumb hold firm in giving directions or suggestions:

1. *Do not give a choice if there is no choice.* "Would you like to help Mrs. Jones?" implies that a "no" response is acceptable. If "Please help Mrs. Jones" is meant, say so. A better alternative for giving choice yet eliciting a positive response is the question, for example, "Would you be willing to help Mrs. Jones?" Many people who do not want to "especially" would be willing to.

2. *When offering suggestions, make certain they are viewed as suggestions and not dictums.* After offering a suggestion, recommend that the person get ideas from others so that he will have a wider choice of options.

3. *When issuing a command or order, make it clear it is an expectation.* "Mrs. Jones' tray is here now" is a simple statement of fact and does not even imply what you want done with that tray. If you wish Mrs. Jones to have her tray while it is hot, say so, for example, "Mrs. Jones' tray just arrived from the kitchen; please take it to her while it is still hot."

4. *Provide choices when choices are possible.* Even a limited amount of freedom of choice is better than no choice at all. "I'm sorry, Mrs. Lucie, you cannot save your break until this afternoon and take off early because there is a meeting that Mrs. Copty and Mrs. Gill must attend at that time, and you and I will be alone for 30 minutes. However, you can alter your schedule either Thursday or Friday—both those days are clear."

PREDICTIVE PRINCIPLE: Opportunity to express expectations of the individual or group, when translated into meaningful terms to members, relates directly to individual identification and invites commitment of members to goal achievement.

Goal setting and evaluation are the lifeblood of nursing effort. Goal setting gives nursing activities meaning; evaluation allows the group to measure fulfillment; success whets the appetite for more achievement and motivates the individual or group to further meaningful activity.

Whether an individual or group goal or process is sufficiently important to exert an effect on a participant's behavior depends on the goal's relationship to the person. The possibilities of what might be expected are many. Confronted with a goal or process, the participant will be uncertain about what to expect but will seek that which has meaning for him. Perceptions and expectations are a selective process and are based on past experiences and present awareness. The participant will attend to those matters and anticipate goals and processes that have a relationship to self or to an extension of the self. Information will affect a person's behavior only to the degree to which he has discovered its personal meaning for himself.

It is important, therefore, that the nurse-leader provide opportunity for the client, individual, or group member to express and clarify his initial expectations. When the individual has the opportunity to participate in setting goals, he is more willing to accept the goals. The more responsive the leader is to the participant's expectations, the less his resistance to the group's intended goals or processes. The effective group leader/manager will structure the situation so that the client or member will express and clarify individual expectations.

To achieve group commitment and resultant behavior a goal must have value and meaning. The goal must be something the members can define, put into their own experience, and accept into their own value system. The following is an example:

Miss Lee, a young graduate, was attempting to interest a group composed primarily of new nursing assistants in foot care for a middle-aged diabetic man. She discussed, at great length, improving circulation, proper shoes, the care of toenails and corns, and bathing and powdering the feet. The group was completely passive until an experienced aide said: "Miss Lee, are you trying to tell us that if we don't do something, Mr. Taylor's sore toe could turn black and he could lose his foot?"

The aide's translation of the objective into something that had meaning for the group and was familiar to them aroused interest and achieved commitment to the goal.

PREDICTIVE PRINCIPLE: Realistic and valid goals promote achievement.

Management by objectives (MBO) is an established format for group participation in goal setting. Setting goals the group can achieve motivates the individual or group to success. Goal setting and record keeping produce gratifying results. With these tools, delegation becomes less difficult and the role of the nurse expands to an amazing degree. The old saying "Goals just beyond reach keep one striving" is false. Goals beyond reach are self-defeating and lead to discouragement and apathy. Realistic means achievable; valid as used here means relevant to the problem. Use of the following three simple, precautionary steps enables the nurse-leader to guide the group in the selection of realistic, valid, attainable goals:

1. *Identify problems.* Descriptions are essential to problem identification. Full, detailed descriptions of the situation and feelings about the situation empower the group to accurately identify the problem.
2. *Set goals.* Accurately identified problems make it possible for the group to

foresee the termination, or at least an alteration, of the problem that would make the situation more tolerable. This imagined absence or alteration of the problem becomes the goal.

EXAMPLE: The goal for a patient who has trouble with contractures is free movement with full range of motion.

Problem	Goal
Contractures	Free movement with full range of motion

3. *Determine ability to accomplish goals.* Determining the group's ability to accomplish the goal establishes whether the goal is realistic. Qualities necessary to the accomplishment of a stated goal would include such things as the following:
   a. *Resources*—either have or can acquire the collective or individual talent, knowledge, and skill appropriate and effective for accomplishment of the goal. When each desired behavior is defined behaviorally in terms of outcome, the learner knows what is expected specifically and can then determine his capability or resources for the tasks.
   b. *Time and energy*—consideration must be given to other tasks facing the group concomitantly.
   c. *Commitment and will of the group.*

PREDICTIVE PRINCIPLE: The extent of involvement of each group member determines the proficiency of the group.

Membership in a group necessitates some degree of personal involvement. Behavior as a group member is guided mainly by the individual's perception of his needs and interests. A member who receives satisfaction from the work experience will be motivated to join inextricably with the group.

Consideration of variables that influence member involvement is essential to understanding the working of groups.

All individuals are members of several groups, any one of which may exert much more influence on the member's life than the work situation does. Family, social clubs, religious and political affiliations, and community projects are examples of group associations that involve the individual.

Membership in a group does not necessarily engage the entire person, but group proficiency requires that each member involve himself fully toward the achievement of group purposes while he is present with the group. A few dedicated persons literally live and breathe nursing and evidence little interest in outside activities. These members have much to contribute, but unless they are carefully controlled, they can dominate the group and destroy its effectiveness. The overly zealous member becomes wearisome to others and eventually creates a backlash of negative reaction that takes its toll in group productivity.

The leader/manager can utilize the devoted member's zeal constructively by channeling some of the worker's energy into activities that can be performed on an individual basis. Keeping the ward library up to date is one way of providing helpful diversion. The interested member could search nursing literature and bring pertinent materials to the station for members of all teams. Another avenue for the individual deeply engrossed in the profession is serving on nursing procedure committees, policy boards, and so on. Care must be taken to ensure broad representation, but usually all who wish to do so have the opportunity to participate in these kinds of activities. There are numerous worthwhile but time-consuming tasks in committee work. The eager member can volunteer to devote as much time and effort as he desires to these responsibilities.

A problem of equal significance is the member who works eight hours a day, five days a week for a paycheck and evidences little or no interest in the endeavors of the nursing group to which he is assigned. This person must be assisted to progress from his dormant or even inhibitory stage to one of productivity, or his position as a group member will become untenable.

Possible reasons for the lack of member involvement might be that conditions in the work setting are not contributing to member satisfaction. Perhaps the staff member does not feel accepted as a necessary part of the group process or rarely has the opportunity to complete assigned tasks without interruption. Perhaps the member does not feel secure in his ability to perform the assigned tasks (tests in management reveal a close relationship between ability and interest). On the other hand, the member may not experience sufficient outlet for his abilities. It is up to group participants to discover conditions that will promote and maintain interest in their work situation to foster member involvement and to pave the way for group proficiency.

Another factor that influences the extent of involvement an individual has in a group is the degree to which the beliefs, values, and attitudes of the group conflict or agree with those of other groups to which he belongs. Conformity pressures may be exerted from both sides, thus forcing the individual to make a choice between the two. This type of conflict occurred when a community health nurse was assigned to head a team in a district that was predominantly populated by Mexican-Americans. The first three-month report revealed very little progress with the families to which the nurse was assigned. On consultation with the nurse the supervisor learned the leader had been indoctrinated since childhood by both family and social groups to believe that "Mexicans are stupid and lazy, do not wish to work, and have as many children as possible in order to collect welfare."

The manager believed the nurse could become a competent and contributing member of the staff. Accordingly, after planning with the nurse, a learning contract was devised and the nurse was assigned to work with a Mexican-American nurse in the district with the provision that a study of Mexican-American culture through a planned program be undertaken. The supervisor reasoned that families could not receive help from a biased leader; therefore a change was necessary. The assignment to attend classes and seminars and read was based on the assumption that, with increased understanding of Mexican-American culture, increased exposure to Mexican-American people, and close work with a Mexican-American nurse, the nurse would have an opportunity to examine her presets and would become able to work on her first assignment.

One primary aim of the nurse-leader is to bring all members of the group having different norms or values into a functioning relationship. Possible means include providing the group members with a role model through exemplary leadership, group discussions, individual conferences, and workshops with continuous exposure of the members to a democratic point of view.

Actions in the interest of the client are to be fostered; if the decision is reached that the member cannot resolve conflict and become involved in the achievement of the group's purposes, the leader may recommend his removal from the work group.

PREDICTIVE PRINCIPLE: Group involvement in goal setting requires the endorsement of the agency and commitment of membership to participate in the outcome.

Group decisions in formulating goals can have a place in employee relations but must be limited to issues that are reasonable and obtainable through the conscientious efforts of all personnel.

Like most business and industrial organizations, health agencies follow established patterns of operation. A governing board gives direction and overall guidance, the administrators furnish the physical environment and services that support the medical and nursing staff, and formulated and stated policies provide guidelines for all administrative action. Ideally, leaders of nursing groups have a part in the formulation of overall policy, but in any case, the leader is governed by the stipulations of the employing agency.

In nursing teams, formation of group goals has more the character of selecting subgoals for procedure. Group aspirations are subordinate to those objectives outlined for all nursing services. Overall goals for the agency are usually stated in general terms such as "To provide nursing care commensurate with the standards established by the American Nurses Association" or "To treat all patients equally." It is important to recognize that although these goals may be desirable and members of the nursing group may wish to become involved in their implementation, they are too vague for specific operation. Examples of goals that imply member involvement are (1) complete a course in cardiac resuscitation, (2) develop a plan that would facilitate interaction among members, and (3) and increase care giver skill in the operation of cardiac monitors. Each of these aims can be worked through operationally and can be successfully accomplished according to the extent of member involvement.

With the kind of objectives just given, participants can work cooperatively to design a plan that will lead to specific realization. The latter objective could be operationally defined by the group in the following way:

Goal: To increase care giver skill in the operation of cardiac monitors.
Operation:
1. Provide each member with a copy of a manual containing necessary background information.
2. Allow two weeks for individual study.
3. Set up a series of five one-hour seminars with in-service director and staff in charge of the cardiac unit.
4. Arrange for practice sessions with equipment. Arrange schedule so that each member has adequate time to attend seminars and practice sessions (equal time does not necessarily have to be given to each member)
5. Have each member take test on theory and practice.
6. Plan additional seminars and practice sessions according to individual need.
7. Allow time for review periods at least once per month.

As the members become involved in planning steps to reach their goal, they will designate the persons who are to assume responsibility for implementation. Total involvement takes place throughout the process, thus committing members to the outcome.

A managerial error is made when a group is allowed to participate in decisions for which there can be no subsequent fulfillment. The following is an example:

Mrs. Beaux, leader of a nursing team, attended a seminar on group dynamics and was particularly impressed with a series of lectures given about employees who were setting their own goals for job fulfillment. The speaker emphasized that if co-workers were given the opportunity, they could meet together to consider intelligently and then formulate goals that would be appropriate to the situation.

Returning to her nursing station, Mrs. Beaux decided to practice some of the principles she had heard. She called together the five members of her team and told them that, in her opinion, the team members would be more satisfied if they decided just how much work they could accomplish in one day. She then gave the team members the opportunity to discuss and to decide among themselves as a group what their work load should be. Mrs. Beaux left the room, believing the group would doubtlessly assess their jobs and establish much higher goals for themselves than she herself would have dared propose.

After the discussion period was over, the group informed Mrs. Beaux they believed they were overworked. Since they had been given the authority to establish their own work load, they would reduce the patient census on their team by two and would relinquish their responsibility for distributing fresh linens to all teams.

The weakness in the original proposal belatedly became clear to Mrs. Beaux. She had allowed individuals to participate in a decision that could not be realized, for she did not have the power to implement the proposal. She had failed to equate her naive assumption with reality and was left with a difficult situation.

The fiasco could have been avoided had the nurse-leader consulted with the head nurse first to see if the plan was feasible and workable. Mrs. Beaux must now use the situation as a bad start toward something better. She can tell the group where the idea originated, what she thought would happen, and the situation she finds herself in now. She can discuss with the group the matter of feelings of overload in work assignment and attempt to work out a solution with them and the head nurse that is mutually satisfactory to both. By this method the nurse-leader's ideas, the group's wishes, and the guidelines and policies of the institution can be blended into a constructive approach.

EFFECTIVE CONFERENCES

Conferences are necessary to the practice of nursing to give and receive information cooperatively and collaboratively.

Grouping persons involved in accomplishing common goals for the purpose of interchange of ideas and solving problems provides a useful tool for building and maintaining mutual understanding.

Nursing conferences are not limited to providers of health services. It is now generally recognized that to attain and maintain optimum mental and physical health, if possible, all significant persons must be included in each phase of client care. Thus in addition to members of the health team, the client, his family, and others who have an interest in the purpose of the conference are included.

A nursing conference is usually called for the purpose of finding out or deciding something. This means there is a reciprocal relationship for the exchange of information. Nurses convene conferences for a variety of purposes. These include (1) direction-giving conferences, in which the leader or client gives information and directions specific to the assignment; (2) patient-centered conferences, in which members identify problems and attempt to arrive at solutions and decide on courses of action; (3) content conferences, in which participants assemble to acquire knowledge about a specific subject; (4) reporting conferences, in which participants give progress reports; (5) general problems conferences, in which individuals express their impressions about the work situation and try to resolve work or personnel problems; and (6) nursing care conferences, in which participants collaborate for problem-oriented nursing care.

Effective communication necessitates a systematic plan for providing and maintaining contact between the leader and group and for person-to-person exchanges. Gathering groups together at specific times for clearly defined purposes will help to realize this goal.

The time for nursing conferences is usually relatively short; therefore the participants must work for brevity and exactness. Conference style is most often informal and more conversational than formal meetings; therefore the group that is cognizant of the need to be purposeful and well organized accomplishes more.

The conference situation is not a "natural" one for the nurse-leaders, and many are tempted to find reasons for not meeting with the entire group at one time. The leader who feels ill at ease in conducting group sessions, for example, may look for reasons to cancel meetings. The excuse may be offered: "There never seems to be a right time to get the group together—when I'm ready, they're not. I would like to have them meet all at one time, but there are just so many hours in a day!" The alternative action is to "catch them on the run" or, worse yet, to trust that the members will discover for themselves what is expected of them.

Time is an important factor, as most care givers spend the greater share of their work period attempting to meet the numerous demands placed on them. It is true, however, that most people find time for activities they deem important and in which they feel comfortable. If one accepts the principle that effort to arrive at group consensus for nursing action cultivates positive outcomes, time must be given to meetings where the process can take place.

The nurse-manager can become adept in the role of conference leader if effort is channeled into acquiring and applying principles of conference technique that will contribute to the realization of effective amalgamation of ideas and feelings.

All conferences have certain commonalities. Accomplishment of purpose is enhanced when members have the opportunity to meet without interruption and come prepared to participate and when behaviors enhance goal accomplishment. Another contributing factor to successful conference sessions is participant understanding of behaviors each individual uses to impart ideas or feelings to others and recognition of the effect specific actions have on the group.

PREDICTIVE PRINCIPLE: Adequate preparation by the leader for all conferences expedites fulfillment of expectations for the conference.

Realities of life make adequate preparation for all situations at all times impossible. Nursing is particularly susceptible to disruptions. New patients are admitted just prior to conference time; substitute staff members are assigned; new procedures are introduced; emergencies occur; and friction occasionally arises among health personnel. In addition to these disruptive elements, the nurse-leader will not necessarily have acquired competency in all phases of nursing. Deviations from the ideal, however, need not deter the nurse-leader from proceeding with preparation as current conditions allow.

Preparation for a conference will depend on the purpose of the meeting. Instructional conferences call for imparting information to members to facilitate completion of assignments. Content and patient-centered conferences require acquisition of knowledge specific to a particular patient or subject. Reporting conferences demand that the reporter know what needs reporting; the content and shared feelings conferences depend on group needs coupled with judicious use of interpersonal relationship skills.

PREDICTIVE PRINCIPLE: Relieving care givers of responsibility while the conference is in session allows members to proceed without interruption.

In most clinical settings, more than one nurse or group is assigned to care for the total patient population. Leaders will want to coordinate their schedules to allow time for necessary meetings and to arrange for the care of patients assigned to them while each group is in session.

Patients cannot be left unattended by nursing staff. This is especially true in acute nursing care units where lack of supervision can have serious consequences. (Intravenous fluids can accelerate or reduce in rate within seconds; patients may require assistance with bodily functions; and there is the ever-present possibility of crises such as hemorrhage, shock, myocardial infarction, or cardiac arrest.)

In structured settings a conference time schedule that considers the needs and desires of all personnel equally will prove to be the most successful. Most leader/managers consider the ideal time for a direction-giving conference to be as soon after the workday has started as possible. The leader will then have the opportunity to give directions to members before the group becomes involved in a multiplicity of tasks. The preferred time for the reporting conference is usually about forty-five minutes before the end of the shift. This arrangement gives members the opportunity to sum up the day's progress before completing last-minute details. Scheduling of content and patient-centered conferences does not usually become an issue other than to find time when members can get together.

Nursing functions cover myriad activities. Each member has a job to do that usually must be done within a certain time limit. Some tasks demand strict compliance to a schedule. Preoperative medications and the collection of specimens illustrate this point. Other assignments, such as the administration of hygienic care, allow for a degree of flexibility. Agency and client routines must be taken into consideration. Serving of meals and provision for treatments given by those other than the nursing personnel further complicate planning care.

Community health agencies work around appointments, clinic-school visits, and other problems. Regardless of setting, all conferences require careful programming.

PREDICTIVE PRINCIPLE: Prior announcement of time, place, purpose, and duration of conferences to all concerned promotes assembly of a group well prepared and ready to focus attention on the purposes of the conference.

The importance of holding conferences for the purpose of giving direction, coordinating activities, and evaluating progress is patent. It is equally evident that each member must know in advance when, where, how long, and for what purpose the conferences will be held.

A written schedule of meeting times is helpful. A printed format may be devised to fit any situation. Information concerning specific conferences can then be filled in easily and posted for all staff members to note. The following is a model of scheduling for an area that has three groups.

Conference	Group I	Group II	Group III
Direction-giving	7:30-7:50 (daily)	8:00-8:20 (daily)	7:30-7:50 (daily)
Patient-centered	1:00-1:30 (Monday)	11:00-11:30 (Tuesday)	1:00-1:30 (Wednesday)
Content	1:00-1:30 (Tuesday)	11:00-11:30 (Wednesday)	1:00-1:30 (Thursday)
Report	2:15-2:35 (daily)	1:40-2:10 (daily)	2:15-2:35 (daily)

When there are three groups, two can meet at one time with careful planning. The head nurse and ward secretary assist the third group in alerting the attending staff to the patients' needs. Leaders in conferences will have informed the covering nurse-leader of any specific needs that require attention during the time of the conference. When there are only two groups, scheduling is simplified. It becomes a matter of one covering for the other while they are in conference and alternating times of meetings from week to week. When only one group is involved, times for meeting together should still be scheduled, but flexibility in timing is more easily managed. In this event, coverage will be arranged on an individual basis.

All members realize there will be occasions when it is impossible to hold to the conference schedule. At such times the situation is usually stressful, often causing the members to forget the times of meetings. If at all possible, however, the leader/manager involved in the disruption should alert another manager to arrange for a trade in times for meetings. If the cause for the delay does not permit this step, the coordinator of nursing services must be alerted to proceed with alteration or trade in the conference schedule with the leader who is detained. Keeping one group waiting for a conference that will not be held is a waste of time, and where more than one group is involved, the time lost is proportionately increased.

In addition to timing, clear purpose and agenda contribute much to successful conferences. People who understand the purpose and agenda can prepare for the meeting and contribute on a higher level.

When a number of people work together in close harmony, it is understandable that they will be interested in one another's lives and will take advantage of opportunities to exchange information and confidences. A few moments can be allotted for this purpose before initiating the conference or while waiting for all members to arrive. Once the meeting has begun, however, participants will need to exercise discipline to keep their attention focused on the purpose for meeting. The leader can assist the group to hold to its mark by recognizing when diversion from the appointed task has occurred and bringing the discussion back into focus by using simple phrases such as "Can we return to . . . ," "You were saying that . . . ," or "Will you explore . . . a little further, please?"

DIRECTION-GIVING CONFERENCE

Direction-giving conferences are meetings called at the beginning of a work shift for the specific purpose of communicating job assignments, delineating areas of responsibility, and imparting information necessary for members to care for patients effectively.

PREDICTIVE PRINCIPLE: Obtaining the most recent data available prior to conference ensures the leader that imparted information is pertinent, inclusive, and accurate.

In settings where there is round-the-clock coverage the nurse-leader will receive a progress report from the person previously responsible for the groups of patients either by word of mouth or via tape recorder while the off-going nurse is completing the assignment. Additional information will be needed before giving instructions to care givers. Leaders or managers will want to check pertinent data, such as preoperative orders, arrangements for tests, and so on, and to visit each patient *before* the time of the conference. This will give the leader opportunity to make a personal assessment of the patient's status.

In active units, frequent attempts will be made to interrupt the time the managing nurse has reserved for personal visits to patients. Most interruptions can be handled by delegating tasks to others. Intercommunication systems prove invaluable to the leader making rounds, allowing the nurse to keep in touch with staff and yet proceed with the intended purpose of allowing client participation in the development of his care plan and providing for client-nurse dialogue. Informal meetings will be conducted by primary care nurses, but the need for careful preparation is not lessened. In many instances the client and his family will engage in preplanning activities by reading, experimenting with procedure, investigating resources, and so on.

PREDICTIVE PRINCIPLE: Information to care givers and/or clients that is paced, systematic, and inclusive allows participants time to assimilate the content and provides them with information necessary to function.

The success or failure of imparting pertinent information to an individual or a group depends on sufficient information and method of presentation. The leader must be sensitive to what information is needed and at what pace the members (client and/or care givers) are able to receive it. In a direction-giving conference, for example, members should not be avalanched with irrelevant information. They want to hear that which will be most useful in the immediate situation.

Much of the information determining routine and time of performance is a part of core information. Routine care, time for meals, procedure for obtaining or imparting information, and so on are best omitted unless there is need for review. New members will require instruction in addition to the routine information, but all members should not be subjected to the instructional part of the newcomer's orientation period.

Routine information that must be transmitted about patients, such as diet, activity, tests, and treatments, can be transcribed on care giver's work sheets by the ward clerk prior to the work period. In group conferences, use of serial order on individual work sheets allows the members to know the routine, thus enabling them to increase speed and effectiveness in writing the things they have just heard.

There is a direct relationship between the requirement for information transmission and task difficulty. The amount of detail necessary in the "how" part of an order depends on how complicated the task is and how experienced the employee is in doing the job. For instance, there is no need to discuss nursing procedures familiar to the listener. But when the situation calls for new knowledge or skills or deeper understanding, the leader must allow time for a clear, understandable explanation.

In giving an order a leader may neglect to explain the reason for the directive. An explanation makes it possible for the worker to use sound judgment if he has a problem, and it often helps to eliminate misunderstanding. The leader may direct an aide to "ambulate Mrs. Sheppard for five minutes every hour." The aide becomes so engrossed in the fulfillment of a heavy assignment that judgments must be made about priority. She decides to omit Mrs. Sheppard's ambulation. A simple statement to the aide at the time of the directive might have ensured proper consideration when priorities were established. The leader could have explained: "Mrs. Sheppard had a vein ligation of both legs yesterday. It is very important that she walk for five minutes every hour to avoid the formation of blood clots in her legs. If one were to form and become dislodged it could travel through the bloodstream directly to her heart and cause her death."

Modern communication technology permits nurses to exchange information necessary to implement care plans in ways that provide for individual timing. Reports, directions, and communications about goal progress may be communicated via tape cassette. The oncoming staff may listen to short reports while off-going care givers continue to work with patients. Any clarification may be done by individuals at their own convenience.

PATIENT-CENTERED CONFERENCES

Patient-centered conferences are meetings in which problem-oriented care is discussed and evaluated. Patient-centered conferences are designed to help overcome the decentralization of the care of patients. The focus of attention is usually on the analysis of one patient or family situation for whom the nurse or group is caring. Patient-centered conferences provide a means whereby all participants will benefit from the experiences of a few. Where possible, the client or other significant people are included in the sessions and the client is the focal point of discussion. The process is a dynamic, interactive, problem-oriented approach, based on a framework operationally sequenced (assessment, problem identification, formulating plans for nursing action, providing for evaluation and implementation).*

In utilizing the nursing process the leader opens the way for consideration of the needs of the whole patient—physiologic, psychologic, spiritual, social, and cultural—to acquire a rationale for nursing action and to devise ways to improve nursing care. The leader has an opportunity to guide members in recognizing individual patient or family needs and in formulating nursing principles that result in nursing prescriptions for action.

Separate meetings about patients or families, which are not in conjunction with another type of conference, allow time for discussion free from interruption. Participants will be more successful in keeping their commitment to purposes if meetings are planned at a time when the major share of the work load has been accomplished and if conferences are well spaced. Frequency of patient-centered conferences depends on the situation. Intensive care units, for example, may not meet more than once a week, whereas an area with a slower pace might have the opportunity to meet more frequently. Thirty-minute to one-hour periods are usually sufficient for the average conference. Problem solving requires at least that much time, and little can be accomplished if the group must work under pressure.

Use of principles of teaching, learning, and leadership will help in assisting the group to become increasingly more skilled in its ability to recognize and to solve specific problems and to make appropriate generalizations in nursing care in similar, although different, nursing situations.

PREDICTIVE PRINCIPLE: Interaction of conference members on an equal basis encourages active participation and leads to usable solutions to the problem.

Conference participants have diverse cultural, educational, and experiential backgrounds. Acceptance of the philosophy that the group together has more knowledge about a subject than any single member does can serve to improve the productivity of the group.

In nursing care conference situations the members make decisions by consensus or majority so that the commitment to such decisions is corporate and not vested in any one individual.

The leader must provide a nonthreatening environment if members are to feel free to share what they have done with others, engage in identification of problems, and give and receive suggestions for further action. If the leader imposes his own opinions on the group prematurely, he, in effect, negates the potential benefits that can be derived from the participation of all members.

*Bower, F. L.: The process of planning nursing care: a model for practice, ed. 2, St. Louis, 1977, The C. V. Mosby Co., p. 10.

In a nursing care conference situation the leader opens the discussion, then invites members to make contributions to the discussion freely. The leader's role is primarily one of facilitating the group work in constructing plans that will benefit a patient or family. Some conferences will require little active participation from the leader, and others will demand a larger contribution. Regardless of who offers content in the conference, each contribution should be given careful consideration. The patient or family and other significant persons may be an integral part of the process.

PREDICTIVE PRINCIPLE: Identification of the nursing problem to be considered expedites the formulation of nursing intervention.

The initial steps in a nursing care conference are (1) to assess the group interest and need, (2) to identify and delineate the problem, (3) to assess the group's knowledge about the problem or prior experiences that relate to the problem, (4) to select and utilize the appropriate content, and (5) to determine ways to evaluate the results of implemented plans.

The following is a sample discussion of a nursing care incident about which a patient-centered conference was conducted. It is not intended to be all inclusive but is used to illustrate how a nurse-leader can conscientiously apply principles of teaching and learning (see Chapter 2) to bring about the desired goal of improving patient care through the use of patient-centered conferences. The participants in the sample conference are members of the nursing team in a newborn nursery setting. Each person participates in ways commensurate with his role and capability. General introductory activities and other material and comments not specifically illustrative have been deleted. What remains is the process and structure.

LVN: I am caring for Baby Lee in 317A. He was born at 2 AM, was full term, and weighed 7 pounds. Everything was going along well until this morning when he began to breathe in a strange way. He became very restless, began to breathe with jerky respirations, and his ribs pulled in with every breath. Right after that he started to grunt, cough, and then turned blue. I was scared to death; I did what I could and called for help. The team leader knew what to do, and he is breathing better now.

Leader: What do you believe are the problems in this situation?

LVN: Well, I'd surely like to know what went wrong with him and I'd like to know if I did the right thing.

Leader: Anything else?

Aide: What I want to know is what do we do if a baby goes bad like that when we are taking care of it!

All: (Indications of consensus.)

Leader: (To LVN) What have you decided is the problem for the group to consider now?

LVN: I think all of us should know what to do in case that happens again.

At this point the group has moved through the preliminary assessment period. The teaching and learning principle that *learner need and readiness influences content and rate of learning* was implemented by the leader. The group was taken through a process that identified their need and readiness to learn.

The nurse-leader then implemented the principles that *participation of the learner in setting learning goals makes learning activities meaningful and useful to the learner and realistic behavioral goal setting enables selection of appropriate and meaningful content.* This was illustrated by the participation of the aide and LVN in stating and delineating the problem and in the group consensus about the topic for the conference. The established goal is realistic and behavioral and indicates to the nurse-leader the body of knowledge necessary to meet the goal. The teaching and learning principles about anxiety and motivation are implemented in this situation because the respiratory distress of Baby Lee has created the anxiety that members may not be able to meet a similar emergency situation.

PREDICTIVE PRINCIPLE: Analyzing nursing care given in the light of established goals enables members to validate their behavior and to devise ways to improve nursing care.

A member confronted with a problem while administering nursing care will react in some way. If the individual can describe his behavior in the nursing situation but is unable to give reasons for the care given, there is evidence of lack of understanding. Nursing care situations are ideal for assisting the members to increase in knowledge and understanding without jeopardizing their sense of personal worth.

There is no better way to implement the teaching and learning principle that *an obvious relationship between learning activities and stated goals increases the motivational value of the activity* than to discuss what was done by the person involved in the situation at the time of the incident.

In the case of Baby Lee the group was well aware of the overall goal areas for the care of all infants—observation, prevention, comfort, and nurturing. When the LVN observed signs and symptoms that deviated from normal, she acted in an attempt to restore the infant to the desired state of being. The immediate crisis for her was over, but unanswered questions remained, causing her to experience anxiety. Through verbal interaction the LVN shared with co-workers her behavior in the time of crisis.

> **Aide:** (To LVN) What did you do when Baby Lee started having trouble?
>
> **LVN:** First, I made sure there was nothing obstructing the air from getting into his lungs.
>
> **Aide:** How did you do that?
>
> **LVN:** I pressed my thumb down on his chin and opened his mouth to see if I could see any signs of obstruction. He had quite a bit of mucus but nothing more. Then I turned him on his side with his head brought forward to relax his throat as much as possible to allow the mucus to run out. By this time the team leader answered my call.
>
> **Leader:** You did the right thing: An open airway is the first thing to look for.

The LVN's actions were a result of her previous knowledge and experience. She acted maturely, demonstrated an ability to function well under stress, and carried out nursing activities based on previously learned materials about the emergency care of the infant who had respiratory distress. The nurse-leader's comment on appropriate action implemented the teaching and learning principle that *rewards of recognition, praise, peer status, or valued gains are motivating and reinforcing factors facilitating learning rate, amount of retention, and degree of behavior change*. The recognition and praise validated and reinforced the appropriate action of the LVN and served as a vehicle for the members to devise ways to meet similar nursing emergencies and thus improve nursing care.

Validation served to help the LVN feel successful about handling the crisis, increased her confidence, lowered her anxiety, and readied the group to acquire additional information and move into the next stage of the learning process.

The LVN has completed the account of her experience. The leader's role now is that of teacher, because the LVN is unable to render the nursing care required in this situation.

Leader: When I arrived, I percussed the baby's posterior chest (illustrates the procedure with hands) before I suctioned him to loosen the secretions. He had quite a lot of thick material in him. This procedure will have to be done every 20 minutes or so.

Aide: Can we do that procedure?

Leader: No, the LVN and I will. Your part is to note if he appears to be in trouble again with his breathing; then call us right away. He is now in an Isolette with oxygen and an IV.

LVN: Baby Lee is suspected of having hyaline membrane disease, which is a condition affecting the lungs. I know that it occurs mostly with premature babies. Baby Lee is full term. I would like to know more about the disease. Can we take it as our subject for the content conference?

Leader: All agreed? Fine. I will get some reading material together and make it available to you. Find out as much as you can before Thursday. In the meantime, I will tell you that Baby Lee's critical period is the next 48 hours. It is very important that he (1) be kept in the warmed Isolette with 40% oxygen, (2) be percussed and suctioned every 20 minutes, (3) have his umbilical catheter kept intact, (4) be watched carefully to see that his IV goes at 10 drops per minute, (5) have his respirations recorded and graphed every 15 minutes (more often if necessary), and (6) be observed for signs of change in color or severe distress.

The LVN and I will assume responsibility for the treatments. We want everyone to help us with observation. Each time you go by his Isolette, will you have a look at him with these things in mind? Should you have occasion to note these same symptoms that the LVN has described in an infant you are caring for, do just as he did. Make sure there is no obstruction, then turn the child on his side, bring his head forward, and call for help.

The nurse-leader has given new information and set limits describing the patient's immediate needs and who is responsible for meeting those needs. This implements the teaching and learning principle that *structure, limits, and feedback provide an environment that promotes security and trust.*

The LVN now takes the lead by giving information he has acquired about the patient but is to him of less importance than was the immediate problem of Baby Lee's compromised respirations.

The group has requested an opportunity to learn more about hyaline membrane disease. The leader has applied the principle that *learning in real rather than contrived situations facilitates ease of learning and retention* and has been consistent in the philosophy of the value of learner participation in goal setting. The nurse-leader (1) made sure the group had enough information to function safely immediately, (2) set group expectations of nursing responsibilities for the next 48 hours to allay anxiety about the course of events before the more long-range goals could be met, and (3) established goals commensurate with group need for the next meeting.

Since the objective for the patient-centered conference was a behavioral goal, the evaluation of the conference is built into the objective itself. If group members demonstrate in their subsequent care of Baby Lee that they can function effectively within the limits and expectations discussed in the conference, learning will have occurred.

PREDICTIVE PRINCIPLE: Formation of written nursing orders or care plans from patient-centered conferences provides a central, continuous source of information.

Nursing orders or care plans are written expressions of the nursing process. They are essential for consistent care. Where advisable, a copy of the care plans may be left with the client, since, ideally at least, he participated in their development. Nursing care plans are best formulated from patient-centered, problem-oriented conferences. Although it is conceivable that the nurse could write a nursing care plan without consulting other persons, it is not recommended. Synthesis of ideas of several people ensures a more comprehensive and accurate care plan. Furthermore, the care plan is more apt to be followed by client and care givers if they participate in its formation.

The patient-centered conference concerning Baby Lee is used as an example of transposing verbal communication into written form where vital content becomes accessible to all personnel involved with his care. Only those headings that have bearing on the case will be explored.

PHYSICIAN'S ORDERS
Warmed Isolette with 40% oxygen
Percuss and suction every 20 minutes or as needed
Heparin-saline solution through umbilical catheter as needed
Sodium bicarbonate, 3.75 gm or 44.6 mEq in 50 ml IV, 10 gtts/minute
Bennett respirator
Record and graph respiratory rate every 15 minutes, every half hour or as needed

NURSE'S ORDERS
Protective measures
Maintain controlled temperature of Isolette
Keep open airway (observe for excessive mucus)
Maintain prescribed flow of IV fluid
Keep arterial catheter in place (may need to inject heparin quickly)
Carefully observe color and breathing
Keep on either side

Physical care
Position on either side with head in forward position
Percuss and suction as needed every 20 minutes or as needed
Observe closely for cyanosis (blueness), dyspnea (difficult breathing)

Family
Mother is highly anxious about child (is hospitalized postpartum in room 342)
Mother may sit by Isolette as desired (physician's permission granted)
Father anxious. Work phone, 282-5486; home, 369-1182
Grandmother, Mrs. Baxter, keeping three small children in their home

It is quite likely that an infant in critical condition might require some religious ritual; in this event the notations would be made under the appropriate heading. Later, as the infant progressed, referrals might be made and other family needs, such as parental teaching, identified that would be worked out through the care plan.

Nursing orders, developed on a systematic basis, derived from careful analysis of patient needs, and structured in collaboration with all concerned individuals and groups, enable clients and agencies better to utilize nursing manpower. The economics involved in planning and implementing patient care are just as important to the agency and patient as is the planning of personnel time and duties. Every coordinator of nursing services expends a considerable length of time planning time schedules for employees, patients, and families. The efficient use of the full abilities and potential of each employee with patient and family will result in maximum services for monies paid.

CONTENT CONFERENCES

Constant input of knowledge enables client and care givers more effectively to perform the tasks expected of them. One way of ensuring participants the opportunity to increase their learning is to provide them with time to meet for the sole purpose of exploring content. Traditionally, content conferences have been reserved for the novice, based on the premise that novices need time set aside to concentrate on specific content. However, when an aide, LVN, or nurse has completed the appropriate basic course, education has just begun. Planned classes or content conferences furnish a vital and necessary link in the continuing growth and education of nursing personnel.

The practice of nursing can be improved in an environment that encourages individuals and groups to investigate ways to prevent problems. The opportunity to improve care entices the member with an inquiring mind and a creative spirit to grow and to innovate better nursing practices. Nursing practiced in a setting where learning is treated as exciting as well as useful reaps the benefits of such an attitude through a continued upgrading of the quality of care given. Individuals who become interested in developing better nursing practices will not only improve in ability but also will, by example, generate interest in others to follow suit.

Content conferences, like patient-centered sessions, are usually held about once a week for a period of thirty minutes to one hour at any convenient time. The scheduling and length of time varies. However, adherence to the scheduled time indicates the importance of and commitment to the need for the conference. When pressures in the work situation occur or some member is not as well prepared as he would like to be, it may seem expedient to drop the meeting from the schedule with the intent of meeting at a "better time." Almost without exception, the more convenient time never arrives. Members who form the habit of keeping their commitments are usually productive.

The goal of a content conference is derived from any aspect of nursing that meets the need of the membership. The field is open to a broad range of subject matter. Medical concerns such as symptoms, pathology, laboratory results, clinical course of a disease, diagnostic tests, and pharmacologic data interest nursing personnel and influence nursing activities and judgments. Nursing content such as patient care or comfort problems, patient teaching needs, new technologic advancements, and preventive care are areas constantly in need of attention. Because of time allotment, all areas cannot be covered; if attempted, the conference would result in a general coverage of a number of problems with no appreciable gain in theoretical and practical understanding of what nursing involves. To ensure a successful content conference the subject matter must be (1) needed by the membership, (2) something that can be considered in the allotted time, and (3) adequately prepared prior to the meeting.

Leadership varies with each conference. As in the patient-centered conference, the initiator of the subject matter usually takes the lead. The amount of guidance and assistance needed to prepare for the conference will depend on the individual's capabilities. Often the leader will suggest sharing the responsibility for presentation of content. All group members are expected to contribute to the discussion. Content conferences need not restrict contributions to the members of the group involved; participation from any person—coordinator of nursing services, physician, social worker, or therapist, including the patient or family—may be included when feasible and appropriate.

PREDICTIVE PRINCIPLE: Member participation in problem-solving processes during content conference results in more meaningful learning.

Participants come to content conferences having acquired a body of antecedent information. They are ready to fit their knowledge and understanding together to form predictive principles that can be used to prescribe nursing actions.

The need to learn more about hyaline membrane disease, expressed by the membership in the patient-centered conference on Baby Lee, will be continued as an example of the theory-building process in a content conference. The following is a model of a problem-solving process in a content conference:

> **LVN:** (After giving a recall of background data about Baby Lee.) The definition of hyaline membrane disease is "a syndrome of neonatal distress, characterized by a hyaline-like material within the alveoli and bronchioles." This disease is very much like emphysema, in which bronchi in the lungs end in thin-walled air spaces (illustrates with chalk drawing).

The LVN has begun the conference by referring to content familiar to the group. Her next step is to introduce new information and then to make it meaningful by relating the facts to the more familiar condition (emphysema). Visual media assist the learning process. The LVN has applied the principle that *content that flows from the familiar to the unfamiliar provides a point of reference and promotes efficient grasping of material.*

> **Aide:** Did you find out why the baby has this disease? I read that babies with hyaline membrane disease are usually premature, and Baby Lee is not.
>
> **LVN:** Yes, I did. The specific cause of the disease is unknown, but it does occur frequently in two conditions. One is with premature babies, as we know, and the other occurs in babies born of mothers who have untreated diabetes mellitus.

Student: What about the mother? Has she been tested?
Leader: The doctor is working with her. She has had a blood test, which proved positive. Mrs. Lee was shocked, to say the least, but is now learning all she can about the problem.

Members in this conference are concerning themselves with a real situation, which is never simple. Extraneous factors will enter in and must be considered if they are pertinent to the subject. These activities actualize the principle that *learning in real rather than contrived situations facilitates ease of learning and retention.*

LVN: Baby Lee's problems center around respirations. I have, with the help of the team leader, placed facts on the blackboard that will help us to see why Baby Lee is having problems. Will you help in deciding what they are? Anything you can add will be welcome.
Student: His carbon dioxide and oxygen combining powers indicate that acidosis is developing.
Aide: What does that mean?
Student: Interference with gas exchange in the lungs causes carbon dioxide retention.

The conference continues in an atmosphere of freedom, allowing facts and concepts to be exchanged and clarification of the learning structure to occur. The problem-solving process continues until the group has formulated principles pertinent to the situation and has developed nursing prescriptions supported by theory. The following is a sample of some of the formalizations as a result of group process.

Predictive principles	Nursing prescription
1. Poor heat regulation center prompts use of external control of temperature.	1. Warm Isolette.
2. Loosening tenacious pulmonary secretions facilitates breathing.	2. Percuss before suctioning to loosen pulmonary secretions.
3. Blood gas measurements indicate changing physiologic state.	3. Keep open arterial catheter (heparin-saline solution can be used).
4. The use of sodium bicarbonate IV combats acidosis.	4. Monitor closely.
5. In respiratory acidosis the use of positive pressure respirator promotes the blowing off of excessive CO_2.	5. Record and graph respiratory rate every half hour or as needed.

PREDICTIVE PRINCIPLE: Conferences held between nurse and client and/or significant others contribute to reciprocal development of care plans and lead to optimal health service for the client and satisfaction for the nurse.

Assessment and maintenance provide the causal elements for primary care conferences. Patient-centered conferences are an effective means to bring together persons who can contribute to and profit from analysis of the care plan. Conferences are usually initiated by the nurse but may originate from any one of the involved persons. The time, place, and length of the meeting depend on several circumstances—needs, urgency, and availability of resources, materials, and personnel. The purpose is to plan together problem-oriented client care. The nursing conference is equally applicable to singular needs and problems of the client as it is to complex situations requiring multiple consideration. The conference may be concerned with an initial assessment process or with an ongoing appraisal of a health situation. Members discuss the health of the client to arrive at a decision of what must be done to help resolve his problem and to delegate responsibility for the maintenance of health, evaluation and management of symptoms, and appropriate referrals.

To function logically and responsibly in an assessment conference the nurse must have knowledge and requisite skills in prescribing, providing care, and making referrals as appropriate.

The nurse-practitioner or nurse clinical specialist has direct access to clients and a one-to-one relationship with the client. Either the nurse or the client can initiate contact. Nursing responsibility includes history and physical examination, patient screening and referrals to appropriate physicians or other health workers, and nursing diagnosis and prescription, including counseling, care, and rehabilitation.

As health care is increasingly valued in our society, nurses are expected to take more responsibility for the delivery of health care, for coordinating preventive services, for initiating or participating in diagnostic screening, and for referring patients who require differential medical diagnoses and medical therapies.

A report* submitted to the Secretary of Health, Education, and Welfare reviewing extended roles for nurses concluded that skills for the nurse-practitioner involve (1) eliciting and recording a health history; (2) making physical and psychosocial assessment, recognizing the range of "normal" and the manifestations of common abnormalities; (3) assessing the environment (family relationships and home, school, and work environments); (4) interpreting selected laboratory findings; (5) making diagnoses and choosing, initiating, and modifying selected therapies; (6) assessing community resources and needs for health care; (7) providing emergency treatment as appropriate, as in cardiac arrest, shock, or hemorrhage; and (8) providing appropriate information to the patient and his family about a diagnosis or plan of therapy.

Primary care nursing, a concept different from the preceding, involves one nurse's being responsible for the total nursing management of a patient or small group of patients. Nursing diagnosis and care plans based on a total and continuing assessment process are the vehicles for continuity and comprehensiveness. Primary care views the client as the center of action and focuses on him as a person, with the nurse having an increased opportunity for individual care.

In primary care, nurses assume considerably greater responsibility for delivery of health care services. Primary care nursing establishes a one-to-one nurse-patient relationship that can be experienced in any setting—home, community, or highly complex care context. The nurse assumes the role of client advocate. Primary care nursing is a self-maintaining care system, open to the environment, with adaptive mechanisms for the single purpose of providing quality services. In this system, direct conferences are held between nurse and client and any other member who has significance to the client and his care.

*Nurs. Outlook **1**:50-51, 1972.

In present practice, utilization of the primary nurse varies extensively. Community health nurses have always functioned with relative independence, but with physician collaboration, assessing problems of individuals and families, treating minor illnesses, referring patients for differential medical diagnosis, arranging for referrals to social service agencies and organizations, giving advice and counsel to promote health and prevent illness, supervising health regimes of normal pregnant women and of children, and working with health-related community action programs.

Team nursing is one of the more common nursing care delivery systems and involves a group of people sharing responsibility for a number of patients. The team conference is the heart of this system. Nursing assessments, diagnosis, and care prescriptions are formulated by the group or team leader and furnish the guidelines for continuity and comprehensive practice. The team member assigned to a given client for a specified period of time is responsible for carrying out the plan and conferring with team members to revise the design.

PREDICTIVE PRINCIPLE: Periodic care review conferences held with colleagues provide a mechanism for the nurse to validate care plans and maintain quality control.

Each nurse, regardless of the system of nursing care delivery, is accountable for overall decisions about how the client is to receive attention. He is a decision maker in control of the quality of nursing care administered during his client contact. Additionally, primary nurses are responsible for the care giver in his absence. With the burgeoning knowledge in nursing, medicine, and related fields, it is necessary to share the knowledge and skills of a number of health experts, each of whom is prepared in a particular area. Together these individuals attempt adequately to meet the comprehensive needs of the client.

Review conferences between the nurse and such colleagues as other care givers, physician, nurse specialist, and supervisory nurse provide an excellent avenue for collegial validation and advisement, with an informal network of peer control and dialogue. During the conference, each nurse presents the information on which the health plan is based and discusses the reasons for nursing prescriptions. Review conferences serve to increase the competency of the nurse, strengthen peer relationships, and maintain quality control necessary for the delivery of this health care system.

Nursing care conferences contribute to a sense of satisfaction in participants. Relationships necessary for a professional level of responsibility and for the comprehensive care of the patient are developed. The dual concept of individual responsibility for the delivery of nursing services and care, with each nurse functioning at his own level of performance and each client participating in the implementation of his care plan to the extent of his motivation and level of competence, makes the practice of nursing challenging and exciting.

Utilization of the problem-solving process has taken a form that allows the learners to compile their facts and concepts into a meaningful pattern that is logical and sensible. Definite guidelines for evaluation of behaviors have been established.

REPORTING CONFERENCES

There is widespread agreement among nursing personnel as to the importance of keeping the nurse-leader informed about ongoing activities. No leader can operate efficiently without sufficient knowledge about member activities. One of the most logical sources of information is the reporting conference, where events of the workday are shared by all those engaged in the administration of care. Members bring to the conference the work sheets on which they have recorded the day's events. They verbally share pertinent information with the group. The coordinator of nursing services attends these sessions, for even though informed of major events throughout the shift, he usually has little opportunity to learn the many details discussed in the reporting conferences.

Reporting conferences have four major goals: (1) to report accurately and objectively relevant information, (2) to give reactions to situations when pertinent, (3) to evaluate the care in the light of objectives, and (4) to update the nursing care plans to ensure continuity of care for the client and family.

Listening is the primary task of the nurse-leader in reporting sessions. He must be a critical listener and be able to make judgments about the material being presented. The tools used to aid in this task are the leader's work sheet; a record of the physician's orders; awareness of client's reactions and nursing prescriptions; and knowledge, understanding, and intuition. As with the instructional conference, each member is encouraged to listen and record appropriate data about all patients or families for whom he is responsible.

The leader will utilize the information received in the reporting conference in finalizing action for the day, in recording data on patients' records, in giving the change-of-shift report to the oncoming staff, and in making plans for the next day.

Many predictive principles that have been proposed for all conferences have direct application to report giving. Prior preparation by all members, attention to behavioral messages, and paced and systematic presentation are of equal importance in the summarizing period.

PREDICTIVE PRINCIPLE: Directions given to conferees before report reveal expectations the leader has for the members.

Because situations vary in nursing, it is difficult to establish a set of criteria for reporting information. In primary care, for example, expectations for client(s) and nurse will be mutually agreed on, with guidance from the leader. In acute situations the member must report many details, whereas in health care centers where the occupants' stay is long-term or in the home, much routine information can be omitted. It is the leader's task to inform the members of the amount and kind of information desired. For example, a nurse-leader might begin by saying, "When I call on you, will you tell us please how the patient ate, his degree of ambulation, how he tolerated his treatments, and anything you believe to be important for us to know?"

This procedure sounds simple, but complications may occur. The average staff member usually gives routine information but may not be clear on what additional data to report. In many cases the worker's past nursing experience and educational background limit the extent of his reporting. Just prior to the conference, for example, an aide may have noted casually one of the patients assigned to him looked a little pale while ambulating in the hall. The worker may not consider this to be significant enough to report. The next day, when the patient is discovered slumped on the floor, the observation becomes significant to the aide and is reported.

There will be occasions when incidents that have proved troublesome to the member will be deleted from the report. The worker may not want to risk criticism, especially if he believes the incident or problem is a result of his mistake or poor judgment.

If something has been omitted from a report, the ultimate accountability lies with the leader. It is his task to prepare the members for their roles and to maintain an atmosphere where free exchange of information can occur. Preoccupation with fixing blame consumes time and energy better spent on solving the problems.

Continuing training, practice, and review, as necessary, will help nurses and clients mature in ability to select appropriate information and to report clearly and accurately.

Reports lend themselves to the use of tape recorders. Clarification and elucidation can be made after listening to the tape and before the reporting nurse departs.

GENERAL PROBLEMS CONFERENCE

One of the more difficult roles for the nurse-leader in conference sessions is to cope with feelings, both his own and those expressed by members. Control of one's feelings is held in personal, social, and cultural esteem by North American society. The individual is expected to maintain "proper" control of his feelings and also must act in a way that enables others to maintain theirs. Participants usually strive to convey precisely the feeling they believe others expect of them at a given time and place. Preoccupation with this can result in letting feelings go unresolved.

Any work assignment has problems and emergencies. The way problems are handled determines the amount and kind of feelings that will be built up in an individual. Many days are filled with one situation after another that builds up tension in the person until he "travels on his nerves."

Members in conference sessions do not always operate as a "happy family." Because of individual interests, clashes occur between the client, the health giving membership, and the management. The nurse is not expected to be a psychiatrist, only to develop the ability to sense feelings and to understand and apply principles of effective interpersonal relationships when they are needed.

PREDICTIVE PRINCIPLE: Sharing of feelings through conferences unifies and integrates the membership and allows work to progress.

In work groups, members sometimes have little in common except that they are drawn together by joint enterprise. The task of becoming spontaneously involved in conference activity when it is a job expectation places the individual in a delicate position. Expressions of feelings will be easier for some than for others.

Problems conferences are directly related to the administration of patient care. They should be scheduled often enough to keep the members in tune with one another. Interpersonal maintenance for goal accomplishment is a legitimate enterprise. A meeting should be called by the leader or any member anytime problems arise that hinder the communication process and therefore reduce work efficiency and effectiveness.

Reasons for tense situations may range from prejudice of one member against another to lack of consideration for the total membership by one individual. For example, problems may be created when a member announces openly that he plans to use all his accrued sick time because he is "never sick." His frequent absences without notice cause gaps in patient care and overloads for the remaining members, and hostility and anger result.

An alternative action for these situations is open expressions of feelings about the behavior and its consequences in a feelings conference. In this way, feelings are expressed openly and handled. Until these feelings are relieved, there will be barriers to communication. Positive relationships need recognition and reinforcement on a continuous basis. It becomes easy to slip into the habit of dealing with crisis situations and to fail to acknowledge those behaviors that keep nursing practice on an even keel.

Expression of feelings becomes easier in the sharing process when one knows what the other is doing and feeling. The "feeling of knowing" is an emotional by-product of communication and makes the difference between the person who feels secure and the one who is anxious.

Development of a climate conducive to fostering collaborative interdependent and independent activity requires time, involvement, and concerted effort by each member. The operation of effective nursing process depends on the maintenance of open, trusting relationships among the participants. If problems are acknowledged and faced frankly, the chances for a remedy are far greater than if ignored and allowed to fester.

PREDICTIVE PRINCIPLE: Understanding and management of group behavior require ability to predict the processes through which feelings and meanings are transmitted among group members.

Investigators of small-group process have found group members address more communication to individuals whose opinions are extreme than to the more conforming members. For instance, an individual group member might believe that the care givers have an obligation to urge hospital management to serve patients their meals on request. If the majority opinion differs greatly from that of the dissenter, the group will exert pressure on the member in an effort to get him to change his opinion. Evidence shows that communication of feelings back to the instigator will reduce the intensity of feelings.

These findings make it possible for the members to pick up cues in behavior when they occur and to recognize the process as it unfolds. Another illustration will prove helpful. Probably the most common feeling expressed in conferences is that of pressure. Nurses seem to be particularly susceptible to pressure because the tasks are numerous, varied, and very often complex. The leader is frequently confronted with a member who is frustrated and angry and who vents his feelings in negative terms. "I have to be everywhere at once and everything to everybody!" "There are not enough hours in the day; I have to do everything around here." "I'm still not caught up; I don't have time to sit in here and talk!" These feelings can be decreased if activities are put on a priority basis and the group shares the responsibility for the necessary ongoing work. Clear identification of anger and attempts to resolve the causes openly can effectively reduce member hostility and give the leader the opportunity to explore feelings with the individual concerned. If the discussion reveals duplication of effort, lack of organization, or, in fact, too large an assignment, adjustments can be made in the structure or perhaps even in the system of care. Failure to change the feelings may result in their intensification and transmission to other members.

The real significance of the "contagion" theory of feelings is that members recognize the impact they have on one another. Feelings of acceptance, caring, trust, and security will be transmitted when they exist, just as feelings of rejection, anger, hate, or hostility will be communicated despite attempts to hide them from the group. It is important to establish the rule among conferees that when feelings are interfering with the work of the group, they must be dealt with.

PREDICTIVE PRINCIPLE: Involvement in group process results in specific gains or losses for the individual member.

Rewards may take the form of such intangibles as prestige, recognition, or affection. The conditions or rules that govern the awarding of the payoff will have important motivational consequences for the members and for the functioning of the group as a whole.

Each person wants to feel that his individual contribution to cooperative endeavor is significant and identifiable. Group work, however, can subjugate some members to others unnecessarily unless steps are taken to offset this possibility.

In group process, "role blurring" is encouraged, in which emphasis is placed on outcomes of the group rather than on the status of the individual. The leader works with health care personnel to provide opportunity for each individual to expand his physical and mental energies to his fullest potential. In the process, personal achievements are recognized and the worth of the person is reinforced, but individual recognition does not take priority over group accomplishment.

If position or salary increments depend on such individual performances as the number of beds made or procedures accomplished, group effort is apt to diminish. If, on the other hand, a group is operating under a policy whereby each person's benefits depend directly on the group's performance, the members will want to engage in whatever behaviors they believe will contribute to this end (working hard, helping others, and making suggestions about ways to improve the group's efficiency).

In industry a reward system of this kind operates most frequently in plant operations where salable items are the end result of effort and dividends include monetary gain. In nursing, patients are the end product; when they have bene-fited from the coordinated efforts of a group, tangible reward to all members, beyond established policy, are not forthcoming. The care giver's motivation, then, centers around achievement of satisfaction in a job well done, acknowledgment by management, and patients' appreciation.

Involvement in group activity does not negate the autonomy and individual accountability reflected in the role of the primary care nurse. This nurse has the freedom to move in and out of groups as necessary to the needs of the client and the dynamics of the nursing care plan.

APPLICATION OF PREDICTIVE PRINCIPLES IN COMMUNICATIONS

RN, Mrs. Turner, recently joined a nursing group in the rehabilitative unit. Her former experience included ten years working with paraplegic patients in another part of the country. She is convinced her knowledge and experience far surpass those of any other members. The RN completes her assignments by herself, communicating as little as possible with the members, who have coun-tered with expressions of hostility.

Problem	Predictive principles	Prescriptions
Noncommunicative member	In retrospect: Preassessment of individual and group knowledges, skills, and expectations estab-lishes baseline data for measurement of progress or change. Perceiving negative feedback enables group members to become aware of others' re-sponses to them and their effects on the group and to modify behavior accordingly. Understanding and management of group be-havior require ability to predict the pro-cesses through which feelings and mean-ings are transmitted among group mem-bers. The interdependent collaborating group fa-cilitates group goal accomplishment. Circumstance and member capability deter-mine the type of directions to be communi-cated. Interaction of conference members on an equal basis encourages active participation and leads to usable solutions to the prob-lem. Integrative positive reinforcement increases individual identification with group goals and the participation level of the individ-ual.	Leader will have confer-ence with RN; state ob-served behavior and problems that have aris-en because of aloofness from others. Assist RN to recognize the influence one member's action has on the entire group and the responsibility of the group to discuss the problem. Arrange meeting with all members; conduct so meeting will be a discus-sion of cause for behav-ior; encourage open communication (not a punitive session). Make positive plans with member for reinforcing positive behavior.

BIBLIOGRAPHY
BOOKS

Amidon, E. J., and Hough, J. B., editors: Interaction analysis: theory, research and application, Reading, Mass., 1967, Addison-Wesley Publishing Co., Inc.

Arndt, C., and Huckabay, L. M. D.: Nursing administration: theory for practice with a systems approach, St. Louis, 1975, The C. V. Mosby Co.

Banathy, B. H.: Instructional systems, Palo Alto, Calif., 1968, Fearon Publishers.

Bell, G. D.: Organizations and human behavior, Englewood Cliffs, N.J., 1967, Prentice-Hall, Inc.

Berne, E.: The structure and dynamics of organizations and groups, New York, 1966, Grove Press, Inc.

Bloom, B. S., editor: Taxonomy of educational objectives: the classification of educational goals. Handbook I. Cognitive domain, New York, 1956, David McKay Co., Inc.

Bloom, B. S., et al.: Handbook on formative and summative evaluation of student learning, New York, 1971, McGraw-Hill Book Co.

Bower, F. L.: The process of planning nursing care: a model for practice, ed. 2, St. Louis, 1977, The C. V. Mosby Co.

Carkhuff, R. R., and Berenson, B. G.: Beyond counseling and therapy, New York, 1967, Holt, Rinehart & Winston, Inc.

Carlson, E.: Learning through games: a new approach to problem solving, Washington, D.C., 1969, Public Affairs Press.

Cartwright, D., and Zander, A., editors: Group dynamics—research and theory, ed. 3, New York, 1968, Harper & Row, Publishers.

Combs, A., et al.: Helping relationships: basic concepts for the helping professions, Boston, 1972, Allyn & Bacon, Inc.

Fast, J.: Body language, New York, 1970, J. B. Lippincott Co.

Gage, N. L., editor: Handbook of research on teaching. A project of the American Research Association, Chicago, 1963, Rand McNally & Co.

Gagne, R. W.: The condition of learning, New York, 1965, Holt, Rinehart & Winston, Inc.

Glasser, W.: Reality therapy: a new approach to psychiatry, New York, 1965, Harper & Row, Publishers.

Glasser, W.: Schools without failure, New York, 1969, Harper & Row, Publishers.

Goffman, E.: Interaction ritual: essays on face-to-face behavior, New York, 1967, Anchor Press.

Gordon, A. K.: Games for growth: educational games in the classroom, Palo Alto, Calif., 1970, Science Research Associates, Inc.

Gulley, H. E.: Discussion, conference, and group process, ed. 2, New York, 1968, Holt, Rinehart & Winston, Inc.

Harris, T. A.: I'm OK—you're OK, New York, 1973, Harper & Row, Publishers.

Hodjetts, R. M.: Management: theory, process and practice, Philadelphia, 1975, W. B. Saunders Co.

Inbar, M., editor: Simulation and games: an international journal of theory, design and research, Beverly Hills, Calif., 1970, Sage Publications, Inc.

Krathwohl, D. R., et al.: Taxonomy of educational objectives: the classification of educational goals. Handbook II. Affective domain, New York, 1964, David McKay Co., Inc.

Litterer, J. A.: Organizations: systems, control and adaptation, ed. 2, New York, 1969, John Wiley & Sons, Inc., vol. 2.

Little, D., and Carnevali, D.: Nursing care planning, 1969, J. B. Lippincott Co.

Luft, J.: Group processes, an introduction to group dynamics, Palo Alto, Calif., 1970, National Press Books.

Mager, R. F.: Developing attitude toward learning, Belmont, Calif., 1968, Fearon Publishers.

Mager, R. F.: Preparing instructional objectives, Palo Alto, Calif., 1962, Fearon Publishers.

Marram, G. D.: The group approach in nursing practice, ed. 2, St. Louis, 1978, The C. V. Mosby Co.

McAshan, H. H.: Writing behavioral objectives: a new approach, New York, 1970, Harper & Row, Publishers.

McGrath, J. E., and Irwin, A.: Small group research, New York, 1966, Holt, Rinehart & Winston, Inc.

McLemore, M., and Bevis, E. O.: Planned change. In Marriner, A., editor: Current perspectives in nursing management, St. Louis, 1979, The C. V. Mosby Co.

Pohl, M. L.: The teaching function of the nursing practitioner, ed. 2, Dubuque, Iowa, 1973, William C. Brown Co., Publishers.

Ruesch, J.: The observer and the observed: human communication theory. In Grinker, R. R., editor: Toward a unified theory of human behavior, New York, 1956, Basic Books, Inc., Publishers.

Ruesch, J.: General theory of communication. In Arieti, S., editor: American handbook of psychiatry, New York, 1961, W. W. Norton & Co., Inc.

Ruesch, J., and Bateson, G.: Communication: the social matrix of psychiatry, New York, 1968, W. W. Norton & Co., Inc.

Ruesch, J., Shannon, A., and Weaver, W.: The methematical theory of communication, Urbana, Ill., 1949, University of Illinois Press.

Simon, A., editor: Classroom interaction newsletter, Philadelphia, 1970, Research for Better Schools.

Tansey, P. J., and Unwin, D.: Simulation and gaming in education, London, 1969, Methuen Educational Ltd.

Twelker, P. A., editor: Instructional simulation systems: an annotated bibliography, Corvallis, Oregon, 1969, Oregon State University Press.

Periodicals

Chopra, A.: Motivation in task oriented groups, J. Nurs. Admin., pp. 55-60, Jan.-Feb. 1973.

Combs, A. W., et al.: Florida studies in the helping professions, University of Florida Social Science Monograph, No. 37, 1969.

Dickoff, P. J., and Wiedenbach, J.: Theory in a practice discipline. Part I. Practice oriented theory, Nurs. Res. **17**(5):415-35, 1968.

Gallagher, J. J., and Aschner, M. J.: A preliminary report on an analysis of classroom interaction, The Merrill Palmer Quarterly of Behavior and Development **9**:3, 1963.

Jehring, J. J.: Motivational problems in the modern hospital, J. Nurs. Admin., pp. 35-47, Nov.-Dec. 1972.

Lewis, G. K.: Communication, a factor in meeting emotional crisis, Nurs. Outlook **13**:36-39, 1965.

Little, D., and Carnevali, D.: The nursing care planning system, Nurs. Outlook **19**:164-167, 1971.

Palmer, M. E.: Patient care conference: an opportunity for meeting staff needs, J. Nurs. Admin., pp. 47-53, March-April 1973.

Smith, D.: Writing objectives as a nursing practice skill, Am. J. Nurs. **71**(2):319-320, 1971.

Steiner, C.: Scripts people live, New York, 1974, Grove Press, Inc.

Stevens, L. F.: Nurse-patient discussion groups, Am. J. Nurs. **63**(12):67-69, 1963.

Teaching patients and use of the self in clinical practice, Nurs. Clin. North Am. **6**:4, Dec. 1971.

Vaill, P. B.: Management language and management action, Calif. Management Rev., pp. 51-58, Oct. 1967.

Veninga, R.: Communications: a patient's eye view, Am. J. Nurs. **73**(2):320-322, 1973.

Zander, A., et al: Unity of group, identification with group and self-esteem of members, J. Pers. **28**: 463-465, 1960.

5 PREDICTIVE PRINCIPLES FOR DELEGATING AUTHORITY

AGENCY STRUCTURE

A working knowledge of the organizational structure of the health agency in which the nurse-manager is employed promotes appropriate delegation of authority, for organizational structure determines the amount and degree of authority that can be delegated.

Delegation of authority to the managerial level closest to the job to be done leads to overall organizational effectiveness and decision making.

Understanding the categories and roles of nursing personnel enables the delegator to select the type and number of personnel appropriate for the job.

JOB DESCRIPTIONS, POLICIES, AND PROCEDURES

Written descriptions of policies, procedures, and/or guidelines by which an employee may handle situations promote ease of operation for the care giver and control of the authority delegated by the nurse-leader/manager.

Staff participation in the formulation of policies, job descriptions, and procedures increases use of policies and improves job satisfaction.

The philosophy and policies of a health agency determine the pattern of nursing care delivery system to be provided.

Guidelines such as established channels, methods, and provision for communication within an agency enable the nurse-leader/manager to delegate tasks and authority appropriately.

Clear lines of communication promote morale among organization members and enhance goal accomplishment.

Reactions to stress influence efficiency of performance in the work situation.

INVESTMENT OF AUTHORITY

The nurse-leader's belief that ultimate accountability lies with him determines the scope and limitations he sets for his leadership.

ASSIGNMENT MAKING

A manager's degree of willingness to be accountable influences the scope, limitations, and style of leadership.

A problem-oriented approach to patient-centered care enables the care giver to develop effective nursing care plans for the client or patient.

The willingness of the nurse-manager to relinquish authority determines the effectiveness of delegating authority to others.

An adequate supply of appropriately prepared personnel enables delegation of authority in response to client and agency needs.

Matching the abilities of care givers to the jobs to be done increases work productivity and individual job satisfaction.

Centralization of information storage and retrieval systems allows for efficient assessment, delegation, and implementation of tasks.

Clear and concise directions enhance task delegation.

A balance between variety and continuity of assignments increases workers' motivation and productivity.

Consideration for each care giver's preferences and areas of expertise influences morale.

A systematic planning process enables effective delegation for work implementation.

MEASURING RESULTS

Assignments that have clearly defined goals, standards, and criteria provide a basis for measurement of outcome.

Frequent evaluation of performance using criteria influences the quality of care and the level of actual performance of care activities.

One of the most important facets of a nurse-leader/manager's job is that of delegating authority. Productivity can be maximized through wise delegation of responsibility to appropriate persons—whether patients, family members, other managers, nurses, or ancillary personnel. Delegation carries with it the responsibility for appropriately guiding and supervising the efforts of others toward the attainment of the tasks delegated. Traditionally, nurses have assumed every conceivable task in the hospital or health agency. In addition to nursing, they have repaired equipment, made supplies, and served as housekeeper, clerks, and secretaries. It is neither realistic nor desirable to assume that a nurse is or should be prepared to function well in all capacities. From an administrative point of view, diversion of the professional nurse's skills to tasks other than nursing is a costly and inefficient use of a professional person's time.

The major responsibility of a nurse-manager is to see that care is provided to a patient (or client) or to a group of patients or to serve with other significant care givers in the roles of validator, catalyst, decision maker, and controller of nursing care quality. The ability to perform these roles assumes that care givers collaborate and accept appropriate shares of responsibility. Inherent in the philosophy of delegating authority is a commitment to the proposition that each nursing care giver must be entrusted with some degree of responsibility for the tasks under his jurisdiction and that he has the authority to act, thus making him accountable for his nursing actions. This assumes that the nurse-manager must possess knowledge and skills commensurate with the responsibility of organizing and directing activities and making nursing care decisions that affect others.

An effective manager is an organizer. Wise delegation of authority can result in an organization that is effective in accomplishing objectives efficiently, cost and time effectively, and with the greatest degree of job satisfaction. The optimal performance of any assignment depends to a large extent on the formulation of definite plans based on the organization's objectives.

AGENCY STRUCTURE

What the employer expects from an employee is based on the policies or objectives that guide the enterprise as determined by the philosophy, or conceptual framework, and standards set by the organization. Most health institutions possess a common basis for existence: to serve the health needs of the public. This goal is reached in accordance with the type of health requirements of the agency's clients. Inherent in meeting health needs are (1) administering patient care, (2) educating health agency personnel and the public, (3) engaging in research, and (4) protecting the health of the public and employees. The type of nursing agency determines the major emphasis, for each kind of agency shapes or sets limits to the type of goals likely to prevail, although there will be much variation among agencies, even of the same type.

PREDICTIVE PRINCIPLE: A working knowledge of the organizational structure of the health agency in which the nurse-manager works promotes appropriate delegation of authority, for organizational structure determines the amount and degree of authority that can be delegated.

There are basically three types of health agencies—official, voluntary, and proprietary. Conceptual frameworks for nursing practice are influenced by the type of agency in which nursing is practiced.

Official agencies operate under federal, state, county, or city direction to provide health benefits for the large segment of the population covered in some way by legislation. Tax monies are the primary source of income. Examples of these agencies are Veterans Administration hospitals, city and county hospitals, city and county health departments, and the U.S. Public Health Service clinics.

Voluntary agencies are nonprofit groups that serve the public according to some special interest group or according to the availability of services to the public through other means. Voluntary agencies depend on monetary gifts for an important part of their capital and operating budget. Since money flows through a special interest group, voluntary agencies may be oriented toward service for a religious, ethnic, economic, or age group. Such orientations have goals that affect standards and techniques of care, priority of services, access to care, relations with other organizations, and directions and rate of development. Examples of these agencies are the Red Cross, Benevolent and Protective Order of Elks hospitals, and the Salvation Army.

Proprietary agencies are privately owned corporations operated for profit by independent owners. Many proprietary agencies receive supplementary funds through private and public funding for provision of health care, research, and special services and are in a position to provide financial assistance to eligible clients. The transplanting of human organs is an example of a service that is financially out of reach for the average citizen but can be made available by special grants and/or fundings.

The type of agency—official, voluntary, or proprietary—influences the following data:

1. Source of funds
2. Cost scales to clients
3. Organizational complexity
4. Number of constraints
    a. Legal
    b. Policy
5. Managerial flexibility and autonomy

Organization

Whenever an enterprise expands beyond the size that can be effectively managed by one person, grouping of activities is necessary and departmentalization occurs. Typical organizational structure of a health agency includes a governing board, a director of the agency, and directors of business affairs, supportive services, and medical and nursing services. As expansion of the facility takes place, organizational structure grows both vertically and horizontally.

Nursing services are set up according to the guidelines established by the agency. The basis for departmentalization usually falls into three categories: territory, function, and service. *Departmentalization by territory* is advocated where nursing measures can best be carried out with economy and expediency of operation by dividing management into geographic areas. Establishment of clinics for migratory workers within their camps is one example; public health supervision by census tract is another. *Departmentalization by function* is usually based on the service to be rendered and the type of care involved, and activities are grouped according to the task being done. The need for specialized skills or equipment makes departmentalization by function desirable. Operating rooms, blood banks, cardiac catheterization units, inhalation therapy, or central supply departments are in this category. *Departmentalization according to medical or nursing specialty or type of nursing service needed* is the most widely accepted practice in health agencies. It is a basis for structuring a complex organization that includes a variety of job activities. Medical, surgical, pediatric, and obstetric areas illustrate departmentalization by medical specialty. Intensive care, ambulatory care, convalescent care, and outpatient services illustrate departmentalization by type of nursing services required.

PREDICTIVE PRINCIPLE: Delegation of authority to the managerial level closest to the job to be done leads to overall organizational effectiveness and decision making.

Delegation of authority can be centralized or decentralized. A *centralized* organization is one in which detailed and comprehensive planning is done by the chief executive or by a group of high-level managers. Under this structure, all nursing assignments are issued from the central nursing office. Centralized organizations tend to deemphasize the human element in favor of efficiency and to encourage close supervision of personnel at every level.

A *decentralized organization* is one in which operating decisions are made by the people closest to the problem. As health agencies move from small, centrally controlled operations to large, complex groups, the need for decentralization of control increases. The intent of decentralized nursing service is to bring decision-making authority, responsibility, and accountability to the operational level. A nurse-manager's major responsibility is to have the client's nursing needs met in a cost-effective manner. This may be accomplished by reducing the degree of vertical control held at the top level and by developing increased horizontal communication at lower levels. A health agency that operates under the philosophy of decentralized power expects the director of nurses to delegate authority to supervisors. The supervisors will place authority in the hands of head nurses, and the head nurses will give staff nurses the opportunity to plan, direct, and guide the operation of nursing care.

Occupations in which individuals traditionally work independently usually carry with them managerial responsibilities. The work done by pathologists, radiologists, directors of medical or nursing services, or supervisors, for example, necessitates hours of individual activity but may also involve a variety of associations with personnel. On the other hand, some situations may dictate a narrow span of management, such as the nurse-leader directing the work of a small group of personnel comprising a nursing team. In all cases the employee's preparation and experience and the type of service to be rendered influence the amount and degree of authority that can be delegated, that is, the degree of centralization of management.

PREDICTIVE PRINCIPLE: Understanding the categories and roles of nursing personnel enables the delegator to select the type and number of personnel appropriate for the job.

Categories of nursing personnel are many and vary with each employing agency. It is impossible to delineate clearly among services rendered by each group because of differences in standards and requirements on the national, state, and local levels and the number of overlapping roles and functions. In general, nursing personnel comprise those who have had both formal and informal preparation. The three main categories of nursing personnel are (1) nurse's aide or assistant, (2) licensed practical (vocational) nurse, and (3) registered nurse.

Nurse's aides are usually trained on the job to perform unskilled services in private homes or health agencies under the supervision of a registered nurse or a physician. Formal preparation usually consists of a few weeks of training in which the aides spend several hours a day learning from classroom demonstration, followed by supervised experience caring for patients in the employing agency. The extent of the training period depends on the philosophy and in-service educational program of the agency. Most nurse's aides administer hygienic care and perform such procedures as taking vital signs and tabulating oral intake and output. As health agencies become aware that nurse's aides are not cost effective, fewer and fewer of them are being employed.

Licensed practical nurses (LPN) or licensed vocational nurses (LVN) may or may not have had formal training in a school designed for that purpose. LPNs or LVNs who are licensed by the state to practice fall into two categories. First, there are those who have received licensure by waiver on proof of a specific number of years of satisfactory nursing practice and have taken a definite number of class hours as prescribed by the licensing board. Vocaticnal or practical nurses who have received licensure by waiver are most often those who worked as nurse's aides for years and were "grandfathered" in when licensure laws went into effect.

The second group of LPNs or LVNs are those who are licensed to practice in their state on completion of a prescribed course of study in an approved vocational school and successful completion of the licensing examination. These courses are offered through an adult education board, in a hospital, or under the auspices of a junior or community college. The LPN or LVN program varies in length from 9 to 18 months and prepares the graduate to function in the home or health agency under the supervision of a physician or registered nurse.

LPNs and LVNs work in highly structured activities under the supervision of nurses and physicians and care for clients with simple nursing problems. They are usually skill or task centered.

Registered nurses are those who are licensed by their state to practice nursing skills in hospitals, military services, offices, clinics, private practice, homes, and the community. Minimal requirements for the RN are that preparation be in a school with an associate of arts or baccalaureate degree program in nursing accredited by the state. According to the National League for Nursing,[*] competencies expected of the *associate of arts degree graduates* on entry into practice include the role of provider of care through the application of the nursing process and management of nursing care for a group of clients with common, well-defined health problems in structured settings. In some places, collaboration with or the supervision of an experienced professional nurse is required.

The beginning practitioner (1) carries out nursing functions directly related to patient care, including participation in implementing the physician's therapeutic

[*]National League for Nursing: Competencies of the associate degree nurse on entry into practice, Nurs. Outlook **26**:346, June 1978. (Developed during workshops conducted in 1977 and 1978 by the Council of Associate Degree Programs.)

plan (for example, by administering medications and treatments); (2) renders direct patient care in nursing situations requiring nursing judgment and recognizes those situations that require a higher degree of nursing expertise; (3) gives patient care that demonstrates knowledge of the nursing principles taught in all courses in the associate degree nursing program; (4) functions as a member of the nursing care team and as such may direct and guide other team members who have less education and experience; and (5) recognizes the client's need for instruction related to health and takes action to provide this instruction.

Diploma program graduates are prepared to (1) function as generalists in hospitals and similar community institutions and (2) provide nursing care to patients and engage in therapeutic, rehabilitative, and preventive activities on behalf of individual patients and groups of patients.*

The graduate of a *baccalaureate degree* program (BS, RN) (1) engages in direct patient care and is a skilled observer and participant; (2) functions as a teacher and a responsible informant of health practices; (3) functions as a leader-supervisor of members of health groups; (4) functions as a collaborator and an effective member of the immediate health team, serves as interpreter of nursing activities to allied professionals in planning optimal health programs, aids other members of the health group in carrying out research, and serves as interpreter of nursing activities to groups outside the professional health groups; and (5) functions as an inquiring person.

There are two postgraduate designations for nurses who practice—the nurse practitioner and the clinical nurse specialist. In general, the nurse practitioner has completed a generic nursing program, is licensed to practice nursing, and has completed either a degree or a nondegree-oriented course structured to provide skills and expanded roles. On the other hand, the clinical nurse specialist is a registered nurse from a generic program who has completed a special program of study leading to a masters degree with an area of concentration designated "clinical nurse specialist." Both of these programs of study prepare the nurse to assume versatile roles with clients with specific nursing and medical problems. These include the following:

1. Obtaining a nursing history
2. Assessing health-illness status
3. Making nursing diagnoses and writing nursing care prescriptions
4. Entering clients into the health care system
5. Providing sustenance, support, counseling, and therapy for clients who are impaired, infirm, or ill and who may be under treatment by others
6. Managing a medical care regime for acutely and chronically ill patients within the protocols of care provided by a licensed physician
7. Preventing illness and teaching how to maintain wellness
8. Teaching and counseling others about health and prevention of illness
9. Supervising and managing care regimens of normal pregnant women

---

* Adapted from a program developed by an ad hoc committee and accepted by the National League for Nursing Council of Diploma Programs, May, 1971.

10. Helping patients in the guidance of children with a view to their optimal physical and emotional development
11. Educating, counseling, and supporting people with regard to the aging process
12. Providing aid and support to patients and their families during the dying process
13. Supervising and teaching other professional people in areas unfamiliar to them

The difference in the practice of the nurse practitioner and that of the clinical nurse specialist is directly related to complexity, scope, and depth. The clinical nurse specialist and the nurse practitioner, who has the benefit of the wider scope of education, can be characterized as follows:

1. Can handle problems of greater complexity and containing more variables
2. Are able to provide more extensive services to families, groups, and communities
3. Practice with greater emphasis on the domain of practice that is nursing rather than medicine
4. Tend to be more holistic in approach
5. Are better prepared to handle the unexpected and to work in unstructured settings

Naturally, individuals differ regardless of their academic preparations. But a broader and more diversified education usually produces a better qualified person able to meet the myriad demands of a modern practice.

Differentiation of roles is in process. Each of the educational programs emphasizes technical competence and skill. Each adds the dimensions of problem solving and judgment. The thread of responsibility is inherent in all statements. But one major weakness is the lack of clarity in delineation of roles in the area of leadership and management. The reality of the nursing situation is that graduates of all LPN or LVN and RN programs are expected to function as nurse-leaders in some capacity. Graduates of programs that do not provide theory and practice in leadership and management find themselves in a difficult situation, for they are expected to assume jobs for which they are unprepared. Some agencies provide leadership and management in-service education programs to alleviate this problem.

JOB DESCRIPTIONS, POLICIES, AND PROCEDURES

Clearly defining the exact nature and the limits of authority for each member in an agency not only provides structure for modes of operation but also promotes role identification by workers, sets boundaries, and avoids the possibility of task duplication.

PREDICTIVE PRINCIPLE: Written descriptions of policies, procedures, and/or guidelines by which an employee may handle situations promote ease of operation for the care giver and control of the authority delegated by the nurse-leader/manager.

PREDICTIVE PRINCIPLE: Staff member participation in the formulation of policies, job descriptions, and procedures increases use of policies and improves job satisfaction.

A sense of personal involvement is created when an individual is given the responsibility for participating in the formulation of policies that concern him. Personal involvement results in a feeling of belonging and a sense of power in the employee. Participation in the establishment of policies helps the member feel his contributions are of value and thus increases commitment. It is not feasible for a health agency to invite each employee to assist with the formulation of all issues, but through the various mechanisms, personnel representing all levels can have a part in most decisions (see Chapter 7). Each department within an agency can send members to policy and procedure meetings to represent the thinking of the group. Members who have had a part in determining both the qualifications required for a job and the procedure for implementing that job are better able to use their capabilities productively and with assurance.

The task of delegating responsibility is lightened for the nurse-manager when affected others have had a part in investing the leader with the right to guide them in the performance of their work. Job descriptions, policies, and procedures become dynamic for working groups when the content is reviewed on a regular basis and changes are made in accordance with increased knowledge and understanding. Investigating current practices and research in comparable settings and studying policies and procedures recommended by licensing associations for professional groups enable the establishment of guidelines to be an ongoing process, that is, one in which guidelines are constantly being revised to reflect current nursing care needs.

PREDICTIVE PRINCIPLE: The philosophy and policies of a health agency determine the pattern of nursing care delivery system to be provided.

There are many ways to deliver nursing care. No one mode of delivery is better than any other because the effectiveness of the delivery system depends on such variables as setting, climate, abilities of the nurse, desires and needs of the client, and philosophy and conceptual framework of the agency.

Basically there are four systems for the delivery of nursing care: (1) functional, (2) team, (3) case, and (4) primary care. Combinations of these methods with new modes for provision of service are continually evolving.

The *functional system* of care involves a method of work organization and personnel assignment in which tasks are divided and assigned to personnel in the interest of time and expediency of service. This mode of operation is the system most often utilized in nursing. Personnel are fitted into fixed slots; one person passes medications, another administers treatments, and others provide hygienic care or do simple tasks such as making beds. Still others may be assigned to such special tasks as helping at the desk by recording for staff and serving as liaison between patients, physicians, family members, and others concerned with the patients.

This task-centered approach to nursing care has been borrowed from industry, where mass production is desired and the assembly line system proves to be the most effective means for achieving goals. As in industry, there are situations and times in nursing when uniformity in work patterns and mass production of nursing services are desirable. However, cost studies indicate other methods are as cost effective as, and sometimes are more so than, functional nursing care. One rationale might be that only one qualified person is available to perform specific tasks (to administer inhalation therapy or to teach a diabetic the administration of insulin), which limits the delegation of special assignments to one individual. Functional nursing is usually viewed by administrators as the most economical way to provide nursing services; however, to achieve true cost effectiveness, many elements must be considered. Recognition of the needs of the client, attention to the satisfactions and dissatisfactions of the care givers, and knowledge of the philosophy and goals of the providers of health services are to be weighed in the light of the selected system. Functional nursing care delivery is probably popular because it is simple, requires no imagination, and involves low levels of commitment to clients.

The *team system* is a mode for providing care developed in the 1950s in which a professional nurse facilitates the efforts of a group of diversified health care personnel to provide for the health needs of an individual or a group of people in either a hospital or a community setting.* In team nursing the leader's primary responsibility is to see that every activity is characterized by mutual sharing of work based on an interest and concern for the individuals served. All efforts are directed toward accomplishing group tasks with as much efficiency and expediency as possible. The thrust of every activity is directed toward delivery of individualized health care. Through the team process the nurse-leader/manager plans, participates in, coordinates, interprets, supervises, and evaluates the care given. Consistent and continuous high-quality care is made possible through written nursing care plans developed by the nurse-leader and co-workers, with evaluation and revision of care plans as new insights are gained.

Team nursing is a philosophy, not simply a methodology. There is nothing new about the idea of assembling a cluster of people to work toward the solution of specific problems. The uniqueness of team nursing becomes apparent when the beliefs and values of the system are understood. The philosophy of team nursing subscribes to the worth of the individual, with priority given to those being served and to those delivering the service, to the need for a prepared person to be the overall coordinator and interpreter of plans for care, to functioning of members as coequals with minimal emphasis on hierarchical lines of authority between the leader and the led, and to a sensitivity and responsiveness to the need for adaptability and change.

To be effective the team plan for nursing requires that care givers be led by one qualified to practice leadership, that all team members be committed to the philosophy of team nursing, that all members possess knowledge and understanding inherent in their roles, that individual members and the group be technically skilled for their assignments, and that the members function collaboratively and cooperatively.

The *case system* is perhaps the oldest method of care delivery. It is used when one-to-one contact is desired. A single individual is assigned to one client where

*See also Douglass, L. M.: Review of leadership in nursing, ed. 2, St. Louis, 1977, The C. V. Mosby Co.

constant care and observation are desired for a specified period of time. In this system the nurse has the responsibility for total nursing care of the patient. In hospitals the case method is most commonly adopted for the care of acutely ill patients, such as those in intensive care units. The one-to-one mode is almost the standard method of assignment for student nurses. In the community the case system is practiced where individual contact is made by public health and mental health nurses. A nurse practitioner's case load can include as many clients as the care giver can handle effectively. There are situations when the client requires or desires seclusion or separation from the general public. In these instances, one-to-one care is usually in practice round the clock. Private duty nurses fill most of these needs and are usually on call for service through a professional registry.

The *primary care system* concept of nursing care was pioneered at Loeb Center by Lydia Hall and developed by Marie Manthey in the 1960s. Primary nursing proposes that nurses have direct access to patient or client with full responsibility for care on a twenty-four–hour basis, produces a more effective method for delivery of nursing care, and thus provides continuous quality care to the patient. The role of the primary nurse requires an ability to form therapeutic relationships with individuals, to make decisions and assume responsibility, to conduct interviews and obtain and assess pertinent data, and to communicate effectively with peers and members of other health care disciplines. The primary nurse has the total responsibility for planning and directing client care for twenty-four hours a day for the duration of the client's need for nursing service. The primary nurse is held accountable for planning comprehensive care and for formulating clear-cut nursing prescriptions for others to continue that care. Each primary nurse coordinates his own activities with clients, physicians, and other personnel. An associate nurse can be assigned to the care of a patient whose primary nurse is off duty. The relief nurse's function is to carry out the care plan designed by the primary nurse. The number of patients a primary nurse can care for depends on such variables as rapidity of patient turnover, amount and kind of medical treatment and nursing services required, number of people involved in client care, and effectiveness and efficiency of the support services.

Primary care can be arranged by contractual agreement between client and nurse or between physician and nurse or can be practiced within the structure of an employing agency. Proponents of the primary nursing delivery system believe this model takes on a whole new concept of caring for a patient and that the individual competence level of each nurse is manifested in respect to performance as a nurse rather than as a manager of people.

All systems designed for the provision of nursing care have strengths and weaknesses that influence achievement of the goals of continuity and comprehensiveness of client care. Factors such as economics, communication, needs of clients, and needs of personnel are to be considered when a system for delivery of nursing care is selected.

PREDICTIVE PRINCIPLE: Guidelines such as established channels, methods, and provision for communication within an agency enable the nurse-leader/manager to delegate tasks and authority appropriately.

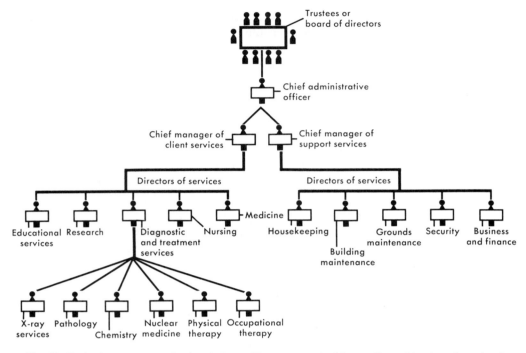

Fig. 12. Typical agency organizational chart with one example (diagnostic and treatment services) of complete hierarchy.

PREDICTIVE PRINCIPLE: Clear lines of communication promote morale among organization members and enhance goal accomplishment.

An organizational chart provides lines of authority and channels of communication. Authority to act in behalf of the person or group at the top of the organizational chart is delegated downward until it rests with the person designated to do specific tasks or fulfill specific roles and functions.

Fig. 12 is a typical agency organizational chart showing channels of authority and communication that progress downward from trustees or board of directors, through a chief administrative officer, to the directors of the various services performed in a health agency.

Fig. 13 is a typical nursing organizational chart showing the lines of authority and the channels of communication from the director, chief executive officer of nursing, who is the top nursing administrative officer, through the various associate directors and supervision or middle management group, to the lower management or head nurses. The effectiveness of an organization depends in part on its having the right information at the right place at the right time.

A model or organizational chart is essential for timely and appropriate communication among individuals linked together in an organization, since it depicts the levels and degrees of authority of all individuals as well as their functions and responsibilities. This is why every bureaucratic organization includes an

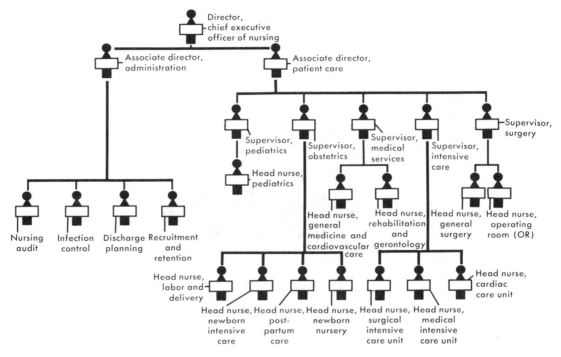

Fig. 13. Typical nursing division organizational chart.

organizational chart in its policy and procedure manual. Additionally, it is invaluable as a visual guide to protocol.

Communication in administration involves provision for major responsibilities: channels, methods, and opportunities for (1) the hierarchy to communicate outwardly, (2) the line and staff to communicate with the hierarchy, (3) the personnel to communicate on interdepartmental levels, and (4) individual clients and nurse to communicate independently with each other.

Channels of communication utilized in the case and functional plans of nursing care are illustrated in Fig. 14. In these systems, assignment of care is made by the charge nurse. A major difference in the systems lies in the area of responsibility. In the case method a single care giver assumes responsibility for the total care of a patient, whereas in the functional method a group of task-oriented persons provides services collectively to a number of patients. In each method the charge nurse remains the authority figure through whom all major communication is channeled.

In the practice of primary care the line of communication (Fig. 15) lies more strongly between one care giver and one or more patients, depending on the variables in the situation. The care giver either chooses or is assigned by a nurse-leader to patients according to the clients' needs and wishes, the nurse's abilities, special interests, and expertise, or the work situation. The nurse assumes full responsibility for administering care to one or more patients twenty-four hours a

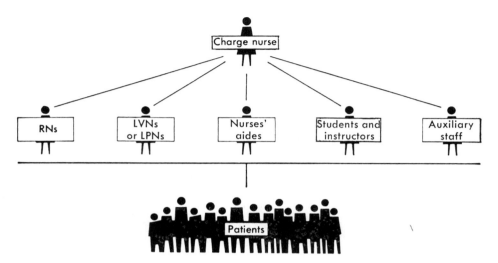

Fig. 14. Channels of communication in case and functional plans of nursing care.

day for the duration of the client's need for nursing services. The primary care nurse views other care givers and the charge nurse as resource persons for validation, suggestions, or assistance. In short, the primary care method incorporates a collegial relationship rather than operating in a hierarchical system.

When team nursing is employed, as illustrated in Fig. 16, channels of communication are established whereby the charge nurse delegates leadership responsibility to a nurse-leader for a group of patients. The team system provides the nurse-leader opportunity to employ any or all methods of assignment according to the assessed needs of the clients and the capabilities and desires of the care givers and receivers. Theoretically, because of the leader's strategic position in terms of influencing and implementing plans, he is influential in motivating personnel and in building a team that will achieve the aims of the group. In this system, team members relate to the nurse-leader, who in turn relates directly to the charge nurse. The charge nurse serves as a resource person and is freer to engage in the promotion and maintenance of comprehensive and continuous care for the clients under the jurisdiction of the nursing teams.

PREDICTIVE PRINCIPLE: Reactions to stress influence efficiency of performance in the work situation.

Sickness in and of itself is stress producing, not only to the people who are ill but also to those who are giving care. Much of nursing still takes place around the sick individual or in critical situations. The critical nature of nursing practice provokes a high stress environment and engenders a feeling of great responsibility within the providers of nursing care. This in itself makes the providers of nursing care of people more vulnerable to additional stresses, which can occur either in the course of their personal lives or in interaction with their colleagues at work. Individuals develop patterns for coping with stress; similarly, groups that work together fall into set ways of dealing with stressful situations. These pat-

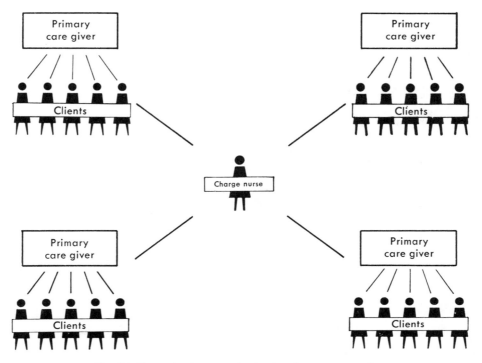

Fig. 15. Channels of communication in primary care nursing.

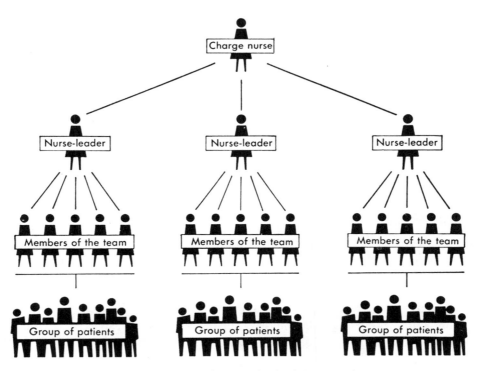

Fig. 16. Channels of communication in team nursing.

terns may or may not be the best way of coping, but at least they allow the individual or group members to perform in the situation. For the individual nurse or group, it is necessary to study and validate appropriate and applicable methods for handling critical situations that create stresses in the work program.

INVESTMENT OF AUTHORITY

Leadership can be given or assumed by an individual or group because of power of personality, position, knowledge, or ability. Management, on the other hand, requires some administrative sanction. Leadership positions can be floating. The assumption of the leadership role carries with it responsibility and authority, whether formalized or not. *Official* authority is invested in a group or a leader by the hierarchy, by the group with which one is working, or both. Then there is *assumed* authority. Assumed authority may be stable, or it may move within the group, one individual at a time being the leader; at other times several individuals lead simultaneously. Difficulty arises only when two participants who have assumed authority are in conflict, resulting in a power struggle. Both official and assumed leadership roles are legitimate sources of authority.

To be effective a manager must be assured of the authority to carry out directives within the agency. Effective delegation of authority depends on the willingness of high level management to release decision-making powers to middle and lower level management and the willingness of those to whom authority is delegated to accept the leadership role with its inherent responsibilities and accountability.

PREDICTIVE PRINCIPLE: The nurse-leader's belief that ultimate accountability lies with him determines the scope and limitations he sets for his leadership.

Delegation of authority never relieves a manager of the basic responsibilities inherent in the position. The nurse-manager takes full responsibility for whatever consequences occur as a result of his delegation of authority. Just as individual members are held accountable to the manager, so the manager is accountable to his immediate supervisor.

Once delegation of authority is made, each care giver will then be held accountable to the delegator. The nurse-manager has a responsibility for maintaining a continuing relationship with care givers to ensure that care is given with continuity, safety, and effectiveness.

ASSIGNMENT MAKING

Development of an assignment-making plan may be rational, deliberative, habitual, purposeful, random, or any combination of these, depending on the knowledge, experience, and skill of the leader or manager. In the case method, assignments change from shift to shift and often from day to day or week to week and are delegated usually by territory. For example, the nurse is directed to take one patient in room 419 or to care for three patients in rooms 420 and 421. In the functional method, assignments are delegated by the tasks to be completed. For example, one is instructed to make beds and another to pass medications. In the team system, groups are divided by territory, and within that territory, assignments are made according to difficulty of patient care and the preparation and/or the abilities of the nurse often in combination with territory. These assignments also tend to change at least weekly.

Primary nursing has no territory. In this system the care giver either chooses or is assigned by a nurse-leader to patients according to the client's needs and wishes and the nurse's abilities, special interests, specific areas, and expertise, as well as according to the individual case load. All care is planned on a twenty-four–hour basis. The nurse works with the patient for the duration of his stay in the hospital and sometimes when he returns at some later date. In some agencies, care is continued into the home.

PREDICTIVE PRINCIPLE: A manager's degree of willingness to be accountable influences the scope, limitations, and style of leadership.

Once authority is delegated, the recipient has the responsibility for carrying through the tasks assigned. Part of the care giver's responsibility can be met through determination of the client's needs and the development of viable care plans. These functions are congruent with the philosophy and conceptual framework of the agency. Bower, in *The Process of Planning Nursing Care,* outlines four phases of planning nursing care: (1) assessment, (2) problem identification, (3) formulation of plans for nursing action, and (4) planning for evaluation.*

PREDICTIVE PRINCIPLE: The willingness of the nurse-manager to relinquish authority determines the effectiveness of delegating authority to others.

The manager who feels secure in his knowledge and ability can develop behavior patterns and an atmosphere that will allow responsible participants to function on a dependent-interdependent relationship with support from the manager. This in no way abridges the nurse's role as leader. The manager still controls the operation in an atmosphere acceptable to everyone. Trust is established, and members are encouraged to develop their capabilities to their maximum potential within the limitations of the job. The manager is concerned about control so that quality is maintained. There are ways to ensure quality of care without restricting the care given in such a manner that his authority and responsibility are weakened or usurped. By serving as a validator and a controller of quality, the nurse-manager (1) is available, (2) makes suggestions, and (3) establishes a peer relationship with the care giver. As a resource person and consultant, the nurse-manager makes relinquishing authority more realistic and easier.

PREDICTIVE PRINCIPLE: An adequate supply of appropriately prepared personnel enables delegation of authority in response to client and agency needs.

PREDICTIVE PRINCIPLE: Matching the abilities of care givers to the jobs to be done increases work productivity and individual job satisfaction.

Administration usually controls the number of workers assigned to any unit. Health agencies determine the categories and numbers of personnel required in their institutions. They seek to maintain a stable nurse-patient ratio that will

---

*Bower, F. L.: The process of planning nursing care: a model for practice, ed. 2, St. Louis, 1977, The C. V. Mosby Co.

ensure the implementation of safe, problem-oriented care. It is obvious that patients with many and varied needs require more nursing services than those who have relatively few problems.

The delegator, a middle or lower management person, is alloted a number of care givers according to the number of personnel available for the work period. It is the nurse-manager's task to assign the members so that the best interests of the patients, staff, and agency are realized.

The manager, for example, may have a client who is placed in reverse isolation and who exhibits many feelings of insecurity. The nurse-manager has three care givers who can practice reverse isolation safely. The manager reasons that one nurse is new to the agency and therefore somewhat unsure; a second is technically skillful but is inclined to be abrupt in the initial approach to patients; a third nurse is capable of caring for physical needs, problem-oriented, and caring in relationships with patients. The leader will, of course, choose the third to care for the patient, realizing that the best interests of patient, staff, and agency will be served.

The primary nurse may also delegate care either to the family or to the patient himself; usually the practitioner in collaboration with the client decides what is to be done and to whom the job will be delegated.

The delegator who knows both the qualifications required for the jobs in the health agency and the abilities and personalities of the care givers is better able to utilize each person's capabilities productively. In any organizational structure, however, personnel factors do not remain constant. Frequently the nurse-leader is assigned a member who is new to the situation and sometimes to the nursing profession. Even if the orientation to the agency is complete and the in-service program extensive, the new employee will require assistance and close supervision from the nurse-manager.

Assigning uncomplicated tasks to a beginner increases his self-confidence and facilitates his progress. The worker can be encouraged to learn and increase his skills, with emphasis on his strengths, so that learning the art of providing quality patient care can be accelerated. Gradually increasing the difficulty of jobs assigned, within job specifications, promotes increased feelings of responsibility and worth and results in optimum productivity.

The nurse-manager can accomplish these tasks, however, only when qualified persons are available in sufficient number. When personnel are not available, the leader must compromise the assignment, which in turn compromises the care of clients. Higher level management must be apprised so that staffing can be increased.

Because of the number of variables associated with provision of care, there is no definitive statement of optimal nurse-patient ratio. One trend in nursing is that the RN to LVN-aide ratio is becoming greater. In some places, as salaries for nursing services increase, fewer RNs are being employed, and LVNs and aides are hired as replacements. Professional nurses have a responsibility to determine the RN to patient ratio they believe necessary for the administration of safe client care and then to work for the maintenance of that essential ratio. In determining the personnel needed, close examination should be given to the various systems of care delivery available. For example, in the team plan, where team leaders are assigned to groups of workers, the supervisory staff is pyramided, thus removing them from the care-giving role. In primary care, more persons are actually giving basic nursing care, making this system more cost effective in the final analysis. Studies are in progress to determine whether nurse's aides are actually cost effective. Because of their limited abilities in some care delivery systems, such as primary care, aides are not considered cost effective. In light of these investigations, some institutions have begun altering their staffing patterns. One way this is being done is by replacing aides with LVNs and RNs as the number of aides decreases through attrition.

PREDICTIVE PRINCIPLE: Centralization of information storage and retrieval systems allows for efficient assessment, delegation, and implementation of tasks.

The care giver is in a key position to obtain and store information concerning the client. A variety of sources are tapped for information. Records, reports, orders, and messages—both written and verbal—provide input for processing information. People are not as efficient or as effective with storage and retrieval of information as are machines. For this reason, many nursing units are incorporating mechanical devices to facilitate the care-giving process. The cassette tape recorder is one medium widely used for transcribing messages and activities. Individual care givers condense their reports to pertinent issues and record them as they have time. The nurse or group coming to the work scene listens to the tape while the worker or group going off completes the assignment. If there is need for clarification or additional information, reporting personnel are accessible for dialogue. New persons who need filling in on details seek out the care giver after he has read the patient's record.

Computers are a major mode of storing information centrally. These are in operation in many health agencies and will become a common adjunct to most nursing arenas within the next few years. An individual can feed the client's data into the system and/or can receive whatever information concerning the client that is needed to facilitate the practice of nursing.

PREDICTIVE PRINCIPLE: Clear and concise directions enhance task delegation.

Assignments for care givers should be both written and verbal. Definite plans should be devised to impart information. Staff members need to know such specifics as whom they will be caring for, where the patients are located, special tasks, coffee and lunch breaks, and any additional commitment. Assignments should be posted in an area easily accessible to staff members early enough to allow the personnel time to arrange individual schedules. Verbal directions can be given through prerecordings, on a one-to-one basis, or in a conference held early in the work period.

Members function better when they know the extent of their assignment. Managers who withhold part of the work assignment to spare the worker the pain of hearing a large assignment or who believe that delegating a task little by little is better than making one large assignment are operating on false assumptions. People who know what the work load for the day is tend to make the best use of their time. Assignments differ when primary care is in progress in that the care givers often arrange their time and tasks around the needs of the client with a central arrangement for relief.

PREDICTIVE PRINCIPLE: A balance between variety and continuity of assignment increases workers' motivation and productivity.

Ideally, a member should be given the same patient assignment at least from one day off until the next. Studies show that assigning primary responsibility to a care giver for the duration of the client's stay is more rewarding to the patient and the nurse and ensures the client of better care, since there is more opportunity to know the patient and to administer quality care on a continuous basis. The only times the client-nurse relationship should be broken are when the nurse and patient have some basic inability to get along, when the care giver finds he cannot meet the patient's needs, or when the nurse has time off. Consistency with assignment allows the worker time to become familiar with the patients and members of the nursing staff. It is well to rotate members from one geographic setting to another to ensure continued flexibility within the department. Occasionally, delegators receive requests from members to remain with the same group or in the same location for long periods of time with such statements as, "I'm more comfortable on the east side," or "I work better with Miss Judd and Mrs. Sampson." Astute leaders will recognize participants' emotional needs but will work with the members to help them understand and accept the rationale of assignments.

Tasks assigned to members are best completed if they are palatable and stimulating. "The work isn't hard," one nurse's aide observed, "It's the never-ending monotony of the job." Routinization is often favored in an effort to facilitate getting the job done and to conserve expense. Too much sameness reduces the degree to which an individual can participate in the organizational affairs of his work and often prevents him from completing a task that is meaningful to him. A nurse assigned to giving preoperative medications day after day and week after week will lose the opportunity to experience the broader implications of nursing care.

If the delegator varies the member's assignments over a period of time to include the total spectrum of care, the member will grow and develop the ability to employ diverse physical, cognitive, and interpersonal skills. In addition, a limited assignment is not economically beneficial to an agency because the employee's training and potential are not being realized.

PREDICTIVE PRINCIPLE: Consideration for each care giver's preferences and areas of expertise influences morale.

Giving thought to members' choices of one assignment over another fosters job satisfaction. Nothing makes a person feel as good about himself as having success in what he is doing; one way to ensure success is to delegate assignments according to the care giver's preferences and expertise, matching these with the needs of the client. Factors that have a bearing on the care giver's preference of assignment include (1) physical characteristics of the job (such as the extent of walking, lifting, and standing) and the type of physical activity involved (such as hygienic care or working with specialized equipment), (2) the degree of independence permitted, (3) the fairness with which the member feels he is being treated, (4) whether he has had a part in policy and procedure making, (5) individual commitment to the decisions, and (6) the degree to which the assignment interests him.

Information concerning preferences should be acquired in a professional and systematic manner to ensure each member equal consideration. The nurse-leader can learn the desires of employees through observation, conferences, and evaluation. Knowledge of a worker's preference for a task does not imply that the member will be given priority. It may be that two or more members wish the same assignment, or an individual may express a desire to engage in work he is incapable of performing. Another may request an assignment in which he excels, not wishing to extend his experience beyond that which he knows to be satisfying. The nurse-leader will consider the wishes of all members and make assignments in the best interests of patient, staff, and agency.

PREDICTIVE PRINCIPLE: A systematic planning process enables effective delegation for work implementation.

One prime quality the nurse-manager must have to delegate assignments effectively is the ability to examine and deal with ever-changing situations. The ability to see problems and issues is not an innate quality. Such insights are cultivated and require consistent practice in uncovering significant facts, weighing evidence, foreseeing contingencies, developing alternatives, and finding the best person for the care to be given.

The delegator can utilize several approaches. He can follow past procedure, observe and copy others, adhere strictly to rules and regulations, adopt the scientific method, or use any combination of these methods.

To model assignments after those methods that have been utilized in the past is stagnation. The follower of standard routines seldom investigates the "why" of an assignment and has little concern with new techniques. "It's always been done this way" provides a satisfactory explanation for the practice in question. For example, in the past a common practice in assigning tasks to others was to determine the number of personnel available for a given day and to divide this figure into the total number of patients to be cared for, with no regard for the patients' individual and priority needs or the workers' capacity to meet them. Such a practice usually leads to casual reorganization of labor by the staff members involved in an effort to correct the inequities of assignment; chaos results.

Another approach to learning the methodology of assignment is through observation and discussion with other nurse-managers in similar situations. The manager selects for his own use what is believed to be the best of his fellow managers' techniques for coordinating group activities. Exchange of experiences among nurse-managers is common practice and can contribute to the improvement of managerial technique, especially if the manager has the opportunity to participate in workshops and institutes that include representatives from a variety of situations. Most managers enjoy discussing their methods and tend to speak of those experiences and practices in which they are successful. There is an element of danger in attempting to apply one manager's methods to another situation, however. A practice that works well for one manager might produce poor results for a person who copies it. Ineffectiveness of the adapted method can be attributed to such variables as differences in goals, personnel, size of department, and composition of nursing groups. Such sharing of experiences, if used as the only source of information, may limit the manager's knowledge and narrow perspective, thus failing to develop the full potential of the nursing delegator's abilities.

A third plan for work distribution is to follow strictly the directives of the agency by adhering to job descriptions, policies, and procedures without concern for individual differences. This manner of delegating keeps the assignments fettered, develops rigid habits for handling work assignments, and prevents the development of flexible attitudes and the full utilization of people.

A methodology patterned on the scientific method is useful for delegating authority. The basic mechanism of the scientific method is to create and test a plan and to evaluate its effectiveness, after which conclusions may be drawn. In pure science a body of knowledge is obtained by means of experiments conducted to confirm or disprove the proposition under consideration. The hypothesis is tested under carefully controlled conditions. During the experiments, observations are made and data kept to record what, when, and how something has happened. Classifications and interpretations of the data are made, and generalizations are drawn. The outcome of such studies may be the formation of a basic law or principle indicating that when certain activities take place under stated conditions, there will be specific consequences.

Scientific knowledge about the management of personnel cannot be considered in the same sense as the pure sciences because of the variables in individuals and their personal social structures. There is, however, a body of knowledge in the field of management from which general principles have been developed. It is feasible to adapt the methods used in the scientific process to delegate responsibility in nursing, but utilization of the problem-solving approach requires that the nurse-manager have a clear understanding of the steps to be taken.

The first prerequisite to coordinated effort is a goal. The overall objective of any group engaged in service is to achieve maximum operational effectiveness in reaching goals. Activity programmed for success leads to accomplishment of goals and results in an awareness and mutual expression of a sense of fulfillment. The delegator of responsibility, in collaboration with others if desirable, observes and analyzes the situation within the context of responsibility to determine what is to be accomplished in a given period of time; this sets the goal.

The American Nurses' Association position paper describes the components of nursing as care, cure, and coordination.* This clearly places responsibility on the nurse for activities other than those usually thought of as patient centered. In this broader definition of care, nurse-leaders formulate goals to include (1) the needs of the client (preventive, sustaining, curative, or rehabilitative care); (2)

---

*Educational preparation for nurse practitioners and assistants to nurses: a position paper, New York, 1965, American Nurses Association, p. 5.

provision for smooth coordination of services (attention to timing when administering care, avoidance of overlap of duties, planning with others for coverage during lunch, coffee break, and conference times, being certain that routine tasks are appropriated, and providing coverage for possible emergencies or unusual circumstances); (3) consideration of the capabilities, limitations, needs, and desires of personnel; and (4) collaboration with others of the health care team.

When the problems and goals are identified, an assignment can be made. At this stage, knowledge, insight, imagination, intuition, and experience are brought to bear to construct a plan that will meet the needs of the situation under consideration. This process involves assessment, problem identification, formulating plans for nursing action, planning for evaluation, and implementation.*

The plan is then observed in action and analyzed. It must be evaluated in terms of the conceptual framework, objectives, and subsequent activities. The variables are measured by the nurse as they operate in the situation (work completed on time, overlap of activities, appreciative patient, discontented staff member, handling of emergency situation). If the nurse-manager establishes that methods of assignment allow the nurses to achieve the goals they have set, there is reason to believe the methods used were valid and can be employed again with assurance. If, on the other hand, it is discovered that the methods of assignment led to undesirable results, the nurse-manager should review the methods employed and establish at which point in the process ineffectiveness began and trouble or failure occurred. The leader will then determine who was involved, what the circumstances were, and when, where, and why the breakdown occurred. He will then go back and rework the method at the point of failure to improve the procedure.

MEASURING RESULTS

Delegation enables one to assign roles, functions, duties, and authority to carry out those roles, functions, and duties. Responsibility can never be delegated; only roles, functions, duties, and authority can be delegated. Responsibility always remains with the delegator. This is why the art of delegation is so crucial to the art of management and leadership. It is in the quality of the decisions made around delegating work that one finds the seeds of success and failure of the enterprise. Evaluation, then, becomes a crucial element in the process of delegation. It is through evaluation that the manager determines whether or not the job was done according to specifications, carried out effectively, and implemented with the greatest possible comfort to the client. The manager attempts to evaluate both the process of doing the job and the product of the job itself. In other words, the evaluation process looks at both the process and the product in order to determine success or failure.

Process evaluation examines the plan itself and how that plan is carried out. Factors examined include the following:

1. Clarity of objectives, time limitations, and availability and use of the equipment

*Bower, F. L.: The process of planning nursing care: a model for practice, ed. 2, St. Louis, 1977, The C. V. Mosby Co.

2. Organization of workers in performing jobs with efficiency and effectiveness
3. Degree of inconvenience to clients or other workers
4. Compliance with safety rules and regulations
5. Use of skillful interpersonal communications
6. Performance of psychomotor skills

There are many other factors that could be considered in the process of delivering client care. These are but a few to provide the evaluator some indications about the process.

Product evaluation is looking at the consequences—the end product of the work. The evaluator goes into a unit, a home, or a nursing area and looks at the finished product. Is the client's bed made properly? Does the room look neat and clean? Is the client resting comfortably? Is the client safe? Is the environment arranged in the proper way? Is all the equipment restored to its proper place? Product evaluation looks only at the consequences, not at the process.

There are many sources of data for the evaluator. The nurse-evaluator may seek data as (1) from his own observations; (2) from clients' observations, feelings, and perceptions; and (3) from key others, for example, family, physicians, supervisors, and other health care providers. The more varied the sources of data for the evaluator, the more accurate the evaluation results are likely to be.

Chapter 6 contains a more extensive discussion of evaluation.

PREDICTIVE PRINCIPLE: Assignments that have clearly defined goals, standards, and criteria provide a basis for measurement of outcome.

The nurse-leader is interested in measuring a diversity of activities within a given assignment. He wants to be sure that individual and group output is of satisfactory quality and quantity and is completed within the prescribed time. The leader desires that resources, people, plant, and equipment are used to the best advantage and that patients receive the full benefit of services. Clearly delineated guidelines are necessary for the evaluation process to function effectively. Guidelines provide an orderly procedure for planning and assessing the caliber and degree of support for health care and for providing institutional services and nursing activities.

Another dimension of the evaluation process is assessment of the contractual agreement. The making of a contract, whether verbal or written, has become an important mode of attaining goals. In lieu of the nurse-leader's delegating specific assignments to personnel, as is the case in the functional or team systems of care, the care giver (examples are the primary care giver or one who is engaged in a special assignment, such as teaching) enters into a contract with the client, with another nurse, or with some other person to carry out the agreement for reaching a specific goal or goals in a specified length of time. The contractual agreement is exemplified in the situation in which a client (the led) and the nurse (the leader) contract with each other for a given amount of instruction in the irrigation and dressing of the patient's leg wound.

The collaborators divide the tasks into realistic stages of accomplishment, using criteria based on quality of performance but keeping in mind that time limits must remain flexible, for health crises do not lend themselves to rigid time schedules. For example, in the first stage the client will observe the nurse in the entire nursing procedure while engaging in purposeful diaglogue about it (how, when, where, what, and why). The patient will read information pertinent to the procedure, supplied by the nurse. In the second stage, with nurse supervision the client will prepare the necessary equipment for irrigation and will remove his dressings, doing both without contamination. He validates actions and understanding with criteria listed in the procedure manual and with his nurse. The third stage will be realized in the client's performance of the wound irrigation. He continues to follow designated procedure (accurate temperature and adequate strength of solution, direction of flow, protection of linens from drainage). In the fourth and final stage the client will learn from the nurse the art of applying a sterile dressing. He opens the dressing without contamination, applies it directly to the wound with sure movement, and fixes it firmly in place with adhesive or bandage.

By such specific agreement and mutual acceptance of responsibility, criteria are established, making the outcomes of this alternative mode as measurable as those within the more traditional systems of care.

Both leader and led must be aware of the goals for the day and must know exactly what is expected of them in terms of quantity, quality, and time if they are to be held responsible for attaining goals. Assignments, leader-participant contact, and group conferences, combined with accessibility of resource people and necessary information, will give the required criteria and data for measuring results.

One cannot discuss assessment of goal achievement without speaking of mastery of the goal. In some instances, there is room for degree of accomplishment, as in the process of bed making, in learning an unsterile technique, or in various levels of communication. At other times no latitude can be allowed. Any break in sterile technique is untenable. Inappropriate counsel or action in crisis intervention may lead to disaster. The nurse-leader builds into the criteria all the contingencies necessary for desired practice and assesses outcomes accordingly. With a clear delineation in the nurse's role the nurse-leader can become the facilitator, validator, collaborator, resource person, and consultant. In this way the leader applies managerial skills largely to direct client care and is interested in that care and in the growing ability of people to provide such service rather than only using these skills to meet the logistical requirements of management. However, the nurse-leader retains the ability and authority to delegate those logistics to another person because logistics and direct client care are interwoven and influence each other.

Some leaders believe they must check personally on all details of an assignment if control of assignment is to be maintained. This autocratic manager feels confident only when he has witnessed the completion of his directions. Such restrictive measures usually result in (1) employee expectation of close supervision; (2) generation of subservient feelings; (3) exhibition of routine, compliant behavior patterns; and (4) lack of assumption of responsibility for the worker's own actions.

The effective leader will find it not only impossible but also undesirable to review all aspects of performance and consequently must select certain critical points that will provide an adequate indication of what is going on. In developing the checking process the leader must consider expenditure of time as well as employee reaction to the evaluative process.

In nursing operation the leader assumes responsibility for the overall functions but in the process of assignment making will delegate the duty of checking certain functions to care givers capable of assuming the role. Responsibility for review of progress can be on an individual basis or may be extended to several members. For example, an experienced member may be given four patients to care for on a primary care basis. The member learns the major needs of the patients and is given freedom to devise his own care plan and schedule for the day.

Another avenue of sharing responsibility for measurement of results is through group effort. The nurse-leader, for instance, may have been informed by group members of a belief that there is wasted effort in each worker's having to interrupt his individual patient assignment to run errands, such as transporting patients, calling for late trays, and locating special pieces of equipment. The delegator could request all care givers to engage in a measuring procedure over a specific period of time to learn who was interrupted, for what purpose, and how frequently. The group could then study the results of the survey to develop a design for greater efficiency. The reader is referred to Chapter 6 for more explicit information concerning the evaluation process.

PREDICTIVE PRINCIPLE: Frequent evaluation of performance using criteria influences the quality of care and the level of actual performance of care activities.

Accurate identification and documentation of behaviors of care givers is difficult. The problem of measurement of clinical competence is compounded because of (1) the variety of clinical problems encountered by the nurse, (2) the number of methods employed to deal with those problems, (3) the paucity of significant and useful research to validate the use of one methodology over another, (4) the difficulty of directly observing all activities, and (5) the tendency on the part of individuals to describe behavior through perceptions that vary greatly from individual to individual.

Evaluation that is left to be done until the end is always product evaluation and process evaluation by hearsay. Evaluation at the end does have value both for the manager and delegatee. However, its value is minimal when compared with frequent evaluations that take place during the process combined with evaluation at the end that views the end product. Frequent evaluation during actual performance of tasks enables the manager to provide supervision, teaching, and help to the delegatee so that corrections can be made during instead of after the activity. Evaluation after the activity can be costly in time, because a worker, proceeding incorrectly, can complete a whole series of tasks that must be redone.

Use of performance criteria enables a manager to determine with accuracy the level of skill being employed by a worker. Performance criteria can be highly specific or fairly general. In working with people who are lower level personnel, for example nurse's aides, orderlies, or other untrained personnel, highly specific criteria are helpful both to the evaluator and to the evaluated. An example of this is the evaluation of an aide's ability to wrap an Ace bandage. A list of criteria for the safe wrapping of an elastic bandage on a leg could provide points such as the following:

1. Tension is placed on the bandage
2. Bandage is wrinkle-free
3. Below-the-knee wrap terminates three fingers below the bend of the knee to prevent compression of the popliteal vein
4. Metal clips holding the end of the bandage are terminated on the shin or the outer lateral portion of the calf, not on the inner aspect, or posterior section, of the calf

A checklist of points such as these comprising highly specific criteria enables the nurse-manager to know how safe, or unsafe, a care giver is. Other criteria—such as gathering all the equipment before a procedure, leaving the area neat and clean, providing comfort for the client during the procedure, and maintaining quality interpersonal relationships during the procedure—enable the nurse-manager to provide specific feedback to workers for both process and product. More general criteria are those found on pp. 204 and 209 to 211.

APPLICATION OF PREDICTIVE PRINCIPLES IN THE DELEGATION OF AUTHORITY

As the nurse-leader, you are responsible for planning and directing the work being done on the unit. You have made the work assignments for the day, and an LVN comes to you with the following statement: "I have had the same assignment for three weeks, and I am tired of it. I would like to learn how to assist with the debridement of burns."

Problem	Predictive principles	Prescription
The LVN is dissatisfied with the work assignment and wishes to increase in knowledge and skills.	Clear lines of communication promote morale among organization members and enhance goal accomplishment.	Encourage LVN to express feelings by listening and giving encouraging motions and words.
	Understanding the categories and roles of nursing personnel enables the delegator to select the type and number of personnel appropriate for the job.	Confirm with LVN that request is legitimate and that the assignment for the day will be unchanged but that plans will be made for change.
	A balance between variety and continuity of assignment increases workers' motivation and productivity.	
	Written descriptions of policies, procedures, and/or guidelines by which an employee may handle situations promote ease of operation for the care giver and control of the authority delegated by the nurse-leader/manager.	Help LVN locate material and resources that will prepare her for the learning episode, for example, procedure manual, books, nurse.

Continued.

Problem	Predictive principles	Prescription
The LVN is dissatisfied with the work assignment—cont'd	Matching the abilities of care givers to the jobs to be done increases work productivity and individual job satisfaction.	Schedule LVN to assist in the care of a burn patient. Arrange for double coverage until LVN is competent.
	Clear and concise directions enhance task delegation.	Inform LVN when and with whom she will be working.
	The willingness of the nurse-manager to relinquish authority determines the effectiveness of delegating authority to others.	Trust LVN to fulfill responsibilities.
	Assignments that have clearly defined goals, standards, and criteria provide a basis for measurement of outcome.	Observe procedure periodically and at strategic times. Obtain feedback from patient, nurse-teacher, physician, and LVN.
	Frequent evaluation of performance using criteria influences the quality of care and the level of actual performance of care activities.	
	Consideration for each care giver's preferences and areas of expertise influences morale.	Be observant for other interests and expertise of LVN. Build into future assignments opportunities for variation.

BIBLIOGRAPHY
Books

Argyris, C.: Management and organizational development, New York, 1971, McGraw-Hill Book Co.

Ayer, R.: Nursing service in transition: a description of organization for classification and utilization of nurse practitioners, Duarte, Calif., 1972, City of Hope Medical Center.

Berne, E.: Structure and dynamics of organizations and groups, Philadelphia, 1963, J. B. Lippincott Co.

Brown, E. L.: Newer dimensions of patient care. Part I. New York, 1961, Russell Sage Foundation.

Department of Health, Education, and Welfare, Secretary's Committee to Study Extended Roles for Nurses: Extending the scope of nursing practice, Washington, D.C., 1971, U.S. Government Printing Office.

French, W.: Personnel management process: human resources administration, ed. 2, Boston, 1970, Houghton Mifflin Co.

Lewis, E. P.: Changing patterns of nursing practice: new needs, new roles, New York, 1971, The American Journal of Nursing Co.

Likert, R.: New patterns in management, New York, 1961, McGraw-Hill Book Co.

Litterer, J. A.: Organizations, systems, control and adaptation, ed. 2, vol. 2, New York, 1969, John Wiley & Sons, Inc.

Lysaught, J. P., editor: National Commission for the Study of Nursing and Nursing Education: an abstract for action, New York, 1970, McGraw-Hill Book Co.

Mann, F. C., Indik, B., and Vroom, V.: The productivity of work groups, Ann Arbor, Mich, 1963, Institute for Social Research, The University of Michigan Press.

National Institutes of Health: Planning for nursing needs and resources, Bethesda, April, 1972, Public Health Service Publication No. 1741-0026, U.S. Department of Health, Education, and Welfare.

Tannenbaum, R., and Weschler, I. D.: Leadership and organization, a behavioral science approach, New York, 1961, McGraw-Hill Book Co.

Taylor, C.: In horizontal orbit, hospitals and cult of efficiency, New York, 1970, Holt, Rinehart & Winston, Inc.

Periodicals

Aydelotte, M.: Standard I, staffing for quality care, J. Nurs. Admin., pp. 33-36, March-April 1973.

Chopra, A.: Motivation in task oriented groups, J. Nurs. Admin., pp. 55-60, Feb.-March 1973.

Cononi, G. A., and Siler, M.: Automated multiphasic health testing in the hospital setting, J. Nurs. Admin., pp. 70-80, Nov.-Dec. 1972.

Department of Health, Education, and Welfare, Secretary's Committee to Study Extended Roles for Nurses: Extending the scope of nursing practice, Am. J. Nurs. 71(12):2346-2351, 1971.

Department of Health, Education, and Welfare, Secretary's Committee to Study Extended Roles for Nurses: Extending the scope of nursing practice, Nurs. Outlook **20**(1):46-52, 1972.

Fielding, V. V.: New team plan frees nurse, Mod. Hosp. **108**(5):122-124, 1967.

Fry, W. F., and Lauer, J.: The planning team: why include nursing leadership? J. Nurs. Admin., pp. 70-78, May 1972.

Graves, H. H.: Can nursing shed bureaucracy? Am. J. Nurs. **71**(3):491-494, 1971.

Hilgar, E. E.: Unit management systems, J. Nurs. Admin., pp. 43-49, Jan.-Feb. 1972.

Howe, G. E.: Decentralization aids coordination of patient care services, Hospitals **43**:53-55, March 1969.

Johnson, N. D.: The professional-bureaucratic conflict, J. Nurs. Admin. pp. 31-39, May-June 1971.

Kinlein, M. L.: Independent nurse practitioner, Nurs. Outlook **20**(1):22-23, 1972.

Knecht, A. A.: Innovation on four tower west/why? Am. J. Nurs. **73**(5):809-810, 1973.

Manthey, M.: Primary care is alive and well in the hospital, Am. J. Nurs. **73**(1):83-87, 1973.

Manthey, M., and Kramer, M.: A dialogue on primary nursing, Nurs. Forum **9**(4):356-379, 1970.

Manthey, M., et al.: Primary nursing, Nurs. Forum **9**(1):65-83, 1970.

Miller, D. I.: Standard II, organization is a process, J. Nurs. Admin. pp. 19-24, March-April 1972.

Murray, D. L.: A case for independent group nursing practice, Nurs. Outlook **20**(1):60-62, 1972.

National League for Nursing: Competencies of the associate degree nurse on entry into practice, Nurs. Outlook **26**:346, June 1978.

Norris, C. M.: Direct access to the patient, Am. J. Nurs. **70**(5):1006-1010, 1970.

Schlegel, M. W.: Innovation on four tower west/ how? Am. J. Nurs. **73**(5):811-816, 1973.

Schwier, M. E., and Gardella, F. A.: Identifying the need for change in nursing service. Part I, Nurs. Outlook **18**(4):56-62, 1970.

Sjarupa, J. A.: Management by objectives: a systematic way to manage change, J. Nurs. Admin., pp. 52-56, March-April 1971.

Smith, M. L.: The clinical specialist: her role in staff development, J. Nurs. Admin., pp. 33-44, Jan.-Feb. 1971.

Somers, J. B.: A computerized nursing care system, Hospitals **45**:93-100, April 1971.

Stevens, B.: Analysis of trends in nursing care management, J. Nurs. Admin., pp. 12-17, Nov.-Dec. 1972.

White, H. C.: Some perceived behavior and attitudes of hospital employees under effective and ineffective supervisors, J. Nurs. Admin., pp. 49-54, Jan.-Feb. 1971.

White, M. B.: Importance of selected nursing activities, Nurs. Res. **21**:4-14, Jan-Feb. 1972.

6 PREDICTIVE PRINCIPLES FOR EVALUATION

CONCEPTUAL FRAMEWORK FOR EVALUATION

COMMITMENT OF ALL CONCERNED

Involvement of personnel in all phases of the evaluatory process increases belief in the fairness and accuracy of the evaluation, establishes a commitment to the evaluation, and increases motivation to utilize the results.

STANDARDS OF PRACTICE AND CRITERIA OF EVALUATION

Clear and concise role delineation and job descriptions enable employee, employer, and client to know the duties and responsibilities of the job.

Clear criteria and standards for measuring performance increase the objectivity and validity of evaluation.

Evaluation of individual and small group activity necessitates establishment of criteria for the evaluation process.

Establishing a clear contract enables the accountable nurse and the client to determine whether the contract has been met.

Use of appropriate assessment tools and sufficient evaluative data gathered from varied situations increases the validity of the conclusions in the assessment of work performance.

Use of the self-evaluation process promotes growth and development of the appraiser and contributes to better quality of care.

Participation of patient or client in evaluation of care contributes to an accurate and composite assessment.

A limited number of incidental observations jeopardizes the accuracy of evaluations.

Informal and formal assessments that are noted and recorded systematically provide significant input to the evaluation process.

Valid interpretation of data depends on equitable evaluation of input.

The evaluator who establishes mutual trust and confidence with the person evaluated and who is familiar with the criteria of evaluation increases the accuracy and usefulness of the evaluation.

The degree to which the value systems of the evaluator and the person evaluated coincide influences their interpersonal relationships and directly affects the evaluation process.

DISPOSITIONAL ACTIVITIES

Frequent feedback on performance by a qualified evaluator, based on appropriate observations, reinforces desired behaviors and increases awareness of areas that need improvement.

Positive and problem-oriented feedback helps the person evaluated to change his behavior to more acceptable levels of performance.

Staff evaluation of nurse-managers reveals general areas of strengths and weaknesses in the leader as perceived by the evaluators and provides the nurse-manager with one means of validation for the effectiveness of the managerial practice.

An evaluation process that includes reciprocal participation both vertically and horizontally provides an avenue for high level morale and job satisfaction.

Evaluation is inherent in all categories of nursing activities and is discussed in each chapter as appropriate. Evaluation is a means to measure the value or amount of something in relationship to specific, desired outcomes or goals. These expectations are either in the form of established criteria or expected outcomes specific to a health agency, care giver, or client.

The term "evaluation," when applied to the personnel appraisal system, involves more than simply recording formal judgments about a person's performance and passing them on to a higher authority. It also involves conveying these judgments directly to the participants in a way that reinforces positive behaviors and leads to improvement of weaknesses or deficiencies in performance. The appraisal system should continue throughout the employee's service to (1) determine whether he should be promoted, demoted, transferred, dismissed, or left at the current level; (2) improve his performance; (3) ascertain potential and uncover hidden abilities; (4) point out continuing education needs; (5) encourage self-development; (6) provide a guide for salary advancement; and (7) test the validity of the personnel selection process.

Traditionally the tendency has been to apply the evaluation procedure sporadically rather than continuously, as a result of pressure outside rather than from within the system, for expediency rather than as an expression of planning, and after the fact rather than as part of preplanned, cumulative, and integrated design. Furthermore, nurses tend to restrict their evaluative views to themselves and to the small functional areas in which nursing care is implemented. Quality control among nurse practitioners is highly significant, but evaluation of other factors, such as agency procedures, organizational structure, record forms, and personnel policies, are of equal importance. Larger units of the health care delivery system, such as the governing board and administration offering institutional services, must provide opportunity periodically and on an equal representation basis for reciprocal evaluation. When this happens, performance of nursing personnel is brought into proper focus and perspective.

In recent years, accountability for the provision of health care has become increasingly important to all care givers. In 1972, Public Law 92-603 authorized the establishment of professional standards review organizations (PSROs) to monitor the quality of medical care financed by federal funds such as Medicare and Medicaid. This legislation has greatly increased efforts among health care providers in all sectors to evaluate and upgrade the quality of care; formalizing the control of quality and cost through PSRO legislation has raised problems. Standardization becomes an issue, as there is no single set of criteria by which quality can be assessed. A second problem is one of measurement, as it is difficult to assess results of care when there are so many people and circumstances that impinge on the care given. A third problem is that of control. Physicians have been charged to assume responsibility for their practice. Time will tell whether or not they accept the responsibility.

The PSRO review procedures as written present a problem to nurses in that the guidelines are geared heavily toward the medical model, addressing the physical care rendered individual clients by individual physicians. They typically do not include those additional aspects of health care that are the essence of nursing practice, that is, attention to the psychologic and social well-being of the client and the degree of knowledge the individual has about his health.

Nursing reactions to PSRO legislation range from fear that governmental regulations will result in restrictive, bureaucratic rules and regulations and medical control of all health professions to enthusiasm because nurses will have the opportunity to strengthen the nursing profession by shaping PSROs in a manner acceptable to nursing.

Section 730 of the *PSRO Program Manual* specifies that nonphysician health care practitioners engage in professional review similar to that required of physicians. A basic assumption of the Department of Health, Education, and Welfare is that review of physicians and nonphysicians should be compatible.

Nursing as a major segment of the health care enterprise recognized that it must be an integral part of the accountability process and needed to formulate appropriate guidelines for the involvement of nurses in review processes and in PSROs. The American Nurses' Association was awarded a contract from the federal government to develop models that could be used for this purpose. Their work was published in 1974 and has served to spark interest among nurses all over the country for evaluation of the profession in terms of accountability.

Evaluation implies a reciprocal process. Organizational theorists affirm the problem of reciprocal evaluation to be one of determining effectiveness, that is, assessing whether the objectives or purposes of the system in process have been attained efficiently. Reciprocal appraisal is a way of saying that assessment has to take place in the context of the circumstances under which the nurse operates, with responsibility for nursing progress being shared by the determiners of those circumstances, including the patient. Accountability rests with all who participate in planning for and providing nursing care. If the hospital requests a tax override or bond issue, the community may choose to defeat it. This is an indicator or part of the evaluative data about community support. If the nursing supervisor or head nurse asks agency administrators for necessary equipment and supplies, the administrators may or may not approve the purchase, which in turn may be an indicator or evaluator of the administrators' support. The nurse-leader may present a well-supported request for an additional staff member to help implement group responsibilities but may or may not have the request sanctioned. This is an indication for evaluation of the administration's responsiveness to nursing needs. The care giver may plan with a client for primary care. The degree to which the client cooperates with the implementation of that care is part of the evaluative data about his commitment to the plan.

Traditionally in nursing, evaluation has been associated with unpleasant experiences during student days when the threat of failure was ever present. Judgments were all too often made with no help given to remedy actions under criticism, leaving the recipient feeling nervous and confused.

Confusion of evaluation with establishing a grade and the negative experiences most nurses have had with activities called "evaluation" have given this device a distasteful aura that is difficult to alter. Some agencies have modified the terminology used to remove negative connotations from the process. The evaluative procedure is sometimes referred to as "efficiency ratings," "performance assessment," and "appraisal." Whatever the term, all nurses evaluate, consciously or unconsciously, and the more nurse-leaders know about what evaluation is and how to evaluate, the more effective will be the use of this tool for improving patient care.

CONCEPTUAL FRAMEWORK FOR EVALUATION

Evaluation of client care and quality control programs is a process and as such requires adoption of a conceptual framework in which to operate. The conceptual bases of all review activities for client care and quality programs are structure, process, and outcomes of care. Evaluation of the *structure* framework involves the study of the agency, concentrating on its mission, organizational characteristics, financial base, management practices, physical facilities and equipment, and status with regard to accreditation, certification, or approval by voluntary or government bodies. Assessment of structure assumes there is a positive relationship between good structural attributes and good care.

Examination of the *process* framework of care inspects and judges what is actually done by the provider of care on behalf of a client. The decision-making process is studied along with therapeutic interventions employed. Major and minor steps taken in the care of a client are reviewed with attention to the rationale for and the sequence of the steps as well as the degree to which they help the client reach specified and attainable goals.

The process of care is directly related to general or specific outcomes of care for the clients. Examples of process criteria would be as follows:

1. To examine a client's record using an instrument that contains specific questions to answer: Are any changes in skin tone noted? Are respiratory rate and quality recorded? Does the record indicate the type and quantity of food eaten?

2. To interview the nurse: Do staff check with one another to ensure that clients are ambulated on schedule? Are precautions taken to protect a client who is in reverse isolation from undue exposure to infection?

3. To observe the care provided: Are clients consulted regarding their care? Are meals served hot and is necessary assistance provided? Are prescribed nursing interventions implemented?

A study of *outcome* refers to the results of care or the client response in terms of changes that can be noted with reference to client-oriented objectives. Variables often tested are disease status, presence or absence of symptoms, physiologic measurements, and ability to engage in activities of daily living. Factors much less often tested are psychologic or emotional responses, knowledge of health status, and compliance with proposed treatment. Examples of outcome criteria for a client postoperatively that are based on client-oriented objectives might be as follows: ambulates without assistance after third postoperative day; surgical wound evidences opening and drainage; is able to void without distress after twenty-four hours; evacuates soft, brown stool between forty-two and seventy-two hours; verbalizes name of surgery; knows about medications he is taking, including side effects; describes restrictions when he returns to work; and expresses emotional and psychologic feelings.

It is very difficult to identify outcome criteria that can be solely attributed to nursing care because the client receives care from other providers, such as physicians and a variety of therapists. Serious work has been in progress among nurses to develop nursing care outcome criteria for the past fifteen years. There are fine reviews in the literature, but the work has just begun. Individual nurses need to apply the process of evaluation that has been developed in their own work settings, make adaptations as necessary, and report their findings so that results can be shared and progress accelerated.

Dr. Bloch, Chief of the Research Grants Section of the Nursing Research Branch, Division of Nursing of the Department of Health, Education, and Welfare, has a vital interest in evaluation of nursing care in terms of process and outcome. She has developed a model of the factors that bear on patient care evaluation.*

Four types of patient problems are proposed: (1) cognitive, such as an obese patient who does not understand the principles of nutrition; (2) psychosocial, such as problems of motivation, attitude, or poverty; (3) behavior, such as excessive drinking or smoking; and (4) health state, such as ulcerative colitis. In this model, these four categories of patient problems make up the basis for evaluation of outcome.

Care providers constitute the structural framework or the system within which all care is provided. Housed between care providers (structure) and care recipient (outcome) is the care given by providers (process). In giving care the problem-solving process is employed, data are collected, the problem is defined, intervention is planned and implemented, and evaluation of the intervention takes place. Dr. Bloch believes that process should be related to outcome in every type of health care evaluation because it provides for review of how providers' actions relate to changes in the recipient of care.

In order for process-outcome evaluation to occur in nursing, certain tasks must be achieved: (1) measurable outcome criteria specific to nursing care provided must be developed (outcomes); (2) reliable and valid methods for measurement of outcomes must be developed (outcomes); (3) measurable process criteria must be known (process); (4) reliable and valid methods for measuring the process of nursing care in all forms, including physical, psychosocial, and cognitive aspects, must be formulated (process); and (5) testing of the various aspects of nursing practice in relation to patient outcomes by applying process as well as outcome measurement must occur (process-outcome).

Dr. Bloch states that the first four steps can be differentiated between process and outcome, but that all five tasks refer to the more inclusive and comprehensive process-outcome type of evaluation. She admits that nursing is not yet prepared to engage in quality control programs based completely on process-outcome evaluation but that the goal should be to work toward the achievement of these tasks through this conceptual framework so that the scientific foundation for nursing can be strengthened.

COMMITMENT OF ALL CONCERNED

Commitment means the act of pledging or binding oneself to a certain course or actions. Commitment first requires a conscious choice among alternatives, then a belief in the ideals that spawned that choice, and finally behaviors that actualize the choice. The strength or degree of the commitment of an individual depends on the amount of belief or faith he has in the choice he made to produce a result he values. For example, a person chooses and commits himself to a political philosophy because he thinks that particular political philosophy will result in the best government; a leader chooses a type of leadership because he believes that type of leadership will result in the best patient care. *Choice* is one of the key

---

*Bloch, D.: Evaluation of nursing care in terms of process and outcome: issues in research and quality assurance, Nurs. Res. **24**(4):257-258, July-Aug. 1975.

activities of commitment. Agencies with policies on personnel evaluation that have been previously established by either the administration or by employees do not offer a choice between "to evaluate" or "not to evaluate." However, within every situation is some element of choice. The choices may be about how evaluations shall be done, who will participate, or the procedure to be used. Within the prescribed policy restrictions, personnel choices made in the full knowledge of limits of choice and options available give the individual or group the beginnings of commitment. Commitment grows through seeing the choices implemented and feeling that the outcome of evaluation will be worthwhile.

PREDICTIVE PRINCIPLE: Involvement of personnel in all phases of the evaluatory process increases belief in the fairness and accuracy of the evaluation, establishes a commitment to the evaluation, and increases motivation to utilize the results.

Within agency structure, each employee cannot be involved in every phase of the evaluation process. Employers usually classify personnel positions based on administrative organization and defined patient and fiscal policies. Job descriptions are usually initially drafted by administrative personnel, but as an agency matures, professional performance committees may be created to represent employees in writing or revising job descriptions, establishing standards of practice, and developing criteria to determine if those standards have been met. Involvement of personnel who are to be affected by the committee's endeavors at all levels of evaluation will give the committee a wider base of support and will enable the committee to receive the necessary feedback to make valid decisions.

Employees can be involved in the formalized process of evaluation through participation activities using prescribed agency tools. Informal, ongoing evaluation is pervasive in all nursing activities whether recognized and labeled or not. Individuals or groups who identify the ongoing nature and use of evaluations, formal or informal, and who can establish self-expectations designed to meet needs will quickly establish commitment to evaluation. The effectiveness of evaluation in improving patient care will become strikingly clear in a short span of time.

STANDARDS OF PRACTICE AND CRITERIA FOR EVALUATION

As quality assurance efforts have progressed, many individuals and groups have become increasingly active in the area of establishing standards to upgrade the quality of care. The most obvious milestone in setting minimum standards of practice was the instigation of the licensure examination, a measure for allowing an individual to practice nursing in a given state. Currently, most agencies have committees composed of representatives of the working group that establishes standards of practice and exercises control over the quality of nursing care in an agency. Quality assurance, criteria, standards of practice and norms for all levels of nursing service personnel and the methods necessary to measure behavior by those standards are the subject of this section.

Isobel Stewart in 1919 first developed guidelines by which a procedure could be effectively standardized. Since that time, these have been modified and adapted by nurses and hospital associations for use in evaluating procedures and personnel. Stewart's criteria are modified here and slightly expanded, but they remain basically as she developed them. These criteria may be applied to any nursing activity and can be useful as guides to develop standards of practice and methods of evaluation for the measurement of quality. *Stewart's criteria (modified)** are as follows:

1. Safe and comfortable for the patient, nurse, and others
2. Technologically and therapeutically as advanced care as modern technology and science permits
3. Efficient and economical in time, energy, and supplies (the degree and priority of economy of time, energy, and supplies are legislated by the demands of criteria 1 and 2)

The three key words "safe," "advanced," and "efficient" must be defined meaningfully for practical everyday use in evaluation. Each evaluating group may wish to discuss and define these words to its own satisfaction. A brief definition for each is suggested here:

1. Safe—will not harm the client or nurse physically or emotionally; does not violate the client's physiologic, emotional, religious, or cultural integrity. Safety implies that the nurse will choose among available alternative actions. These actions will have the greatest potential for accomplishing the desired goal with the least risk of an undesirable consequence.
2. Advanced—uses skills and equipment and involves making decisions or exercising judgment based on the latest available knowledge in physical, biologic, behavioral, and social sciences.
3. Efficient—produces the greatest amount of results with the least waste. Efficient does not mean merely "fast." It means effective, productive, and adequately fulfilling a purpose with the best possible use of the energy, time, and materials available.

PREDICTIVE PRINCIPLE: Clear and concise role delineation and job descriptions enable employee, employer, and client to know the duties and responsibilities of the job.

Role delineation and job descriptions are discussed in Chapter 4 and will not be repeated here.

Employees need copies of job descriptions available to them for all job classifications. Job descriptions help all employees know what every other employee was hired to do. It is equally important for a care giver to know what his job *is not* as well as to know what it *is*. Nursing roles and job descriptions, clearly described in terms of relevance of each item to nursing practice, provide an objective way to ascertain if goals have been reached. If the job description is vague or if it ends with "and such other duties as may be required," the employee will not know what direction to take or what goals and objectives will be considered as most significant when outcomes are surveyed.

In addition to role delineation and job description, where management by objectives (MBO) is in effect, individuals will be appraised on the basis of individual objectives mutually set by the participant(s) and the immediate supervisor.

---

*Stewart, I. M.: Possibilities of standardization in nursing techniques, Mod. Hosp., June 1919.

Usually these objectives fall into the categories of routine duties, problem-solving goals, creative goals, and personal goals. They are always consistent with the larger goals of the agency.

Vagueness in setting up job descriptions leads to a guessing game. Participants need to know areas of overlapping responsibility and areas of differing responsibility. Clear job descriptions and objectives are the nucleus of all subsequent evaluative activities.

PREDICTIVE PRINCIPLE: Clear criteria and standards for measuring performance increase the objectivity and validity of evaluation.

The difference between performance standards and evaluation criteria can be unclear. *Performance standards* are usually general minimal standards established to govern the quality of nursing care. These standards definitively describe safety and expertise necessary for acceptable performance of the job. *Evaluation criteria* enable the evaluator (care giver, client, nurse-leader, supervisor, or worker) to establish categories for review and to determine the *degree* and *extent* to which the person evaluated is performing in relationship to the established minimal standard.

Objectivity and validity in evaluation of performance are ideals that are never completely attained. *Objectivity* means unprejudiced, based on real evidence, and uninvolved with self or at least minimally influenced by subjective involvement. Objectivity, although not completely attainable, can be controlled to some extent through the use of criteria as guides for making judgments and by remaining sensitive to and aware of biases and feelings.

Validity is the degree and extent to which the evaluation tool measures what it was intended to measure. Validity has two basic elements: (1) *reliability,* the degree and extent that an evaluation measures something, and (2) *relevance,* the degree and extent that it actually does measure what it is intended to measure. A criterion can measure reliably without measuring relevantly, and vice versa. However, a criterion must be both reliable and relevant for it to be valid.

The following is an example in which job classification, qualifications, standards of practice, and criteria of evaluation are followed through for one area of responsibility.

The Cedar Valley Visiting Nurse Association employs several levels of personnel who give nursing care on a team basis. LVNs are employed to perform specified functions. The following information is taken from performance materials provided to all personnel. One small area has been chosen to simplify the process. These items are not to be construed as complete.

Job classification: Licensed vocational nurse.

Job qualifications: Licensure by the state and one year of hospital or nursing home experience.

Other requirements: Two character references, two professional performance references, and two formal interviews with designees of the Visiting Nurse Association.

Job description: Will, under the supervision of a registered nurse, give basic care to designated patients. This includes appropriate hygienic care; special mouth, pubic, and foot care; and oral medications and specified treatments.

Standards of practice: Will exercise safety in the care of patients and will seek assistance or guidance when needed. Will collaborate with the team leader in making decisions about procedure. Hygienic care is expected to be performed to the following standards: Mouth—mucosa and teeth clean, breath fresh, etc.

Criteria of evaluation: Mouth care: Gives routine mouth care to appropriate patients. Observes when other than routine mouth care is needed.

Administers special mouth care procedures when necessary.

Uses equipment appropriate to the type of mouth care to be given.

Exercises safety precautions to protect the patient from injury (aspiration, gum or buccal abrasions).

Protects self from contamination or contagion.

Uses procedures requiring minimum expenditure of effort for both patient and nurse with maximum amount of comfort for both.

Follows latest and most up-to-date directives about procedure.

Displays economical use of time and equipment (for both agency and patient).

Use of a model similar to this one for all nursing activities will provide participants with evaluative structure. (Note that the criteria for evaluations spelled out in behavioral terms facilitate the assessment process.)

This kind of structure provides a measure of safety for both the evaluator and the person evaluated by making objectivity more achievable. A nurse-leader can have positive or negative feelings about the LVN but if the procedure has been performed and the criteria met as written, personal feelings are less likely to influence evaluative judgment.

The standard of performance "mucosa and teeth clean, breath fresh" could be labeled a "relevant criterion." If an evaluator looked at the mouth of the patient and it exhibited clean mucosa and teeth and the patient's breath was odorless, the evaluator could unequivocally state that the standard had been achieved. The clean mouth indicates only that the desired result has been attained. Accurate evaluation of the practice used to accomplish the standard must be obtained by other means. The *list of criteria* is both relevant and reliable if, when used, the criteria measure the fact that a clean mouth was achieved (the criteria are relevant) and that the procedure was done with the appropriate equipment, the use of safety precautions, the least amount of effort, the latest technology, and the greatest economy (the criteria are reliable).

The American Nurses' Association, the American Medical Association, PSROs, and combinations of nurses, physicians, and other health care providers are working diligently to develop models that assist with the identification of criteria, establishment of standards and determination of norms for the evaluation of health care. It is necessary for the reader to understand the way in which these terms are used.

Criteria in this context refer to the names or descriptions of variables without any quantification or value judgment. "Pulse," "respiration," "degree and kind of movement," and "extent of knowledge" each represent a criterion. Criteria should be developed by knowledgeable and expert practitioners for specific groups of populations, such as those who have had a certain type of surgery, who are paraplegic, or who are anxious or in crisis. It may be important in criterion development to designate other factors such as age, sex, religion, and culture.

Nursing process criteria can be developed on the basis of the nursing process model—assessing, planning, implementing, and evaluating nursing care—with components of each part of the process delineated in detail. Data can be acquired from numerous sources and methods: (1) information from client records, (2) observation of the client, (3) interview with the client, (4) interview with the nursing personnel, (5) observation of the nursing personnel, (6) observation of the client's environment, (7) observation of unit management, and (8) observer inference.

A *standard* is a desired and achievable level of performance that can be compared with the criterion. Before a standard can be tested the method(s) to be used must be identified and spelled out as to the precise means for measurement. Again, these values will have to be determined by experts, depending on the population served. They will then be compared when the criterion variable is measured. For example, the standard for the criterion of "pulse" could be "between 70 and 90"; for "respiration" the standard may be "between 14 and 20"; for degree and kind of movement the standard may be "wheel chair—manipulates self with use of upper torso"; and for "extent of knowledge" the standard may be described as "changes own dressing without contamination." Seldom does a client or practitioner achieve optimal level in all categories. Unless perfection is acquired, there always is latitude in performance. Also, standards for assessment of nursing care are still incomplete. Most of those developed lack specificity in quantitative terms, making measurement of the criteria difficult.

Norm is defined as a level or range of performance regarded as typical or normal for any individual(s) or situation(s). It refers to a conclusion reached as a result of empiric study of present conditions or circumstances. Norms are fairly easily determined for some criteria, such as "length of hospitalization," "amount of medication taken," or "morbidity." A problem appears in that norms for a vast number of criteria in the assessment of nursing care are unknown. For example, "level of stress," "amount of pain," "degree of motivation," or "sufficient number and kinds of nursing personnel" remain undetermined. It is only through research that reliable norms can be developed to test criteria. In the meantime, hypothetic norms can be used, based on present knowledge and experience.

In this framework, clear criteria, standards of performance, and norms for measuring performance provide both the evaluator and the person evaluated with guidelines for what constitutes good patient care. With these guidelines, value judgments can be made and the criteria for evaluation can unequivocally establish specific behavior expectations for excellence of nursing care.

The appraisal system for personnel should consider such criteria as job knowledge, ability to carry through on assignments, judgment, attitude, cooperation, dependability, and production. Carefully thought-out criteria and standards for performance help the evaluator and the person evaluated take all relevant factors into account when assessing performance, thus minimizing the effect of personal bias.

PREDICTIVE PRINCIPLE: Evaluation of individual and small group activity necessitates establishment of criteria for the evaluation process.

Nurse practitioners who function independently or in small groups are accountable for both the tangibles and the intangibles of nursing and are expected to engage in a broad spectrum of roles, demonstrating the degree of expertise inherent in each of the roles.

The criteria used to evaluate the profession as a whole can be applied to individual or group practice. Following are some pivotal questions posed for making evaluative judgments.

1. Is the care giver or group leader legally qualified for the role?
2. Does authority for individual or group action lie with the participants, and if group effort is in process, is there an interdependent relationship?
3. Is there provision for individuals to pursue independent practice and to utilize one another as resource persons?
4. Are goals designed to meet the needs of the client or patient and practitioner?
5. Do care givers have a part in the development of goals, and are they committed to their fulfillment?
6. Are policies and job descriptions available that explain what is expected of each member, are the members cognizant of their meaning, and are the expectations fulfilled?
7. Are nursing care plans formulated and implemented?
8. Does the care giver receive self-improvement and professional development through a well-designed educational program?
9. Do nurse members manifest behaviors indicating attitudes of satisfaction with their roles?
10. Is there evidence of nondiscriminatory behavior?
11. Is there a systematic design for evaluation of personnel and nursing care with respect to themselves and the total organization?

PREDICTIVE PRINCIPLE: Establishing a clear contract enables the accountable nurse and the client to determine whether the contract has been met.

Nurses who are directly accountable to their patients and families, such as in the practice of primary care, bear responsibility for their services. Agreements for nursing care may be entered into between the patient and nurse, the health agency and the care giver, or the physician and nurse. Implicit in the concept of accountability is obligation, liability, and trustworthiness. At the onset of employment a client and/or his family confers with the nurse for the purpose of mutual assessment, sharing of philosophy and expectations, and review of policies and procedures held by the employing person or agency. This is the time for the care giver and client to negotiate and to make the decision to accept or reject the conditions as they are delineated. Inherent in the agreement is reciprocal accountability to see that on-going processes for alteration of plans and evaluation as necessary for meeting expectations are implemented.

The nurse-practitioner will (1) determine and accept responsibility for the leadership role; (2) identify his own and the client's capabilities and limitations; (3) set realistic scope and limitations of performance for self and client; (4) promote a climate for collaborative and cooperative communication; (5) make self available to patients, families, and other interested members of the health team for reporting; (6) develop problem-oriented care plans with the client and/or family; (7) carry prescribed plan into action and receive feedback from client and others about the results of the service; (8) seek assistance from appropriate resources when necessary; and (9) evaluate quality of performance and initiate steps for necessary changes or modification.

PREDICTIVE PRINCIPLE: Use of appropriate assessment tools and sufficient evaluative data gathered from varied situations increases the validity of the conclusions in the assessment of work performance.

The modern theory of performance appraisal is based on important concepts: (1) that the foundation of performance appraisal rests on the criteria and standards established for various health care positions, (2) that there is participation in the process by all concerned, (3) that there is emphasis on obtaining factual information about specific achievements as they relate to criteria and standards, and (4) that the appraisal process can facilitate change in individual behavior in order to achieve personal and organizational goals.

Nursing practice is validated through informal and formal means. No single style has been found to be consistently superior to another. Most individuals and health agencies utilize more than one technique, depending on (1) the purpose of the evaluation, (2) the availability of resources, and (3) the expertise and preference of those involved in the appraisal process.

Evaluation is both intuitive and subjective. The evaluation process takes the form of informal and formal evaluation. *Informal evaluation* may consist of (1) observation of an individual's work performance while he is engaged in nursing functions; (2) on the job, incidental face-to-face work and/or collaboration; (3) reflections offered during a meeting or conference; (4) reactions of an involved person, such as a patient, family member, or staff person; or (5) notation of the effects of a worker's actions on patients, families, personnel, or environment. *Formal assessment* includes many methods. Nurses most often utilize (1) anecdotal recordings, (2) checklists based on preestablished criteria, (3) dialogue based on one-to-one and group exchange, (4) rating scales, and (5) cumulative records of activities engaged in for professional growth and/or advancement. Nurses may avail themselves of other methods, such as written and computer tests and other technologic testing devices. Practitioners can test their evaluative skills individually and collectively by viewing a filmed or taped nursing action and then assessing the situation. Videotaping with instant replay is a most appropriate device for the assessment of some nursing activities. Microtelevision can be used in actual or simulated settings. Evaluation of verbal and nonverbal interaction is particularly subject to this method.

All these avenues are most effective when there is commitment to the evaluation process by the evaluator, the person being evaluated, and the receiver of the information.

Anecdotal recording. An anecdote is a brief account of an incident and is an important means of illuminating evidence for evaluation. The anecdotal note has both advantages and disadvantages. The device is useful for frequent brief observations where variations in situations and personalities preclude advance determination of behavior. With this mechanism, it is possible to discover trends of conditions and behavior over a period of time. In many ways the anecdotal notes are superior to checklists or rating scales because observers are not forced into rigid structure in describing behavior. However, it is the very latitude of anecdotal notes that often leads to difficulty. The tool also provides a means for recording a description of a specific situation that could not have been anticipated and to tell how the individual acted in the situation. The anecdotal note is a means for describing a nurse's experience with a person or group. The anecdotal method is useful for recording and evaluating patient progress. Essentially, nurses' notes are one form of anecdotal record, since they outline serially factual information with definite reference to the patient's progress. Other uses for this mode include validating technical skills, dialogue, and interpersonal relationships.

In any of these areas the behavioral pattern may vary from person to person and situation to situation. Although the general conditions and behaviors can be prescribed beforehand, the specific activities will be determined by circumstances incident to the occasion.

For maximum clarity, an anecdotal notation should include (1) a description of the particular occasion; (2) a delineation of the behavior noted, indicating who, what, why, when, where, and how; and (3) the evaluator's opinion or estimate of the incident and/or behavior. Decisions concerning what to observe and record are made on the basis of previously determined criteria, formal and informal. For expediency the evaluator will develop a code or an abbreviated system for recording to facilitate speedy and accurate memorandums.

Perhaps the greatest difficulty in the use of anecdotal notes is the matter of developing some relationship among the various notations. Before it is possible to get impressions of the overall behavior in a given period of time, it is necessary to organize the descriptive notes. Often the notes bear little or no relationship to one another, and for this reason it is difficult to use them. The burden of organizing the notes falls on the observer or on the person who is attempting to interpret the meaning of the notes in relation to the behavior of the person evaluated.

Checklist. By definition a checklist is a grouping of items by which something may be confirmed or verified. The checklist could be called a behavioral inventory. The checking process implies that standards and criteria are available for gauging items. The inspection procedure requires scrutiny of behavior under investigation. Checklists are most useful for determining the status of tangible items, such as inventory and maintenance of equipment and supplies. They have the advantage that items to be observed can be determined in advance and will be the same criteria used in each situation. Checklists are of some use as yardsticks for appraisal of nursing skills and techniques. There is no guarantee, however, that the observed behavior is a persistent one and that the procedure will provide a representative picture of the individual being evaluated.

Checklists applied in nursing attempt to itemize behaviors that are considered important elements of a task. One approach is to list satisfactory behaviors in a column, then determine the worker's overall performance on the basis of the items. For example, in observing administration of medications, the evaluator looks to see if the person being evaluated (1) checks physician's orders against nursing medication cards, (2) prepares the medication accurately using prescribed procedure, (3) identifies the patient and checks the medication card against the patient's wristband, (4) administers the medication, and (5) accurately charts medication given. It is recommended that only significant behaviors essential for a successful performance be included on the checklist. Only those behaviors that, if omitted or performed incorrectly, would make the difference between successful and unsuccessful performance should be included. The checklist does not lend itself well to evaluating patient progress, dialogue, or interpersonal relationships.

Rating scale. The rating scale, quite similar to the checklist, is another type of evaluation tool used in describing observed skills and performance. The basis of the rating device consists of such items as descriptive paragraphs, sentences, or phrases to serve as guidelines for the evaluator. Unlike the checklist, the rating scale may involve judgments as to quantitative and qualitative abilities. Such rating scales at the lower end might range from "incapable of performing a given task" to "poor" or "unsatisfactory." The scale will at its higher limits use such descriptive terms as "excellent," "outstanding," or "exceptional."

Some scales for the rating of performance employ the numeric system, using "one" to indicate the lowest behavioral pattern and "ten" or more to indicate the highest. The evaluator may fabricate a scale according to his own design and check behavioral patterns as occurring "consistently," "frequently," "sometimes," or "never." These numbers or words are ill defined, and only the evaluator may know what an individual's level of performance and achievement is.

The rating scale is usually reserved for formal evaluation procedures, such as periodic assessment of an employee and is frequently associated with retention, promotion, and tenure. The device is comparative in nature. The rating is based on retrospective recordings and observations and is subject to human errors associated with recall and interpretation. This tool is most useful when each unit on the rating scale is identified and listed in terms of specific behaviors or circumstances.

A well-calibrated rating scale will consider (1) individual preparation for the role, (2) work setting and environment, (3) functions in relation to agency criteria, and (4) interpersonal relationships. Maximal utilization of the assessment tool depends on involved individuals having prior knowledge of, participation in, acceptance of, and commitment to the content and use of the rating scale.

PREDICTIVE PRINCIPLE: Use of the self-evaluation process promotes growth and development of the appraiser and contributes to better quality of care.

Self-evaluation is used by everyone from childhood to senescence. The ability to be critical in assessing one's own performance is a mark of maturity and an integral part of nursing practice. Self-evaluation is implicit and continuous in the nursing process at every level of care giving. Self-evaluation has many valuable effects. The one engaged in introspection seeks to (1) obtain estimates of his level of achievement; (2) acquire meaningful information to assist with improvement in nursing practice; (3) gain information for self-improvement, growth and development, and the achievement of personal goals in a socially acceptable manner; and (4) enhance and improve human relations.

Self-rating can be heavily influenced by the individual's tendencies to overestimate or underestimate his own capabilities or achievements. Much success of self-evaluation programs depends on the preliminary preparation of the participants to recognize their own strengths and weaknesses and to be as objective as possible in rating personal performance. Provided with adequate and procedural criteria for the assessment process and with various other appropriate tools, the individual can evaluate his progress in relation to these objectives, subject to constant reexamination and feedback. Self-evaluation is connected with personal goals, self-perception, self-confidence, and feelings of competence or incompetence. Most people have a fairly accurate picture of themselves and their abilities, but communication of self-evaluation is overlaid with many factors. Some of these are (1) who is reading the evaluation, (2) how the evaluation will be used, (3) the social acceptability of the self-judgment, and (4) peer pressures. If the care giver's self-appraisal threatens a job, promotion, salary increase, or prestige or peer regard, it is unlikely that the assessment will be articulated and communicated. If, as is often the case, social pressure decries extremely high self-appraisals and the individual values social appraisal, the care giver's self-evaluation is not likely to reflect areas of high competence. If (1) the evaluation is geared to citing goals for self, degrees to which goals have been realized, and plans for goal attainment, (2) the self-evaluation is to be used as a record of and provision for growth and not as a means for punishment or reward, and (3) the self-evaluation report is confidential within preestablished limits and constraints, then self-evaluation is an accurate and useful tool and is likely to be effective when used in conjunction with other devices.

PREDICTIVE PRINCIPLE: Participation of patient or client in evaluation of care contributes to an accurate and composite assessment.

As the recipient of care, the patient or client is in a strategic position to become involved in the verification of the effectiveness of his care. Basic to this concept is the belief that (1) care givers and recipients will have a vested interest in outcomes, (2) they will want to assume reciprocal responsibility for the implementation and revision of plans for care administered, (3) plans and evaluations will have a greater depth and increased objectivity when more than one person is involved, and (4) participation in the development and assessment of his care expedites and individualizes the patient's treatment and well-being.

Some clients are unable or simply do not wish to participate in planning for their health needs. This factor does not negate the feasibility of client contribution to the collection of evaluative data. The nurse observes the client's behavior and verbalizes subjective data. If the patient demonstrates that the objectives have been fulfilled, the desired evidence is acquired.

One approach to client evaluation is to establish the process on a continuum basis and to develop collaboratively with him a care plan that considers all phases of the process—assessment, problem identification, formulation of plans for nursing action, and planning for evaluation and implementation.* Nursing prescriptions are prepared with the client or patient and his family and with the

---

*Bower, F. L.: The process of planning nursing care: a model for practice, ed. 2, St. Louis, 1977, The C. V. Mosby Co.

help of other members of the health team if needed. A copy is left with the patient. Updating and changing the care program are continuous and are done in conjunction with the client. This participatory mechanism provides an uncomplicated system for client evaluation. It is simple to assess the quality of various aspects of patient care, taking into consideration his knowledge of the treatment and the realization that it has been completed.

A checklist or questionnaire is another means of obtaining client data. Information gleaned from these tools usually refers to care already given, for example, "Did you feel nursing service was adequate?" "What more would you have liked for the nurse to do?" "Were your medications and treatments administered according to plan?" "Were you taught how to use the exchange plan in preparing your meals?" "Can you use the exchange plan now that you are home?" These serve as input for assessing nursing action in general. The questionnaire or checklist designed to determine the discharged patient's understanding of his home care plan elicits information that assists the primary nurse in maintaining a continuous and comprehensive follow-up.

Although the client is encouraged to contribute ideas and approaches to problem-oriented treatment, the responsibility for developing, maintaining, implementing, and evaluating care rests with a particular nurse, who is held accountable for this service.

PREDICTIVE PRINCIPLE: A limited number of incidental observations jeopardizes the accuracy of evaluations.

PREDICTIVE PRINCIPLE: Informal and formal assessments that are noted and recorded systematically provide significant input to the evaluation process.

Observations of completed tasks can give an unreliable picture of performance. For example, the nurse-leader walks into a patient's room one hour after the change of the morning shift and finds the patient clean and neatly groomed, the bed freshly made, and the unit straight and uncluttered. Without additional data the nurse-leader could conclude that the nurse assigned to this patient was efficient and thorough. More complete data might reveal (1) that this patient was first on the list and therefore was cared for first regardless of the fact that another patient wanted early care so that he would be ready for a long-awaited visit from a loved one; (2) that the patient's receiving such efficient and thorough care was at the expense of the patient's breakfast, which became cold while waiting for the care giver to complete the care; (3) that the linen was piled on the floor while the bed was being changed; or (4) that the patient was bathed in one small pan of water, which was not changed during the bath.

Value judgments made on one performance, the end product of a performance without reference to the process, or on many performances in the same situation can be erroneous because of lack of a variety of observations that would validate or refute previous judgments. For instance, a practitioner may use aseptic technique smoothly, correctly, and consistently when emptying catheter bags but may contaminate unknowingly when changing a sterile dressing. The criterion "practices sterile technique with a high degree of skill" may be true when the nurse is performing one task and not true when performing another.

Both informal and formal input becomes significant if noted systematically and recorded as consistently as possible. The evaluation process is a means of determining the professional characteristics of an individual or a group. Similar behaviors as recorded in the evaluator's notes or tabulations indicate that a set of actions is predominately exhibited. Desirable behaviors that are rarely manifested are not given high priority when assessments are made; however, isolated achievements might become significant when motivation and potential are discussed.

Undesirable behaviors are important to consider. Again, isolated incidences are not used as conclusive data unless they become significant to the safety or welfare of the client. The right to be "human," or to improve, includes provision for making some mistakes without penalty or guilt. The evaluator's primary responsibility is to observe and note those behaviors exhibited most frequently and to deal with them. The aggregate of these samples gives a more reliable basis for determining a trend of behavior.

PREDICTIVE PRINCIPLE: Valid interpretation of data depends on equitable evaluation of input.

Factors used in performance evaluation programs vary widely from one appraisal plan to another. Information gleaned from evaluation procedures may be meaningful only if it is used constructively and interpreted correctly. Judgments about the assignment of relative weight or value of each factor under consideration often become the responsibility of the nurse-leader, who will follow prescribed guidelines*: (1) client and nurse safety, (2) advanced knowledge and technology, (3) client comfort, (4) efficient use of time, and (5) cost effectiveness.

Other factors of an equitable evaluation of input for consideration are as follows:

1. Whatever the specific criteria used, they should relate to the job description and performance standards.
2. Objective assessments should receive greater weight than subjective judgments.
3. When one person is evaluated and more than one individual is involved, the evaluators' impressions of the incident are diluted because it is difficult to determine the extent of each member's participation and the qualitative assistance obtained from extraneous sources.
4. Time is a factor in calibrating certain skills.
5. No single methodology should constitute the basis for success or failure in any nursing effort.

PREDICTIVE PRINCIPLE: The evaluator who establishes mutual trust and confidence with the person evaluated and who is familiar with the criteria of evaluation increases the accuracy and usefulness of the evaluation.

When the evaluator and the person evaluated have a trusting relationship, anxiety about evaluation is somewhat reduced. The extent to which evaluation activities cause anxiety, however, is directly related to what the person being evaluated stands to gain or lose. Evaluation that is constant and ongoing and has as its objective the improvement of patient care through the upgrading of perfor-

---

*Stewart, I. M.: Possibilities of standardization in nursing techniques, Mod. Hosp., June 1919.

mance becomes so much a part of routine and everyday nursing relationships that threat is reduced.

Reasons individuals may resist attempts to evaluate or control them are (1) danger of being removed from the job, suspended, relieved of responsibilities, or demoted; (2) disruption of self-image; (3) incongruence in individual and organizational objectives; (4) belief that the expected standard of performance is absent, too low, too high, or not important; (5) dislike of designated leader or manager; and (6) existence of an informal individual or group control that is more important to the person being evaluated.

Evaluations resulting from cooperative effort and accompanied by qualitative explanations that elucidate conclusions enable behavioral changes to be effected. Job descriptions, standards of practice, and criteria of evaluations all contribute to the ability to participate in evaluations. An employee who knows what constitutes a "good" or "bad" activity can recognize his own success or failure and take the initiative in corrective action. Consistently accurate self-evaluation is the ultimate achievement of evaluative activities, for it enables self-perpetuating growth.

The effect of evaluative comments on member behavior is related to the manner and intent of the message. Positive comments such as "You did a very good job on that" or "That was a fine bit of work you just did" serve to boost the morale of the worker and encourage continued high level performance. Negative remarks create varied feelings ranging from the desire to improve to deep hostility toward the evaluator without a change in the undesirable behavior. Negative comments are very likely to be accompanied by an explanation of the reason for the criticism, whereas positive comments are seldom accompanied by explanation. It is important for the person being evaluated to have information about *why* a behavior is "good" or "bad" so that the characteristics of the behavior can be either identified and repeated or changed.

Whether the evaluation is informal or formal, the evaluator bears in mind the need to preserve the integrity of the person or group being evaluated. Positive feedback, earned and given appropriately, contributes to the morale of each individual involved in the evaluation procedure.

Negative feedback is also essential for growth, as is positive feedback, and although it is often more difficult to give and to receive, it provides necessary data. Withholding feedback of any kind, positive or negative, is an ultimately hostile act because it robs another person of data he needs to make intelligent choices and behavioral changes. In terms of personal acceptance of evaluation procedures, it is generally true that the more familiar a person is with the criteria used for evaluation, the more likely it is that he will accept and support those criteria.

PREDICTIVE PRINCIPLE: The degree to which the value systems of the evaluator and the person evaluated coincide influences their interpersonal relationships and directly affects the evaluation process.

The dynamics of personal interaction and decisions are not wholly shaped by policies, job descriptions, and agreements. The conditions under which an individual operates and his perception of himself and others are the result of his value system. Value systems affect attitudes, which permeate and influence all contacts and have a direct effect on the task of evaluation. The bulk of administrative science literature in recent years emphasizes interpersonal relationships and the manner in which informal relations affected by values enhance or subvert interaction and organizational structure.

Interpersonal relationships are broad in scope, complex in nature, and constantly shifting. An attitudinal survey is a helpful part of the evaluation procedure. A cluster of attitudes recorded over a period of time assists the nurseleader in guiding members toward positive directional goals. When guidelines are vague, evaluators may rely on discriminatory behaviors and may tend to introduce ascriptive criteria such as race, religion, sex, age, social background, personal connections, and friendships (Chapter 1).

A major industrial firm supported the need for a well-defined and clearly understood policy to avoid discriminatory reaction. It was concluded that interpersonal pressures have their greatest impact on a manager's decisions when he is not fully aware of policy; also the manager's personality and values have their greatest impact on his decisions when he is not certain of procedural format.* Assessments become ability oriented when objective criteria for the administration of patient care are considered, and knowledge, creativity, and job performance take precedence. Values are a part of each person and therefore influence evaluation. Clarity about one's own standards and those of the person evaluated help keep value systems in perspective.

DISPOSITIONAL ACTIVITIES

Dispositional activities are those functions that channel the evaluative information to the appropriate source. Not all evaluation activities are such that a formal disposition is required.

Most evaluative feedback is verbal or behavioral and occurs between the evaluator and the person evaluated. This type of evaluation is incidental and frequent throughout a working day; it is seldom translated into a formal report. Behaviors, such as a frown from a co-nurse when a requested diabetic urine sample is obtained late or a smile when the diabetic urine results are obtained on time, are evaluative in nature and act as reinforcers of desired behaviors.

Evaluations that are more formal, but still not written or reported, take place in the form of conferences. Unwritten and informal evaluations not reported to others should be based on the same criteria used for written reports. The evaluator has some purpose for scheduling such conferences, which necessitates preplanning of procedures that will facilitate accomplishment of the goal. The form and timing of the formal evaluative information depends on how the evaluation is to be used. Evaluative information may be dispensed to any person involved in primary care, in independent nursing practice or in the organization who has official access to the information or his designee. Among these may be any one or all of the following:

1. Client
2. Individual employee

*Quinn, R. P., Tabor, J. M., and Gordon, L. K.: The decision to discriminate: a study of executive selection, Ann Arbor, Mich., 1968, Institute for Social Research, The University of Michigan Press.

3. Person evaluated
4. Head nurse
5. Supervisor
6. Nursing service personnel
7. Official committees of the agency
   a. retention committee
   b. professional standards committees
   c. personnel promotion committees
   d. research or data collection committees
8. Personnel office

The form the dispositional activity takes can be in any one or a combination of the following:

1. Verbal feedback
2. Behavioral feedback
3. Written memo
4. Formal evaluation using prescribed form
5. Signed official or personal letter

All evaluations, regardless of the form used, must be substantiated and qualified with first-hand evidence of the application of established criteria.

PREDICTIVE PRINCIPLE: Frequent feedback on performance by a qualified evaluator, based on appropriate observations, reinforces desired behaviors and increases awareness of areas that need improvement.

PREDICTIVE PRINCIPLE: Positive and problem-oriented feedback helps the person evaluated to change his behavior to more acceptable levels of performance.

Feedback is defined as the return of a portion of the output of any process or system to the input. Broadly, feedback is any information that results from a process; it is checking out what message the other individual or group has to convey so that the information can be used in a constructive way.

Feedback is the most important factor influencing behavioral change. The most effective evaluative feedback is given at the time the incident occurs. The closer the feedback occurs to the time of the incident, the more nearly the participants can place it in context and the more meaningful it will be.

There are many applications of the feedback process in nursing leadership and management. With feedback the nurse-manager is better able to devise, to make necessary changes in present plans, and to make appropriate adaptations for the future. In the feedback process the nurse-leader works with personnel to assess past performance, to make judgments on actions, and to determine whether messages and instructions are clearly understood for the present.

The feedback process in evaluation involves positive, negative, and problem-solving feedback. *Positive feedback* is tremendously important in the evaluation process. So often a person's inference about evaluation is negative; he expects to hear about only that which is wrong. Informing an individual that his work and presence in the organization are valued is very important.

The following comments exemplify positive feedback and provide descriptive data for evaluation of the worker: "I noticed that you planned Mr. B's care with him very carefully, providing him with several choices. He expressed pleasure that you consulted him," or "You reorganized your work schedule very well despite the emergency this morning. That action demonstrated a cool head and good judgment," or "The teaching plan you developed for Mrs. Y was based on her needs and abilities. She is learning well."

Negative feedback is expressing a message of disapproval about a circumstance or behavior. "I did not like the way you spoke to Mr. C's family" and "You contaminated the site of incision when you changed the dressing" describe negative feedback. Although there may be times when negative feedback is needed, negative statements should be avoided as much as possible.

Problem-solving feedback can be applied in most situations where answers are needed. The nurse-manager could consult with the nurse about his dialogue with Mrs. C's family. "I saw sparks flying between you and Mr. C's family. Could we discuss the issues and see if there is another way to approach them?" With the nurse who contaminated the incision an approach might be "Mrs. B, I noticed you were having some trouble with dressings today. I have freed you for an hour tomorrow so that you may take an in-service class in this procedure." The problems are identified, but with the problem-solving approach the probability of hostility is lessened.

Time should be budgeted for feedback conferences between the nurse-manager and workers. A time investment is required but the payoff is worth the effort in terms of increased understanding and fewer mistakes. The conferences should focus on task and process based on agency job description, standards of practice developed for the area, and criteria of evaluation. If all these are not available, attempts can be made to acquire other evaluative tools. The American Nurses' Association, National League of Nursing, and American Hospital Association are reliable sources for assistance.

PREDICTIVE PRINCIPLE: Staff evaluation of nurse-managers reveals general areas of strengths and weaknesses in the leader as perceived by the evaluators and provides the nurse-manager with one means of validation for the effectiveness of the managerial practice.

Although many nurses in leadership and management positions believe wholeheartedly in the process of evaluation for their staff, it becomes an uncomfortable matter when their performance is under scrutiny. The usual procedure is for the immediate supervisor to evaluate the leader or manager, with only incidental input from the staff supervised.

Staff evaluation of the leader occurs on an informal basis through many ways. The leader/manager assumes staff assessment is high when there is cooperation, willingness to receive and follow orders, freedom to ask questions, and the goals of the group are achieved at a desired level. Conversely, the nurse-leader/manager senses evaluation of the role is unsatisfactory when there is quarreling, distrust, unwillingness to participate in planning and implementing care, and evidence that goals are not achieved.

The nurse-manager cannot ascertain objectively the reactions to the leader by those who are led unless the led are given the opportunity to respond anonymously. It is suggested that each staff member receive an evaluation form on which he can rank items that pertain to the nurse-leader/manager role. The tool should reflect the standards of care and criteria developed for the agency and the specified work area. Examples that may be included are "Gives appropriate answers to my questions," "Provides help when needed," and "Listens to me when I discuss nursing care problems." The leader's behavior is evaluated on a scale that indicates ranges of reaction such as "always," "almost always," "usually," "sometimes," and "never." Numeric responses are used sometimes, with an explanation as to their meaning. In addition to responses to items, comments and suggestions should always be asked for. The evaluations should be given to a person outside the clinical area for tabulation and typing of comments.

The results may then be given to the nurse-leader/manager. It is proposed that the first evaluation not be shared with anyone other than the leader/manager. This provides the nurse-manager with the opportunity to (1) obtain an overall assessment of himself in terms of strengths and weaknesses, (2) validate his own assessment with that of those led, (3) identify and deal with staff problems that might not otherwise have been known, and (4) make changes or adaptations in his own behavior.

Future evaluations by the staff could be included in the formal evaluation process of the nurse-leader/manager.

There are many benefits derived from positive and problem-oriented feedback. Open communication between leader and followers fosters trust and respect. When workers feel their work, attitudes, and comments are considered important by their leader, they are better able to value themselves as persons and as contributing members of the enterprise. When appreciation of the person evaluated is incorporated into the formal evaluation process, there is tangible evidence that this individual is worthy of recognition and reward.

With continuous feedback the evaluator avoids surprises. There is opportunity to check out with the worker areas where there may be misunderstanding. This averts the painful circumstance wherein a member is evaluated poorly without opportunity to offer defense or to make changes in behavior.

PREDICTIVE PRINCIPLE: An evaluation process that includes reciprocal participation both vertically and horizontally provides an avenue for high level morale and job satisfaction.

Assumption of responsibility for one's actions and individual growth and development requires feedback data. There is no way to equate the democratic process with secrecy. Employees want to know how they stand in the eyes of the evaluator and management because status in the organization, raises, promotion, and seniority depend to an extent on assessment of individual performance. Counseling after performance appraisal that invites a reciprocal process is an indispensable step in the evaluation process. Not only are the individual's strengths recognized and areas that need improvement identified, but a feeling of self-worth and value is nurtured that serves to promote a high level of job satisfaction.

The individual or group in question not only should see the progress report but also should actually be involved in the assessment process. The evaluator can then validate actions as they occur and are later discussed and recorded. Unresolved differences of opinion in appraisal may remain even after attempts at clarification. In a fair manner and with the right to appeal in due process, opportunity should be provided for opposing views to be heard and recorded. The group or person being reviewed may request a third party report in defense of stated opinion. The evaluator may also wish to elicit assistance from outside sources, such as an immediate supervisor, nurse-leader, or allied health personnel, in gathering data and preparing the report.

All written evaluations should be read and signed by the person evaluated in the presence of the evaluators, and any rebuttal or confirmation that the person evaluated wishes to enclose can then be attached and forwarded to the appropriate agency official or committee.

APPLICATION OF PREDICTIVE PRINCIPLES IN EVALUATION OF PERSONNEL

An LVN encounters the head nurse in the hall and says, "I wish you'd place Mrs. Mitchell (an aide) somewhere else. I can't stand to work with her another minute!" The nurse asks, "What is going on?" After clarification the head nurse determines the LVN believes Mrs. Mitchell is "not doing her job."

Problem	Principles	Prescription
To validate whether Mrs. Mitchell is performing job requirements.	Clear criteria and standards for measuring performance increase the objectivity and validity of evaluation.	Make preliminary observations and assessments based on standards of performance and criteria.
	Involvement of personnel in all phases of the evaluatory process increases belief in the fairness and accuracy of the evaluation, establishes a commitment to the evaluation, and increases motivation to utilize the results.	Inform Mrs. Mitchell that she is going to be evaluated. Determine if Mrs. Mitchell has job descriptions, standards of practice, and criteria and initiate cooperative activities of evaluation.
	Clear and concise role delineation and job descriptions enable employee, employer, and client to know the duties and responsibilities of the job.	
	Use of appropriate assessment tools and sufficient evaluative data gathered from varied situations increases the validity of the conclusions in the assessment of work performance.	Collect behavioral notations about Mrs. Mitchell's work; Mrs. Mitchell's evaluation about herself; and evaluation of patients cared for by her (made at various times of the work period, observing for the use of safety precautions, comfort measures, and efficiency).
	Frequent feedback on performance by a qualified evaluator, based on appropriate observations, reinforces desired behaviors and increases awareness of areas that need improvement.	Set time aside to compare data, draw conclusions, and design ways to improve. Record evaluation and make appropriate disposition of the information.
	Positive and problem-oriented feedback helps the person evaluated to change his behavior to more acceptable levels of performance.	

BIBLIOGRAPHY
Books

Alexander, E. L.: Nursing administration in the hospital health care system, ed. 2, St. Louis, 1978, The C. V. Mosby Co.

Armstrong, R. J., et al.: The development and evaluation of behavioral objectives, Worthington, Ohio, 1970, Charles A. Jones Publishing Co.

Biehler, R. F.: Psychology applied to teaching, Boston, 1971, Houghton Mifflin Co.

Durbin, R. L., and Springall, W. H.: Organization and administration of health care: theory, practice, environment, ed. 2, St. Louis, 1974, The C. V. Mosby Co.

Flanders, N. A.: Analyzing teaching behavior, Reading, Mass., 1970, Addison-Wesley Publishing Co., Inc.

Gagné, R. M.: Perspectives of curriculum evaluation, Chicago, 1967, Rand McNally & Co.

Haussman, R., and Hegyvary, S.: Monitoring quality of nursing care. Part III. Professional review for nursing: an empirical investigation, Washington, D.C., 1977, DHEW Pub. No. HRA, U.S. Government Printing Office.

Havelock, R. G.: A guide to innovation in education, Ann Arbor, Mich., 1970, Center for Research on Utilization of Scientific Knowledge, Institute for Social Research, The University of Michigan Press.

Hough, J. B., and Duncan, J. K.: Teaching: description and analysis, Reading, Mass., 1970, Addison-Wesley Publishing Co., Inc.

Litwack, S. R., and Wykle, M.: Counseling, evaluation and student development in nursing education, Philadelphia, 1972, W. B. Saunders Co.

Longest, B.: Management practices for the health professional, Reston, Va., 1976, Reston Publishing Co.

Mager, R. F., and Pipe, P.: Analyzing performance problems, Belmont, Calif., 1970, Fearon Publishers.

Schweer, J. E., and Gebbie, K. M.: Creative teaching in clinical nursing, ed. 3, St. Louis, 1976, The C. V. Mosby Company.

Shaffer, S. M., Indorato, K. L., and Deneselya, J. A.: Teaching in schools of nursing, St. Louis, 1972, The C. V. Mosby Company.

Stevens, B.: The nurse evaluator in education and service, New York, 1978, McGraw-Hill Book Co.

Warren, R. L.: Studying your community, New York, 1965, The Free Press.

Periodicals

Aiken, L., and Aiken, J.: A systematic approach to the evaluation of interpersonal relationships, Am. J. Nurs. 70(4):863-867, 1970.

Bare, C. E.: Behavioral changes through effective evaluation, J. Nurs. Educ. 6(11):7-9, 1967.

Bidwell, C., and Froebe, D.: Development of an instrument for evaluating hospital nursing performance, J. Nurs. Admin., pp. 10-15, Sept.-Oct. 1971.

Bloch, D.: Evaluation of nursing care in terms of process and outcome: issues in research and quality assurance, Nurs. Res. 24(4):256-263, 1975.

Bloch, D.: Criteria, standards, norms—crucial terms in quality assurance, J. Nurs. Admin., pp. 20-30, Sept. 1977.

Boe, G., and Cleveland, R.: Performance appraisal: an upbeat approach, Health Serv. Manager 9(7): 1-4, 1976.

Cantor, M.: Standard V: education for quality care, J. Nurs. Admin., pp. 48-54, Feb.-March 1973.

Clissold, G. K., and Metz, E. A.: Evaluation—a tangible process, Nurs. Outlook 14(3):41-45, 1966.

Cochran, T. C., and Ransen, P. J.: Developing an evaluation tool by group action, Am. J. Nurs. 62(3):94-97, 1962.

De Tornyay, R.: Measuring problem-solving skills by means of the simulated clinical nursing problem test, J. Nurs. Educ. 7(10):3-8, 1968.

Diddie, P.: Quality assurance—a general hospital meets the challenge, J. Nurs. Admin., pp. 6-16, July-Aug. 1976.

Ginter, P., and Rucks, A.: Performance measurement and control: try two approaches, Health Serv. Manager 10(10):1-3, 5, 1977.

Haar, L., and Hicks, J.: Performance appraisal: derivation of effective assessment tools, Nurs. Digest 5(3):38-47, Fall 1977.

Hamric, A., Gresham, L., and Eccard, M.: Staff evaluation of clinical leaders, J. Nurs. Admin., pp. 18-26, Jan. 1978.

Kirsch, A. I.: Planning for a sensible health care system, Nurs. Outlook 20(10):640-647, 1972.

Kopelke, C.: The nominal group approach as an evaluation tool, J. Nurs. Admin., pp. 32-34, Dec. 1976.

Long, K. R.: Consumer controlled nursing, Nurs. Outlook 17(9):51-54, 1969.

Marram, G. D.: Patients' evaluation of their care: importance to the nurse, Nurs. Outlook 21(5):322-324, 1973.

McClure, M.: The long road to accountability, Nurs. Outlook 26(1):47-50, 1978.

McGregor, D., and Smith, M.: An uneasy look at performance appraisal, J. Nurs. Admin., pp. 27-31, Sept. 1975.

Moore, M. A.: Philosophy, purpose and objectives: why do we have them? J. Nurs. Admin., pp. 9-14, May-June 1971.

Nelson, C., and Arford, P.: Strategy for clinical advancement, J. Nurs. Admin., pp. 46-51, April 1977.

N. L. N. Testing Services: Let's examine, an annotated bibliography on measurement and evaluation. Part II. Nurs. Outlook **16**(6):52-53, 1968.

Ortelt, J.: The development of a scale for rating clinical performance, J. Nurs. Educ. **5**(1):15-17, 1966.

Palmer, M. E.: Cumulative record of personal and professional growth, Nurs. Outlook **14**(6):39-41, 1967.

Pardee, G., et al.: Patient care evaluation is every nurse's job, Am. J. Nurs. **71**(10):1958-1960, 1971.

Peterson, G. G.: Evaluating the assignments head nurses make, Am. J. Nurs. **73**(4):641-644, 1973.

Rieder, G.: Performance review—a mixed bag, J. Nurs. Admin., pp. 20-24, May-June 1974.

Rosen, A., and Abraham, G. E.: Evaluation of a procedure for assessing the performance of staff nurses, Nurs. Res. **12**:78-82, Spring 1963.

Slee, V. N.: How to know if you have quality control, Hosp. Prog. **53**(1):38-43, 1972.

South, J.: The performance profile: a technique for using appraisals effectively, J. Nurs. Admin., pp. 27-31, Jan. 1978.

Topf, M.: A behavioral checklist for estimating the development of communication skills, J. Nurs. Educ. **8**(11):29-34, 1969.

Veninga, R.: Interpersonal feedback: a cost-benefit analysis, J. Nurs. Admin., pp. 40-43, Feb. 1975.

Wooley, A.: The long and tortured history of clinical evaluation, Nurs. Outlook **25**(5):308-315, 1977.

7 PREDICTIVE PRINCIPLES FOR CHANGING

BASIC GROUND RULES

Using clear communication and ground rules facilitates the interpersonal exchanges necessary for planned changes to occur.

Sharing ideas and opinions and using interpersonal communication predictive principles develop trust in the group process and facilitate effective problem solving.

CONDITIONS NECESSARY TO CHANGING

Failure of a nursing care delivery system to meet the needs of its practitioners, clients, and/or employers ensures changes in or the death of the system.

The breakdown of effectiveness of standard procedures and traditional organization patterns causes an increase in anxiety of the individual nursing care giver.

Experiencing high anxiety levels provides a need for change or adaptation, accompanied by an increase in individual and collective energy.

Need for change or adaptation stimulates personal fantasies of solutions or anticipation of the achievement of objectives.

Free exchange of ideas about goals and subgoals enables the establishment of specific and legitimate goals and collaboration for their achievement.

Explicit participation and support of the administration for change ensures that the changing group has the power and authority to implement plans for change.

Creating environmental and operational conditions that nurture the change process supports the potential success of the change effort.

Group commitment to the change process itself instead of to specific changes enables continuing investigation, growth, and improvement.

BASIC ORGANIZATIONAL PATTERNS FOR CHANGING

Use of an organizational pattern for changing that utilizes a framework for guiding the logistics of human resources in a task-oriented system promotes effective and efficient use of energy toward attainment of the goal.

BASIC PLANNING STRATEGIES FOR CHANGING

An explicit and definitive task analysis supports the ability of the client system to have an overall view of the subgoals and tasks to accomplish these goals.

Formation and assignment of task groups according to the task, time limitations, and capabilities of the change participants enable each member to contribute optimally.

Organization of change participants around components of task analysis decreases "power" and increases goal orientation of work groups.

Feedback from an alter group during the planning phase increases the probability that the group product will meet the staff needs, fulfill the task charge, and be useful to the target system.

Generating several solutions to a problem to achieve a goal enables the group to select an option most nearly in keeping with group needs.

Explicit rewards or recognition of individual or group achievement reinforces changing behaviors and promotes continuing efforts toward realization of goals.

Stability is a mirage or a nirvana for which one yearns or dreams. Individuals move through life seeking stability as knights sought the mythical Holy Grail. But life consists of balancing forces that tug and push in powerful energy fields. Nurses often feel caught in these forces, tossed and helpless in their grasp. The feeling of loss of control is frightening, and the energy drain in simply attempting to cope is tremendous. Energy exerted toward controlling self and others is often wasted because the forces of life's changes buffet people like a volleyball floating on a river. The resultant sense of powerlessness is a devastating feeling, and anger, aggression, frustration, and depression are high correlates of this powerlessness.

Control is the key. To affect, influence, and facilitate changes rather than be tossed hopelessly by them, one must focus the energy of control on the *forces causing change,* not the *people who are buffeted* or caught in the forces. This strange paradox can be likened again to the volleyball on the river. The force, speed, direction, and temperature of the water in the river directly influence the inflation pressure within the ball and the direction and rapidity with which it moves. If the change agent wishes to control the ball, his most reasonable approach is to control the flow of water in the river. Volleyballs do not lend themselves to having rudders, sails, or engines placed on them for control of movement; neither do people. Volleyballs can be tethered to a rope or string, but such control severely limits their movement and makes them single direction oriented. Real, free-moving direction is exerted by controlling the forces that regulate the flow of water. This can be accomplished by removing or adding rocks and boulders, leveling the terrain, smoothing the river bed, rechanneling a curve, damming up tributaries and reducing the water volume, or even altering the water temperature by adding a power plant. Similarly, energy directed toward identifying and isolating the forces causing change, examining the consequences of controlling each of these forces, wisely selecting which consequence is desirable, and manipulating the force field is energy that has a payoff in a directly controlled and effective change program.

The context of nursing and its influence on nursing change

Nursing is a process or system and is subject to influences of other processes. Alterations in other processes or systems act as stimuli to nursing, and nursing responds to them either adaptively or maladaptively. The system that does not respond will not remain viable. The system that responds maladaptively may cease to be functional and thus become outmoded or unused. Nursing is an open system and is linked with other living processes. Nursing is influenced by and is responsive to stresses from such other operant systems as the political system, the social system, and the technologic system.

1. *The political system.* Funding patterns, such legislated matters as national health insurance, licensure and accreditation laws, nurse and other health worker practice acts, and educational legislation affecting nursing care delivery, client receipt, and nursing manpower production and distribution constitute the political system or arena. This arena is the basic battleground for nursing care quality control, education and development, and delivery system funding. A system of universal health insurance is just a step away. Nursing leaders need to address themselves to the politics of health care and the subsequent cash flow patterns, which are derived from legislation on the community, state, and federal levels. Management of nursing care delivery will be influenced by political trends.

2. *The social system.* The characteristics of populations in social systems and their needs change. For instance, the values in the United States have shifted from the melting pot dream of complete amalgamation of ethnic and racial population to pridefully organized groups, with emphasis on cultural, racial, and ethnic uniqueness. The need system shifted when the value system changed. Population characteristics are constantly changing, both nationally and in the specific environment of any nursing care group. The shift may be to concentrations of senior citizens in particular locations as retirement villages become popular. There may be high density areas for specific ethnic groups or for great num-

bers of young people, as around colleges and universities. As mental hospitals empty and halfway houses, board and care homes, and other such group-living situations become more prevalent and preferred, concentrations of the disabled or socially maladapted will be more common. Other alterations are evidenced by changes in marriage patterns, the role of women, family dynamics, organizations and power groups, and trends in social values.

3. *The technologic system.* The technologic system affects nursing through various avenues. The equipment developed for health care giving and teaching makes nursing care pattern changes necessary. Transportation patterns are causing health care delivery modes to adapt. Mobile clinics, increasingly efficient urban transportation, satellite centers, and other nonhospital-oriented care systems are the direct result of increased transportation technology. *Computer technology* perhaps offers the largest untapped potential for influencing modifications in nursing care. This potential is being implemented in some health care centers on trial bases with varying success. The near future will see computer banks utilized for central recording and instant retrieval of client information for solving nursing problems. The client's chart will be a tape in a computer; his social security number will be the magic key to his cumulative health record, which will be easily transferred, with his permission, from one health arena to another, enabling the client's health care to become integrated. Nurses needing information relevant to the situation, from preoperative procedures to the order and sequence of diagnostic tests, may obtain this information with greatest efficiency by computerized instant data control.

Because of these and other forces, changes in nursing are gathering speed and nurses are learning to respond to the needs for alteration, to control some of the variables influencing change, and thus to affect the direction, speed, and quality of innovations. The problem with modification is that change is not permanent; each ensuing experience brings another set of circumstances to be viewed, dealt with, and recycled into the change format.

Nurses cannot usually affect all the forces that make up the context of nursing and thereby influence nursing response to those forces. However, nurses can attain enough influence over the immediate variables affecting nursing care to govern the direction, rate, and expression of change in nursing. This chapter addresses itself to those areas over which nursing leaders can exercise influence and effect change.

The process of changing*

The process of changing is a process of leadership and accountability. It is a method of organizational structure and management and a means of adaptation and problem solving. In the process of changing, the interdependent and mutually inclusive nature of all processes meaningful to nursing is obvious. Planned change is change with a purpose, devised to solve problems of nursing care through the use of behavioral science technologies. Planned change is a type of

---

*The remainder of this chapter is adapted from Bevis, E. O.: Curriculum building in nursing: a process, ed. 2, St. Louis, 1978, The C. V. Mosby Co., chap. 5 and 8.

human engineering where theories of human behavior are applied so that intelligent choices and actions are made. *The process of changing deals with alterations by choice and deliberation and is distinctly different from change by indoctrination, coercion, natural growth, and accident. In all facets of nursing, appropriate application of behavioral science techniques can produce changes that are the result of collective and collaborative choice, that is, participatory changing.*

For any nursing care system to change and grow, practitioners must respond through participation and collaboration to the vast number of variables in the health needs system with constructive deliberate changes in ways and means of coping with health problems. The use of theories of change with all recipients of nursing care—individual client, family group, and community—is necessary to the creative element of nursing processes.

One of the most difficult problems facing change agents is the lack of a conclusive theory on how to implement changes. Many studies have been done on the mechanics, the dynamics of change. According to Bennis,* there is no theory of changing. However, there are some propositions about effecting social change that can be used as guides for change in nursing.

Change theorists commonly refer to the components of the change process as follows:

Agent: Facilitator, social scientist, nurse (trained in the science of change)
Rate: Speed at which change takes place (evolutionary, slow, revolutionary, galloping)
Arena: Organization, institution (the place in which the change occurs, the environment of change)
Person: Target of change (client of change, the client system; may be an individual or a group)

The bureaucratic way in which nursing care agencies are organized—the use of authoritative patterns of organization, the use of committee structure, and the use of parliamentary law for decision making—locks nursing care systems into stable and sometimes inflexible patterns of unproductive behavior. These practices mitigate against optimal participation, generation of the most workable alternatives, and maximum use of all participants' talents in planning for changes.

Nursing agencies, like most institutions, are organized around the military model of authoritarian structure. Employees fit into a line organization that stacks in groups or units toward people with more and more power and authority.

All authoritarian organizations use some modification of this military pattern. There are many variations of format, but basically each person is responsible, at least in name, for all that occurs beneath his level in the hierarchical setup. In this way, decisions are delayed while they are passed up the line for someone with "more authority to make decisions" to act on. When groups organized in the traditional bureaucratic or hierarchical form deny that the authoritarian pattern exists, managers are placed in the position of having to maintain the responsibility because of institutional organization but with little or no authority because of the nursing group organization. Attempting to change the system can absorb energy that would be better used in making changes in nursing care and can

---

*Bennis, W. G.: Changing organizations, New York, 1966, McGraw-Hill Book Co., pp. 81-94 and 99-108.

effectively delay work to that end. Since the objective is usually nursing care improvement rather than institutional reorganization, a group can (for that objective) create a nursing organization that will facilitate work; for example, the staff can agree to try a different organizational mode for planning, creating, building, and testing change. Formal lines of operation can be maintained for other business and activities. The organizational problem is twofold: (1) how to get maximum participation by the total group involved with change and (2) how to make the changes flexible and responsive to society's or clients' needs. There are four categories of change factors that facilitate the two goals listed: (1) basic ground rules, (2) conditions necessary to changing, (3) basic organizational patterns for changing, and (4) basic planning strategies for changing. "Basic" is used because the suggestions here are beginning ones; for each phase of change activities the group may wish to modify, add to, delete, or suspend some of the organizational modes, ground rules, or planning strategies, depending on immediate needs.

BASIC GROUND RULES

During change, people become somewhat frightened of the future because it is an unknown. Change participants easily become suspicious that something is being put "over on them." People often feel isolated and powerless. Their usual power bases are dissolved, familiar landmarks disappear, and fear of having no influence over the changes often underlies some of the resistive behavior seen in groups. There are ways a change agent can avoid some of the difficulties resulting from the nebulosity of change. Ground rules for the group interaction involved in planning for and implementing changes can, when used consistently, help to decrease communication problems.

PREDICTIVE PRINCIPLE: Using clear communication and ground rules facilitates the interpersonal exchanges necessary for planned changes to occur.

Group work toward changing is facilitated if there are some basic operational ground rules for the accomplishment of objectives. Nurses working together for change need to develop ground rules that facilitate change and promote healthy group relationships. It is possible to achieve both ends. Most often, nursing staff working relationships have established patterns of interaction—some patterns that facilitate and some that inhibit functional communications. On any nursing staff there are committees or groups that are powerful. Immediately on the opening of an issue, pro and con groups draw their battle lines, and win-lose conflicts are generated. With people who have worked together for long periods of time, the "red flags" or "buttons" that will elicit known predictable reactions are familiar and assessable. Button pushing and red flag waving can be a favorite pastime or a smooth way to sidetrack an issue. There are no easy answers to the problem of establishing communication patterns that are more supportive, productive, and useful for facilitating change. An outside communication facilitator is invaluable to any group that considers approaching change. Neutral, uninvolved facilitators can help group members look at transactions and interactions, analyze the communication factors, and establish more effective ways of communicating. The following list provides a sample of items that groups might like to consider for operational ground rules. Each group will evolve its own list and supplement it as it is used. Following are some prescriptive interpersonal ground rules for change communications:

1. Try to have no surprises. Let everyone know in advance plans that are under way; peep previews, preliminary reports, and agreements to check out rumors will keep surprises to a minimum.

2. Provide as much informational input as possible. Part of the backbone of any planned change is the collection of data phase. "Handouts," consultation with experts, training sessions, television, movies, and other audiovisual materials, circulation of helpful articles, and data discussion sessions prior to the time the information must be used help to provide the data base necessary to planned changes.

3. Make conflicts explicit and legitimate. Bring out hidden agenda items so that real issues can be handled. Legitimacy of conflict makes it possible to look for alternatives that meet every group's goals rather than locking into win-lose power struggles.

4. Identify high investment areas (areas of high feelings) and elicit the help of a neutral facilitator either from within the group or from a source unrelated to the problem or issue itself. This enables all factions to struggle or "fight fair," for a facilitator will ensure each participant's rights.

5. Make risks legitimate and failure salvageable and acceptable. Operating in small task areas or "bits and pieces" allows greater risks to be taken because if one small part fails, the whole system of changes is not likely to fall apart. Back-up systems are other options for handling the problem if an original plan fails.

6. Make change in the middle of a trial run acceptable. Then if a plan being instituted is not working, alterations in the plan can be made without violating the group's preconceived notion that a trial run *must* be made all the way through.

7. Try to make it necessary to analyze failure or the reasons a part of a program is not working so that alterations and changes are not precipitous or without fair trial and so that the parts of a plan that may be causing the problems can be changed.

8. Agree to respond to each other's contributions to the group—comments, needs, and behaviors. Acknowledgment of entering into the group process reinforces and encourages continuing contributions and provides feedback. To be unacknowledged or consistently erased leaves one having few behavioral cues, having a feeling of impotence and powerlessness, and feeling very alone in the group. Other participants are aware of nonresponsiveness and are reluctant to risk contributing and not being responded to. A simple agreement to say "amen" or use some "body language" that is an obvious acknowledgment is necessary to a developing sense of being important to the group.

9. When complete win-lose deadlocks occur, agree to some form of action that will allow unlocking and saving of pride. Delay the issue or shuttle it to another time if necessary so the group can be explicitly charged to look for options to meet criteria for a solution that pleases all. One way is to say "What do we want in the solution that will fulfill the needs of both groups?" Then brainstorm for criteria. Try never to make a voting decision while in win-lose situations.

10. Delay making "final" decisions. Make tentative decisions, take a consensus, decide on a "trial" basis or accept something as a "provisional" or "working copy." Voting and recording in the minutes create a feeling of finality that makes it more difficult for members of the change group to accept alterations. Minutes become "laws," and members refer to them to "win" battles. If records are needed, call them "notes on the conference" or "record of discussion."

PREDICTIVE PRINCIPLE: Sharing ideas and opinions and using interpersonal communication predictive principles develop trust in the group process and facilitate effective problem solving.

Free exchange of ideas is not possible without an atmosphere of trust. Trust is basic to the mechanisms of planned change and is developed through consistently respecting the rights and limits of others and through meeting the needs of individuals and the group as a whole. Continuing communication requires a set of changing, evolving, colleague-oriented, equally participative ground rules. In autocratic systems, loyalty is given to the institution or group, the employer, "boss," or the supervising personnel. Peer group relations are marked by competition and a win-lose attitude in setting goals or generating solutions.

In a group in which the safeguards of ground rules have been established, in which each group member assumes the responsibilities for the group's work and is accountable for the quality of the group's communications, several things occur:

1. Individual faith in the ability of the group to produce successfully increases.
2. Individual respect for members' ability to participate increases.
3. Trust in the group process increases.
4. Group skill in problem solving increases.
5. Win-lose discussions decrease as the group becomes increasingly skillful at designing a multiplicity of options that are win-win.
6. Essential support for individuals becomes possible without sacrificing the goals of the group.
7. Loyalty to the profession of nursing and to colleagues begins to replace loyalty to agency or authority people.

CONDITIONS NECESSARY TO CHANGING

The rapid changes occurring in society cause change "waves" that affect all facets of life. Rigid structures, like seawalls, take the brunt of change waves and crack under the constant battering. Flexibility enables people and institutions to survive battering by altered needs that make change inevitable.

PREDICTIVE PRINCIPLE: Failure of a nursing care delivery system to meet the needs of its practitioners, clients, and/or employers ensures changes in or the death of the system.

Change occurs when needs arise that standard procedures and modes of behavior cannot meet. When new factors appear and many variables become part of a formally stable organization, new adaptive mechanisms are necessary to ensure continuity, quality, and efficiency of nursing care responses. Organizations, institutions, and individuals having found a modus operandi that works for them tend to "fix" or "solidify" that operational system, because the very fact that it works is reinforcing. Thus when factors in the environment or some of the needs of consumers of the nursing care delivery system change, the system fails to respond by modifying its standard mode of operation, causing a decrease in efficiency, unmet needs, unachieved purposes, a decrease in quality care, and a reduction in nurse and employer satisfaction.

For instance, when the quality expectations of clients change, the nursing care delivery system may or may not respond to that change. If the system does not alter with each new need or new variable, the problems begin to accrue and affect the relevancy of the whole care system. Eventually the variables accrue— changes in the ethnic composition of the client group, shifting emphasis in the numbers of clients cared for at home rather than in the hospital, number of clients seeking nursing care, changing laws affecting nursing education and service, and greater participation of clients in their own health care. The system of nursing must either respond to these changes or remain rigidly unresponsive and thereby become increasingly irrelevant. Subsequently, the majority of the nurse's time is spent in coping with a series of crises generated by poor adaptation. Nursing historically has had very few variables, for many factors were stable and dependable, and standard procedures and stylized care systems were the ways used to cope with those conditions. Now health care as a national concern is a focus of the energy of consumers, legislators, and health professionals. The variables are so many and the stable factors so few that standard, previously learned modes of operation will no longer serve. The cues in the nursing world that were formerly considered stable points of reference no longer exist. Nursing will either decline as a discipline or devise more flexible and versatile programs of service and education.

PREDICTIVE PRINCIPLE: The breakdown of effectiveness of standard procedures and traditional organization patterns causes an increase in anxiety of the individual nursing care giver.

Anxiety is the signal of readiness to change. Even though mild anxiety is the natural state of an organism, a rise in the normal level of anxiety makes for discomfort, and nurses often seek to return to a more comfortable state of being. If change procedures that will enable better coping with the new factors are not instituted, anxiety will continue to increase until total efficiency is affected. Some nursing groups do not institute plans for changing until there are a limited number of choices; change is then a matter of crisis. In this instance, change that is planned for long-term goals must be delayed while crisis intervention occurs, panic is controlled, or extreme anxiety states are lowered.

Crisis is a time when intense learning can occur and rapid changes can be made. A change agent must be available during crisis to participate with the nursing group in crisis intervention activities. Changes are easier when nurses preplan and work out changes in advance. But when a care delivery crisis occurs because of legislation, administrative edict, client demands, or changes in the nursing care group composition, crisis can become the useful vehicle for change.

PREDICTIVE PRINCIPLE: Experiencing high anxiety levels provides a need for change or adaptation, accompanied by an increase in individual and collective energy.

People in the anxiety–need-to-change sequence exhibit greater work output. However, if there is no articulation of goals, the work output takes on the form of "busy work," of trying to make the obsolete system work successfully, of vicious circles, or of activities designed to control self and others. If the next phase of planned change is instituted, energy is available for work toward planning change. Nurses experiencing anxiety are open to alternatives and can learn new behaviors both for planning and for implementing changes. Change agents who can provide options, models, cues and stimulants and otherwise facilitate solution-directed activities during anxiety help the group use their energy in positive ways. This phase of anxiety, when the energy output level is increased, is "prime time" for changing.

PREDICTIVE PRINCIPLE: Need for change or adaptation stimulates personal fantasies of solutions or anticipation of the achievement of objectives.

Everyone who is troubled dreams a dream of "trouble free." Fantasies occur, such as "If only this and that were so, all would be right with heaven and earth" and "If we had this or that in our agency, the millennium would be here." Everyone anticipates longingly the achievement of his private vision of how things could be better. One of the difficulties is that visions of improvement, visions of *how* things could be improved, and visions of "objectives" are *private*. As private objectives, they have the connotation of illegitimacy, or being unacceptable. People fear offending other people—"power" people, vested interest groups, and friends. If the goals are shared at all, they are shared with a few chosen associates. When nurses share ideas and goals, they find others in the group have common dreams and goals. Aloneness is decreased, and objectives become legitimate.

PREDICTIVE PRINCIPLE: Free exchange of ideas about goals and subgoals enables the establishment of specific and legitimate goals and collaboration for their achievement.

Visions of the future can be translated into group objectives only if the group provides a time or a mechanism for articulating ideas and fantasies about the future so that goals for work and criteria for changes can be established.

Change can be just a "happening," that is, a product of chance. Chance brings many alterations—some toward a desired end, some away from it. The ability to talk freely together as a group involved in changing promotes the realization of group goals through the mechanism of *making goals and means for reaching them legitimate, explicit topics for discussion.* Participation of those affected by change at every level—administration, head nurses, staff nurses, LVNs, aides, and students—generates a commitment to the change process itself and makes collaboration for specific tasks possible and desirable.

PREDICTIVE PRINCIPLE: Explicit participation and support of the administration for change ensures that the changing group has the power and authority to implement plans for change.

Every nursing organization has an administrator, a supervisor, a chief, a chairman, or a director. This person, in the eyes of the institution, is accountable to his superior for the activities of the staff, the delivery of care, and the success or failure of the developing change enterprise. Thus no changes of major dimensions can occur without the consent and participation of the ranking persons. Because authority figures have and can exercise veto power or can influence administrators up the line to exercise veto power, the veto ability needs to be made explicit to the planning group. Inclusion of high level management people in work (task groups, heuristics, findings) decreases surprise, keeps them involved with the changes being planned, and reduces the chance that vetoes will occur.

PREDICTIVE PRINCIPLE: Creating environmental and operational conditions that nurture the change process supports the potential success of the change effort.

For change to occur, certain conditions must be provided. The change agent or manager seeks, in collaboration with others, to establish these conditions so that planned change can proceed. These conditions are as follows:

1. *Key organizational people must support and participate in the change.* In nursing care delivery system change, administrators, directors, committee chairmen, in-service education coordinators, physicians, and other key power people must support the idea of planned change as a total group effort. Since this means relinquishing some power to the group and exposing oneself in the group on a peer basis, it is at first a beginning acquiescence but one designed to become a growing commitment. Dignified retirements, transfers, and resignations are not necessary except in rare instances. Trust, collaboration, peer relationships, and free exchange of ideas are *learned* phenomena, and, with a skilled change agent, any group can learn these behaviors.

2. *The processes employed in change must be congruent with the philosophy, processes, and goals of change.* The ends do not justify the means, and the means employed for change must be of the same kind and caliber as the desired change. People learn as much from models as they learn from any other learning mode, and the means for obtaining change furnish a behavior model for groups in the process of change. If an authority figure resists change, and if subterfuge, underground tactics, deviousness, and dishonesty are used to obviate the authority structure, the planned change will contain the same group tactics; thus the seeds of failure for the new attainments are sown.

3. *Participation in change is a voluntary commitment, as is opposition to change, and the battle must be freely and overtly fought.* The implications of this condition are (1) that the only pressures existing on individual participants are peer group pressures and (2) that only in discussions where differences are aired openly without authority pressure for a particular, previously determined outcome can there be true resolution through the examination of available alternatives. In addition, mutual agreement must be reached within the change group and not imposed by an authority figure.

4. *All relevant or interdependent units are involved or oriented to the fact that the process of change is occurring in one of the groups so that change does not damage, shock, or interrupt other contingent units.* For instance, if nurses wish to change the delivery pattern in a section of an agency to make their care of better quality, then nurses of other sections, physicians, other departments (x-ray, laboratory, and dietary), and all authority people involved should be

notified so that shock, threat, and articulation problems are anticipated and minimized. Organizational patterns undergoing change in a nursing care situation need to be communicated to other departments interconnected with nursing so that others can aid the change instead of blocking it and so that the changes do not interrupt or decrease the effectiveness of others or of services to the client. The administration could question the feasibility or workability of the new plan or the plan could fail, not because the change is ineffective but because the proper "other" people were not consulted, alerted, oriented, or included in the planning phase.

PREDICTIVE PRINCIPLE: Group commitment to the change process itself instead of to specific changes enables continuing investigation, growth, and improvement.

Groups who organize for change and who proceed to plan and implement change can devise a desired change that gets frozen into decisions of total commitment. Commitment to the specific change, rather than to changing, is a trap. Using words like "provisional," "tentative," "trial," and "interim" communicates the concept of change as a process—continuing and progressing forever. Nurse commitment to flexibility, innovation, and creativity becomes real only with use. The process-of-change concept is actualized by building a framework for change that provides for and necessitates constant use of feedback for making continuous alterations to the whole nursing care system. For instance, no public health nurse would make a plan for a visit to be acted on regardless of the conditions encountered on the visit. The conditions encountered on arriving at the client's home would become rapidly gathered data that would probably be utilized quickly to alter the preconceived plan. The same habit of gathering and utilizing data and feedback and altering plans becomes a habit, whether one is dealing with nursing care delivery system, individual patient care, or organizational structure.

BASIC ORGANIZATIONAL PATTERNS FOR CHANGING

Most health agencies are organized for stability. Standing committees, steering committees, executive committees, and ad hoc committees are the avenues through which the work of the agency is accomplished. Normal bureaucratic agencies are structured to change slowly. They do change, but their response to the forces causing the need to change is slowed by the very mechanisms that provide them with stability and permanency. To speed change to make agencies more responsive to social forces, new, sometimes temporary, and sometimes permanent alterations must be made in the organizational structure.

PREDICTIVE PRINCIPLE: Use of an organizational pattern for changing that utilizes a framework for guiding the logistics of human resources in a task-oriented system promotes effective and efficient use of energy toward attainment of the goal.

Organizations can take a variety of organizational patterns or structures. The types described here will be traditional (bureaucratic) nursing agency organization, modified traditional or "linking pin," collegia, and functional team.

Traditional or bureaucratic systems are typical of nursing service organizations. Hospitals, colleges, most businesses, and governmental agencies in the United States function under a hierarchial structure. Committee structure

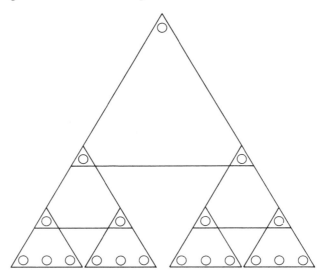

Fig. 17. Traditional pyramid type committee structure of bureaucracies.

pyramids toward the top chairmanships, which are awarded by rank and tenure. A committee superstructure of "chairpersons" meets and plans the work other committees are to do. Fig. 17 illustrates this organizational format. Changes are slow and difficult to make when using this organizational pattern. Response time is delayed while decisions are filtered through a maze of official channels.

Nursing organizations usually have all six characteristics listed by Bennis as typical of authoritarian organizations[*]:

1. They have a division of work based on functional specialization (often medical model clinical specialization).
2. They have clear-cut channels of communication and hierarchy of authority and responsibility.
3. They are characterized by rules and bylaws and job descriptions that cover the rights, duties, responsibilities, and relationships of members.
4. They have specific and predetermined procedural specifications and directions for handling work situations.
5. There is a certain amount of impersonality in the relationships between levels of the hierarchy.
6. Tenure and promotion are based on job or technical competence.

The modified traditional or "linking pin" organizational system has many of the characteristics of the preceding list. It varies somewhat in that the groups within the organization have some autonomy; leaders may be appointed or elected and are not necessarily chosen because they are ranking members of the hierarchy; leadership can rotate periodically; and one or more members of each group belong either to another group or to a central "executive or advisory" board or group, thus linking each group and providing continuity, liaison, and communication. Procedure manuals, job descriptions, and other marks of bureaucratic organization are still in evidence. However, in linking pin organizational structure, committees are small, task oriented, and organized so that one member of a

[*]Bennis, W. G.: Changing organizations, New York, 1966, McGraw-Hill Book Co., p. 5.

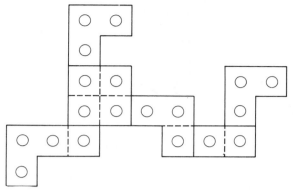

Fig. 18. Linking pin organizational structure. One person on a given task group serves on another task group working on a related task, thus furnishing a communication link and enabling the tasks to complement each other.

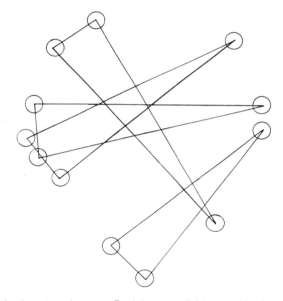

Fig. 19. Collegia. Objectives are clear cut. Participants collaborate with whom they need to at the time to achieve the goal. Lines are temporal. Membership in group is by ability. (From Bevis, E. O.: Curriculum building in nursing process, ed. 2, St. Louis, 1978, The C. V. Mosby Co.)

task committee serves on a related committee and is the communication pathway that enables work to be complementary and supportive toward goal attainment. Authority people may or may not be the "link" (Fig. 18).

On the opposite side of the continuum is a very loosely knit organizational pattern called a collegium. Individual accountability is an earmark of a collegial organization; roles are almost completely blurred and can shift and change with the task to be accomplished (Fig. 19). Small groups assemble and shift in membership based on the needs of the group to accomplish an objective. Group membership is temporal, as is group leadership. Leadership is almost always by ability to facilitate the task, knowledge of the part of the task being worked on, sudden inspiration or insights, and other phenomena. Investment of energy is toward the

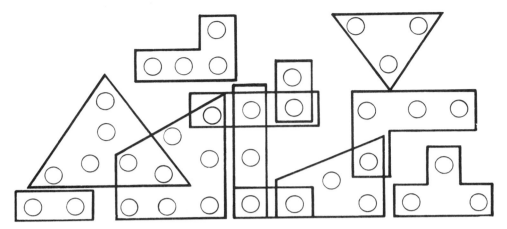

Fig. 20. Functional team. Groups are established and dissolved around tasks that need doing. Membership is by ability to contribute to the task. Role blurring occurs. Rank, position, and tenure are unimportant. All participate equally. (From Bevis, E. O.: Curriculum building in nursing: a process, ed. 2, St. Louis, 1978, The C. V. Mosby Co.)

task, and no energy is committed to stabilizing the group. The "job" or "task" to be accomplished can be envisioned as being like a basketball passed back and forth among the players according to their place on the court, the pattern of play, or their particular talents. The group moves the ball down the court, throwing it from one person or small group to another until at last someone puts it in the basket and the job is finished. If the ball hits the backboard and bounces back into play (feedback), reworking occurs until the ball is finally put through the basket and the goal is attained.

The type of organization that offers the most for change in nursing is a modification and synthesis of the collegium and linking pin approaches—the functional team or task group organization.

In functional teams (Fig. 20), groups or task forces of from two to five participants are organized around specific tasks. Membership on the task force lasts for the duration of the job. Once the job is accomplished, the task force dissolves. Role blurring occurs, and task force members contribute on equal footing according to their ability. Leadership in the group evolves from group needs and is not imposed on the group from without. Ground rules may change from task to task or from day to day within the same task force, for they, too, are generated in response to the needs of the task and not on a permanent basis. Completed work can either be sent to another task group for a critique—called an alter group or a feedback group (Fig. 21)—or submitted to the whole group. Reworking, revising, or altering based on the feedback may be done by the same task force or may be altered by the critiquing group, depending on the agreement between the groups. The difference between a collegium and a functional team is the degree of structure. Functional teams are highly structured, that is, they are given clear directions, time binds, checks and balances, a quality control or feedback mechanism, and a person or group with whom to communicate. Collegia work as a "happening."

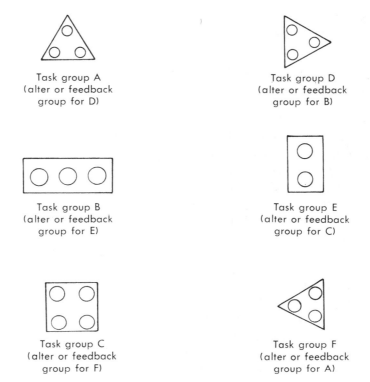

Fig. 21. Typical task group organization pattern with feedback or alter group assignments. (From Bevis, E. O.: Curriculum building in nursing: a process, ed. 2, St. Louis, 1978, The C. V. Mosby Co.)

BASIC PLANNING STRATEGIES FOR CHANGING

An altered organizational pattern for change preserves an altered way of looking at the task of changing. Often nursing care groups do not know what they wish to change to. They just know what they wish to change from. The goals and the content of changing can be separated from the process of changing. The change process can follow any number of patterns. The most effective patterns use a task analysis framework. Task analysis is a methodology that arose from systems analysis. Systems analysis was used during World War II to ensure the delivery of weapons to the fighting forces by specific times. Systems analysis has been most commonly associated with the space program and has been highly successful in enabling many companies manufacturing a small component of a space system to complete their work and deliver their component at the time specified with confidence that the component would work effectively when interlinked with the other components being produced. These same methods are now component tasks. These tasks are then assigned to small groups. The completed product is used as a basis for the next stage of work, forming a systemic linkage of work designed to achieve goals.

PREDICTIVE PRINCIPLE: An explicit and definitive task analysis supports the ability of the client system to have an overall view of the subgoals and tasks to accomplish these goals.

PREDICTIVE PRINCIPLE: Formation and assignment of task groups according to the task, time limitations, and capabilities of the change participants enable each member to contribute optimally.

PREDICTIVE PRINCIPLE: Organization of change participants around components of task analysis decreases "power" plays and increases goal orientation of work groups.

The traditional way of organizing for change involves the establishment of committees. Committees, subcommittees, and ad hoc committees are the modes used in most bureaucratic organizations that rely on parliamentary law, parliamentary procedures, and parliamentary organizational forms. Committees have several characteristics that make them poor means for achieving change:

1. Committees tend to be power bases for individuals and factions in an organization. Much effort then goes into maintaining the power group, obtaining more power, and exercising power.
2. Power struggles tend to develop over traditional "red flag" issues, and individuals lock into a win-lose situation. The parliamentary procedures then tend to inhibit the search for alternatives that are win-win. The very act of voting locks people into win-lose modes.
3. Once power struggles arise in a committee and power lines are drawn, each new issue perpetuates the power struggle. This causes compromises to be made in ways that may pull the teeth from changes. This is done over the issue of power and influence and not often over the issues inherent in change.
4. Committee membership becomes a prestige item, and changes that threaten the prestige, power, or existence of membership are resisted. Thus the committee tends to structure in order to perpetuate its own existence. Energy that could go into accomplishing goals is funneled off into committee maintenance.

The first major planning strategy for change is to opt for a structure that enables nurses and interested others to form small, loosely knit task groups. These groups are formed of individuals who have an interest in or expertise for a specific task to achieve a specific goal. A task group organizational pattern assumes a task analysis format. Task analysis is a method of taking a large goal or "piece" of desired change and breaking it down into the steps, subgoals, or "tasks" that will ensure the reaching of the overall objective. Often the sheer size and magnitude of a change is frightening. Task analysis is reassuring in that groups can see the probability of succeeding in a small given task, where the overall job may be overwhelming. Small tasks or jobs are easier to achieve, and success is fairly quick, clear, and definitive. Success then breeds successes, and the reinforcement of completing one small bit of the total job motivates and energizes the nursing group to go on to the next task group and the next task. New people, new working relationships, and a new task dissipate the potential for developing power plays that siphon energy from the job to be done.

Every change goal can be reached by the simple expedient measure of analyzing the steps necessary to reach the goal. In each of the steps or sequence components there is a group of tasks for that component that must occur before that phase of development can be successfully organized and accomplished. Each group will need to analyze the tasks that are necessary to the change patterns of each individual nursing group. The following is an example of a task analysis.

Example of a task analysis

Goal: To create a better nursing care record or charting form and system.

Task analysis:
1. Devise criteria for a desirable charting form.
2. Imagine components of a format that would meet those criteria.
3. Generate two or three alternative plans for using the components.
4. Choose a plan or synthesize from the ones presented.
5. Measure synthesized plan against established criteria.
6. Plan and select ways and means for testing a sample run of the new charting forms.
7. Institute the test run.
8. Get feedback from testers and share with all work groups.
9. Alter plan, using feedback.
10. Retest.
11. Confirm and implement or revise and retest the plan until perfected.
12. Establish regular evaluation and review so change is ongoing.

Example of task analysis for task 1: Devise criteria for a desirable charting form.
1. List the purposes of the nursing care record.
2. List the content necessary to accomplish the purposes.
3. Survey target group: What do participants like about present forms? What is disliked about them? What would the members prefer in a form? Do the present forms accomplish the purposes as listed? Categorize and sort findings and provide summary.
4. Survey similar agencies over the country for sample forms and analyze for strengths and limitations. Categorize and sort findings; provide a summary.
5. Survey the literature on nursing record formats. Distribute useful articles or annotated notes or summaries to target group.
6. Obtain summaries and findings from all task groups. Ask three different task groups working independently to present the criteria by which they would evaluate a charting form and system.
7. Each of the three groups presents its criteria to three different alter groups for critique and feedback.
8. Select and use the feedback felt appropriate to improve criteria.
9. Present criteria of all three task groups to the target population. Obtain feedback and suggestions.
10. Assign one task group to use feedback to make one criteria list to create a charting form and system.

The task force organizational pattern allows implementation of a format for change that facilitates optimal participation by all people involved in change. A task analysis framework for organizing nursing care systems change enables tasks small enough to be handled in a short time span to be assigned to a specific group for a specific purpose. The tasks listed can be divided among small task forces and the work accomplished efficiently.

By using the task group format, power struggles have little time to develop and compromise is often delayed until adequate numbers of choices have been generated. Groups are small enough so that each member can generate possibilities and choices and bring them to the group for a critique. The group can then put together the desired product from individual contributions.

Task groups are transitory, membership expectations are for a temporary existence, work is task oriented with no energy given to maintaining the group, and dissolution is natural when the task is completed.

Working in task groups using a task analysis as a basis for organizing for change accomplishes some of the following:

1. Explicit and definitive task analysis provides client systems with an overall view of goals and steps that must be taken to reach the goals.
2. Established target dates enable change participants to pace their work realistically.
3. Temporary organization keeps the faculty and students job or task oriented and decreases focus on power.
4. Participating in task groups outside the area of immediate skill widens the horizon of individual members' views of nursing, decreases tunnel vision, provides scope, and brings fresh ideas from people not necessarily "locked into" a single system or way of accomplishing a goal or viewing a concept.
5. Working with people outside of usual committee structure broadens the base of working relationships and decreases fantasies about what colleagues are like; it establishes new communication habits and patterns.

PREDICTIVE PRINCIPLE: Feedback from an alter group during the planning phase increases the probability that the group product will meet the staff needs, fulfill the task charge, and be useful to the target system.

The second planning strategy that is most useful is to provide for feedback prior to total staff and management consideration. Feedback is provided by task groups called alter groups (Fig. 16). These critique groups provide checks and balances so that the creators of an idea, or task, can have the benefit of objective feedback, for example, a disinterested perspective for examining the work, asking questions, suggesting clarification of specific parts, looking at congruencies between parts, suggesting revision, addition, or deletion in the work, and any other functions of feedback. The use of an alter group not only improves the product of the task group and helps to prepare it for total group discussion, but also widens the base of support through investment. When the second group becomes involved, it has already participated in the accomplishing of the task and therefore is prepared to speak to it and to support, at least in some measure, the group originally assigned to that task. The more people who participate in the creation of an idea or the completion of a task, the more balanced the discussion of that suggested alternative is likely to be.

PREDICTIVE PRINCIPLE: Generating several solutions to a problem to achieve a goal enables the group to select an option most nearly in keeping with group needs.

The third basic planning strategy suggested here is the generation of more than one choice for every phase of, or task in, change building (see example task analysis). Choice is perhaps the most important aspect of facilitating change. One of the reasons preplanned change can be so effective is that groups need not be faced with having to accept an option because it is the only one available. Group planning for change includes, at every phase, the assigning of more than one task group to a task, with directions to work independently of each other, and the offering of more than one alternative plan to the total group. The consequences of having a choice are that (1) groups tend to be more stimulated as they look at options and discuss the potentialities and liabilities of each plan; (2) congruence or incongruence of parts of the plans with the theoretical base of the total plan are brought to light; and (3) the best parts of the options can be pooled for developing a plan that meets the needs of the group.

PREDICTIVE PRINCIPLE: Explicit rewards or recognition of individual or group achievement reinforces changing behaviors and promotes continuing efforts toward realization of goals.

The last important strategy for change to be discussed here involves an obvious and explicit reward system. There is reward inherent in creating workable changes, which are tangible manifestations of visions. The more emphasis that can be placed on the continuity of the road from the past (what individuals wished to accomplish) to the present (what the total group has accomplished), the greater will be the feeling of success. Beyond the reinforcement of accomplishing goals is the individual group member's contribution to that goal. Often work becomes such a synthesis of so many people's ideas that individual contributions are lost, and an anonymity develops that makes the work itself impersonal and easy to disown as not being a part of each person as an individual. There are some things that change agents can do to keep the personal element in the changes without destroying the group feeling. For instance, when members of a task group, three or four people, collaborate on a special project and generate a piece of the puzzle appropriate for distribution to others or for publication, it is reinforcing to give recognition to the people preparing the product. By-lines, such as "prepared by Dianne Nicholson and Lucy Miller, in collaboration with other members of the nursing staff of Hillview Health Center," are expressive of the individual work and the contribution of the "whole," and thus give special credit to the authors without detracting from the general credit due the group. Following are other reinforcing activities:

1. Encourage and facilitate publication of materials generated.
2. Provide letters, encouragement, and active support for efficiency evaluations and promotions.
3. Speak to "power" people, for example, head nurses, supervisors, and other managers, of specific contributions individuals have made.
4. Promote publicity for innovative endeavors through local newspapers, agency newsletters, and so on.
5. Celebrate milestones of accomplishment with small parties (this activity interrupts flow and marks progress and thus provides a point of reference).
6. Save early work as a starting point marker to make comparisons and provide perspectives on how far the group has come in achieving changes.
7. Distribute general congratulatory letters periodically when particularly effective results have been achieved.

These activities are useful for role modeling the process of valuing the contributions of individuals. Too often nurses tend to devalue their own work and value that of outsiders. Any activity that provides patterns of behavior establishing the value of "home town prophets" builds self-confidence and helps the group make it legitimate to use each other as consultants.

APPLICATION OF PREDICTIVE PRINCIPLES OF CHANGING

A representative from the evening shift approaches the head nurse and states: "The afternoon personnel have asked me to represent them. They wish to discontinue charting on evening shift patients. It is a meaningless bit of busy work and a waste of time. We could just check off medications and sign the nursing record page that we've seen the patient."

Problem	Principles	Prescription
How to enable the group to determine what changes in charting and charting policies will best meet the needs of patients and staff.	Failure of a nursing care delivery system to meet the needs of its practitioners, clients, and/or employers ensures changes in or the death of the system.	Make critique of the system legitimate and elicit consensus that change is needed.
	The breakdown of effectiveness of standard procedures and traditional organization patterns causes an increase in anxiety of the individual nursing care giver.	Elicit agreement to participate in work toward finding workable solution to problem.
	Experiencing high anxiety levels provides a need for change or adaptation accompanied by an increase in individual and collective energy.	Channel energy into task groups, goal setting, and goal attainment.
	Need for change or adaptation stimulates personal fantasies of solutions or anticipation of the achievement of objectives.	Involve group in brainstorming about problems and possible workable nursing recording forms and procedures.
	Free exchange of ideas about goals and subgoals enables the establishment of specific and legitimate goals and collaboration for their achievement.	Brainstorm about a process for change that would involve all concerned and accomplish goals; brainstorm about goals and steps or tasks necessary to achieve goals.
	Explicit participation and support of the administration for change ensures that the changing group has the power and authority to implement plans for change.	Invite appropriate power people to take part in the discussions from the first or have regular appointments; be sure power people condone or consent to potential change.
	Creating environmental and operational conditions that nurture the change process supports the potential success of the change effort.	
	Use of an organizational pattern for changing that utilizes a framework for guiding the logistics of human resources in a task-oriented system promotes effective and efficient use of energy toward attainment of the goal.	Get consensus for an organization for change that uses everyone's potential without regard to status, rank, or position—transient task groups of some kind.
	An explicit and definitive task analysis supports the ability of the client system to have an overall view of the subgoals and tasks to accomplish these goals.	Assign a task group to do a task analysis on overall goal.

Problem	Principles	Prescription
	Formation and assignment of task groups according to the task, time limitations, and capabilities of the change participants enables each member to contribute optimally.	Assign task groups to tasks identified by the analysis group.
	Feedback from an alter group during the planning phase increases the probability that the group product will meet the staff needs, fulfill the task charge, and be useful to the target system.	When tasks are completed, give to feedback group; rework task, based on feedback.
	Generating several solutions to a problem to achieve a goal enables the group to select an option most nearly in keeping with group needs.	Be sure that several task groups work on alternative solutions so group will have a choice.
	Explicit rewards or recognition of individual or group achievement reinforces changing behaviors and promotes continuing efforts toward realization of goals.	Acknowledge groups' and participants' contribution; write notes for change participants; acknowledge ideas; give reinforcement for participation; set up mechanism for continued review, testing, and evaluation of planned program of change.

BIBLIOGRAPHY
Books

Alexander, E. L.: Nursing administration in the hospital health care system, ed. 2, St. Louis, 1978, The·C. V. Mosby Co.

Bennis, W. G.: Changing organizations, New York, 1966, McGraw-Hill Book Co.

Bennis, W. G., Benne, K. D., and Chin, R.: The planning of change, ed. 2, New York, 1969, Holt, Rinehart & Winston, Inc.

Bevis, E. O.: Curriculum building in nursing: a process, ed. 2, St. Louis, 1978, The C. V. Mosby Co.

Havelock, R. G.: A guide to innovation in education, Ann Arbor, Mich., 1970, Center for Research on Utilization of Scientific Knowledge, Institute of Social Research, The University of Michigan Press.

Saunders, L.: Permanence and change. In Lewis, E. P.: Changing patterns of nursing practice, New York, 1971, The American Journal of Nursing Co.

Seiler, J. A.: Systems analysis in organizational behavior, Homewood, Ill., 1967, The Dorsey Press, Inc.

Periodicals

Simms, L. L.: Administrative changes and implications for nursing practice in the hospital, Nurs. Clin. North Am. **8**(2):227-234, June 1973.

8 PREDICTIVE PRINCIPLES OF LEADERSHIP BEHAVIOR

FUNDAMENTALS OF LEADERSHIP

Understanding various managerial systems and the work environment provides the leader with a basis for determining a suitable type of leadership for the situation or for developing congruent adaptive behaviors within the environment.

A clear operational definition of leadership expectations expedites role definition and role enactment.

Knowledge of theory levels and ability to formulate valid predictive principles promote the leader's ability to identify the levels on which members are functioning to facilitate growth in problem solving and goal attainment.

Identification of leadership traits associated with managerial climates facilitates the conversion of traits into operational behaviors.

AWARENESS OF SELF

Knowledge and understanding of factors that contribute to mental health permit self-assessment of one's state of mental health.

Identification of the leader's own needs aids in the identification of needs of others.

Accurate appraisal of self promotes healthy emotional organization.

Acceptance of self creates a climate for the acceptance of others.

Accomplishing goals through assertive behavior enables a nurse-leader to exercise the rights of self without denying the rights and feelings of others.

Consistent use of nonassertive behavior ignores personal rights of the nurse-leader and leads to lowered self-esteem and maladaptive behaviors.

Achievement of one's goals through aggressive acts violates another person's rights and results in feelings of domination, humiliation, and hostility.

KNOWLEDGE OF THE JOB

The demands of the situation in which a leader is to function influence the qualities, characteristics, knowledge, and skills necessary for successful leadership.

The degree to which the leader is clinically knowledgeable and competent directly influences feelings of security about the appropriateness of nursing activity.

MUTUAL RESPECT

Understanding and practicing the basic elements of mutual respect facilitate effective leadership.

Expressions of respect for others by the leader precipitate acts of mutual respect among members.

OPEN CHANNELS OF COMMUNICATION

Knowledge of appropriate channels of communication facilitates efficient utilization of line organization.

The nurse working in an expanded role provides leadership initiative in establishing channels of communication congruent with the role.

KNOWLEDGE OF PARTICIPANTS' CAPABILITIES

An understanding of sociocultural backgrounds of members helps the leader assess job capabilities.

Reactions to stress influence efficiency of performance in the work situation.

Knowledge of a care giver's preparation and experience promotes fullest use of skills and provides a basis for continued growth.

ENVIRONMENT

A work environment that is open and amenable to valid change assists in personal and professional growth and development.

Leadership and management have many similarities. Leadership differs from management in the sense that leadership means to lead or guide others, whereas management is the act of handling, controlling, directing, and supervising. Effective leaders may utilize elements of management in the leadership process, but it is not always necessary to their success as leaders. A leader is successful in his role only if he has followers who are willing to be influenced in goal setting and achievement.

The practice of professional nursing carries with it the responsibility to lead, manage, and/or facilitate others.

Leadership is not automatic. Effective leadership is a learned process; it is the ability to mobilize behaviors toward the achievement of a purpose through the investiture and acceptance of authority. The culmination of all nursing activity is in the delivery of patient care. Scientifically based, problem-oriented behavior in the client's interest will produce quality care and is likely to be administered at less cost to the consumer of health services.

The outcome of nursing leadership function is some aspect of nursing practice. Administrative emphasis is on clinical competency, proficiency in nursing performance, management of clinical nursing activities and patient advocacy, as well as operation of a unit. Health care delivery groups with varying responsibilities for patient care need to interact with each other for better patient care in a systematic and collaborative fashion. Communication between administration, medicine, other health care givers, consumers, and nurses concerning health care will increase the effectiveness of that care. The overall quality of patient care is effective and efficient only to the degree that nurse-leaders relate to the environment in which they perform in a significant and organizational manner.

This chapter discusses the fundamentals of leadership, awareness of self, and knowledge of the tasks to be performed. Similarly, it is concerned with the capabilities of the leader, as well as with the environment in which nursing care is rendered. Most of these concepts have been integrated into the content of the preceding chapters.

FUNDAMENTALS OF LEADERSHIP

Historically, leadership was awarded to the strong. From primitive man to the present, rule of the powerful has been felt on all levels. Cunning and brain power have replaced brute strength, but the system still exists in some milieus. It is a hallmark of an advanced civilization that leaders receive their authority from the groups they lead and maintain their leadership only as long as they meet the needs of the groups they are guiding.

Even in the most democratic of leadership situations, authority and power struggles exist. In nursing, for example, for too long the capable nurse-leaders have not been delegated authority and power commensurate with responsibility for planning and decision making. Traditional management practices reflect the belief that nurses at the operational level require close supervision and control; therefore someone else must retain the power. The divestment of authority from those nurses on operational levels has led to power struggles. If ignored, these power struggles dissipate energy, divide and demoralize the participants, and result in decreased productivity.

It is necessary for clear understanding to define what is meant by the terms "authority," "power," and "influence." *Authority* means the right to give commands, enforce laws, or exact obedience. The one who has authority generally is considered to have the knowledge and expertise in a given field necessary to make judgments and to direct others. Formally, authority is commonly viewed as originating at the top of an organizational hierarchy and flowing downward via delegation. However, authority must be accepted by its subjects before it becomes a reality.

Power implies the ability or capacity to act or perform effectively. It is the ability to impose the will of one person or group so as to bring about certain behaviors of other persons or groups. In interpersonal relationships, power is defined as the ability to satisfy or not to satisfy the needs of another person or group and as a result to affect behavior. The ultimate means of securing power is the use of force. This can be in subtle forms of speech or covert acts or in forceful acts, such as witholding salary or other rewards.

Power implies a relationship of interdependency. The effective leader will honor this concept, knowing that success in any venture rests in collaborative effort of the participants. The use of aggressive, assertive, or passive behavior becomes vitally important in power relationships.

Influence is a relationship in which the behavior of an individual or group is affected by another individual or group. Influence can come from direct or indirect sources. It can be exerted because of certain role expectations of a position, individual(s), or a group. Nurse-worker, nurse-client, or nurse-physician are examples of direct influence. Indirect influence is far more subtle in nature, as the major base of influence is intangible. One does not need to have authority and power to exercise influence over another. Motivation for influencing others is couched in terms of gains and costs to be expected. The influencing process utilized by the leader may be in the form of advice, suggestion, discussion, persuasion, or role modeling. The outcome of influence is uncertain because one cannot predict with assurance the effects of influence. Influence can be said to be operational when response by others to the one who influences occurs voluntarily and without coercion.

In summary, authority, influence, and power are distinguishable, but they are interdependent. Each is vital to the leadership role. A professional nurse-leader must have the authority to make decisions affecting the behavior of others. Leaders must have the power and ability to satisfy or not to satisfy human needs, and they must exercise influence directly and indirectly to effect change.

Sociologists Lewen, Lippitt, and White describe three generally accepted styles of leadership: autocratic, democratic, and laissez-faire. Other styles closely related to these are paternalistic and participative. *Autocratic leadership* means that one person has supreme power to make decisions for others. Paternalistic leadership is closely related to autocratic. The group depends on the leader, who makes all the decisions, but the paternal leader considers the welfare of his group more than the autocrat does. *Democratic leadership* means authority is vested in the leader by the group, and the group has a part in decision making. Participative leadership is similar to democratic leadership except that the leader ultimately makes decisions for the group. The members are allowed and encouraged to make suggestions, discuss issues, and participate in problem solving, but the leader decides. *Laissez-faire leadership* means that group members do as they please, and neither the group members nor the leader accepts the responsibility for decision making.

One style of leadership is rarely practiced alone. Combinations of different styles are used, depending on the situation, the group, and the characteristics of the leader. A leader tends to practice a process of leadership dictated by his personality, background, experience, and knowledge and the context of the nursing situations. The old axiom "leaders are born, not made" is not true. Leadership is learned. The nurse can acquire leadership ability through the educational process and by the consistent application of appropriate leadership principles to everyday nursing situations.

PREDICTIVE PRINCIPLE: Understanding various managerial systems and the work environment provides the leader with a basis for determining a suitable type of leadership for the situation or for developing congruent adaptive behaviors within the environment.

Autocratic leadership

Autocratic (authoritarian) leadership is a directive style of supervision. Common characteristics found in autocracy are a low degree of participation by the people involved, a high degree of punitiveness, a high degree of pressure placed on the worker for output of work, much emphasis on structure and policy, and minimal emphasis on consideration, mutual trust, respect, or warmth for the employee. The focus is on working, with greater emphasis on the system than on the client. Decisions are made by the leader, or responsibility for making them is delegated by him.

Autocratic leadership is the traditional forte of nursing. Historically the chain of command from supervisor, head nurse, staff nurse, senior student to beginning student carried with it status that commanded awe of and unquestioning obedience to those in charge. In this organizational structure the physician was omnipotent, and the existence of nurse functions based on nursing knowledge and independent of physicians' orders was all but unrecognized. The subservient attitude exemplified by "I'm not paid to think, I'm paid to follow orders" marked this type of organization. Decisions were made by designated people, and few dared question their authority. The autocratic leader speaks in terms of *I, me, my,* and *mine* even when referring to group effort. *We, us,* and *our* seem lost from his vocabulary. Individualism is sacrified for the sake of organizational goals.

The autocrat is stern, strict, or just, according to his own established principles and guidelines for action. He gives praise or criticism to each member on his own initiative and remains aloof from people most of the time. His principles and guidelines may be effective, but they may not be in the best interest of the individuals involved. He has no one to turn to for validation; therefore, since the autocratic leader makes all decisions and plots all directives, he retains all authority, as well as all responsibility. Since there is minimal group participation, there is limited commitment to the results of group behavior, little feeling of responsibility for the success or failure of the enterprise, and always someone else for the group to blame—the leader or another scapegoat.

Authoritarian leadership implies frustration of significant needs in the followers. Because there is no safe outlet for the expression of feelings, morale and sometimes productivity are lowered, and reactions of hostility, apathy, or blind obedience can occur. The led are usually unwilling to exercise initiative for fear that innovation will increase the chance for error and will result in punitive measures. In terms of service to clients, the followers tend to seek satisfaction from the abstract values of the enterprise, such as monetary remuneration or promotion, rather than from the value of service to people.

When nurses in practice situations have fixed rules established for them and feel they have no recourse, one avenue of retaliation is to comply with the demands made on them but to retreat personally. Apathy spreads throughout the membership, resulting in demoralization, decreased effectiveness, and poor care for the patients.

Blind obedience to autocracy may result because some nurses prefer to be followers, they fear responsibility, or they have other interests or needs that take precedence over the job at hand. They take the path of least resistance on the job because their energies are expended elsewhere. Other nurses may believe they do not possess the qualities necessary for leadership and are satisfied to function under others. Some nurses, however, modify the environment in ways that allow them to be effective regardless of bureaucratic leadership.

Laissez-faire leadership

Laissez-faire leadership is described as open and permissive, abdicating, frustrating, confusing, and uncontrolled. Laissez-faire leadership is leadership in which each group member sets goals independently. It is the least efficient of the three types of leadership and exists either in rebellion against autocratic leadership or because no leader is invested with responsibility and no one assumes the role. It exists when a leader is too weak or too threatened to exercise the functions of leadership or when lack of trust within the group prevents unity.

Hostility generated by autocratic leadership can produce a nurse who is determined to be the opposite of all that was despised in the autocratic system and thereby withholds leadership activities and functions in a laissez-faire manner. Because of lack of information, this nurse practices laissez-faire leadership in the mistaken belief that democratic rule is being practiced. Guidelines, rules and regulations, limit setting, and decisions are not seen as safeguards for the individual group member, the patient, and the agency but as infringements on the rights and dignity of the worker.

The staff nurse who has great need of approval may practice laissez-faire leadership out of fear of offending group members. This leader wants to please everyone and, in the attempt, fails to give strength and direction, to set limits, and to conduct open and honest discussions.

Democratic leadership

Democratic and participatory leadership is employed with the consent and support of those who are led. The leader's security does not depend on the maintenance of the existing conditions. A democratic climate is conducive to the process of exploration and discovery of the individual. People sense that their own feelings and thoughts, as well as those of others, are important. Democracy is authority invested in the leader by individuals or a group, with the right to make certain decisions and judgments and to take action. Democracy does not mean an investment of *all* power in the leader, nor does it imply that a vote is taken on everything.

Democracy is the power to act sometimes in behalf of others. In this system it is legitimate to express controversial beliefs and to give and receive feedback so that behaviors may be altered. Ultimately in the democratic system the leader may be stripped of the power invested in him by the group. In other instances, channels of administration can be bypassed. Jeffersonian democracy is classless. Each individual has equal rights and opportunities to become the leader; thus leadership exists on all levels.

Inherent in democracy is the major element of *trust,* confidence by the group that the leader will function in the best interest of all concerned—client, community, the nursing group, and agency—and by the leader that the membership will support him.

For trust and support to exist, both leader and members must possess successful experiences in having their needs and expectations met by each other. Free and open communication using appropriate channels can promote a feeling of security; the leader is confident in his ability to work with people and resources available to him for the benefit of his clients. He accepts responsibility for his failures rather than projecting them onto individuals or an organization. Because he knows his only limitation to be his level of competence, he is committed to growth as a professional. Assessment of each care giver's ability and optimal use of his knowledge and skills will develop individual and group potential to the maximum. Within the democratic or consulting framework, meaningful goals can be established and the participants can develop ways for objectively evaluating their own accomplishment.

It is not possible to specify the type of management that will be the most productive in any given situation. The democratic approach is proposed as the ideal method of operation, but occasions will arise when the authoritarian or even the laissez-faire approach will be desirable. In most instances, leadership style is a mixture of the three types of leadership. For nursing at the present time, autocracy modified by some democratic operations is the general rule.

PREDICTIVE PRINCIPLE: A clear operational definition of leadership expectations expedites role definition and role enactment.

Nursing leadership is the ability to use the processes of life to facilitate the movement of a person, a group, a family, or a community toward the establishment and attainment of a goal (see Chapter 1). The strength of the leader's influence depends on the interactive variables of the task, the clients to be served, the organizational structure, the external environment, and the characteristics of the leader and the followers. Leadership is a learned behavior pattern; therefore utilizing leadership role enactment theories is necessary for making the leadership process operational.

Critical attention should be given to the selection of nurse-leaders who are best able to learn and systematically utilize sound principles in the leadership process from the point of goal determination to goal achievement. Communication will permeate all components of the process. With feedback the leader can evaluate the realization of goals and can reactivate the components of the problem-solving process as demanded by the situation to achieve fully that which is desired. This problem-solving behavior will equip the nurse-leader to cope with the ever-changing processes in the health scene as administrator, nurse-clinician, counselor, teacher, and resource person whenever and whomever he serves.

PREDICTIVE PRINCIPLE: Knowledge of theory levels and ability to formulate valid predictive principles promote the leader's ability to identify the levels on which members are functioning to facilitate growth in problem solving and goal attainment.

The formulation of a valid theory is described fully in Chapter 1. Level I is composed of *naming,* or *labeling,* and *classifying,* or *categorizing,* the result. Level II also has two phases: *depicting,* or describing, and *factor relating.* The third level is *situation relating,* concerned with causal relationships. The fourth level in theory building is *situation producing,* comprising the formulation of prescriptive theories. When situation-producing theories are analyzed, they consist of three aspects: (1) a definable goal, (2) a prescription, and (3) a study or diagram of specific activities and directions, which, if followed, produce a predicted result or attain preset goals. The final component in the fourth level is a survey list of resources, techniques, and behavioral patterns that can be structured into goal-producing activities. At this stage the wider the nurse-leader's knowledge of experiences of related situations, treatment, and results produced, the more reliable the results. In addition, the nurse's behaviors will reflect more effectively the acquired principles or predictive theories, which predict desired outcomes. This knowledge of theory levels equips the leader with the tools necessary for identifying the level at which individuals and groups are operating and to provide guidance that will promote growth up through the levels.

PREDICTIVE PRINCIPLE: Identification of leadership traits associated with managerial climates facilitates the conversion of traits into operational behaviors.

The trait theory of leadership proposes that there are certain traits or qualities that can make an effective leader. Trait theory emerged in the nineteenth and early twentieth centuries when it was thought that if traits of great men could be identified, then people could be trained in the acquisition of the traits and thus become leaders.

A leadership trait is an attribute, quality, characteristic, or distinguishing mark of an individual. Leadership traits also imply a distinctive temperament or mood and include that which is outstanding in one's personality. This may be physical, mental, or social. A physical trait can be described as a peculiarity or walk or posture that sets the individual apart and makes him unique. It may also become an idiosyncrasy or a mannerism. Some leadership traits identified by researchers have included striking physique, strong body and character, articulate, sympathetic, understanding, honest, courageous, and on and on, naming almost every trait known to man. The trait theory as a single explanation for leader behavior is no longer recognized as valid. It has become apparent that one trait could act to determine success or failure of leadership efforts, depending on conditions, circumstances, and behaviors present in the situation.

The term "climate" in this book does not refer to temperature, such as humidity or other natural climatic conditions, but rather to the general context or overall picture of conditions in which one operates. Climate is thought of as a social condition or mood or a generality of opinion or attitude held by a group. This then becomes the climate of that group. In totality, climate includes opinions peculiar to a stated group of individuals or a society. One may speak of the social climate of a certain group as being warm or friendly. The converse is also true. The climate of a health agency may be open or closed toward those not initiated into the agency. For instance, those giving nursing care or medical treatment can create a climate of concern for the general welfare of the patient.

The following outline affords a partial comparative summary of the various climates that could exist in a health agency, divided into three major categories.

Democratic	Authoritarian	Laissez-faire
Responsible and accountable	Accountable	Uncontrolled
Open	Defensive	Open
Facilitating	Restricting	Permissive
Freeing	Coercing	Abdicating
Encouraging	Discouraging	Frustrating
Accepting	Accepting and rejecting	Accepting and rejecting
Differences valued	Conforming valued	Indifferent
Variety	Uniformity	Variety
Equality	Inequality	Equality
Participative	Individual	Participative and individual
Self-legislative	Imposed legislation	Indifferent to legislation
Trusting	Fearing	Indifference
Available	Controlled availability	Available and unavilable
Encouraging	Forcing	Lacking in direction
Freedom of choice	Limited choice	Freedom of choice
Led by choice	Leader imposed	Led by choice
Cooperation	Competition	Confusion
Equal opportunity	Controlled opportunity	Open to opportunity
Opportunity	Exploitation	Uncontrolled
Challenge	Threat	Permissive
Recognition	Praise	Acceptance
Self-disciplined	Punishment	Lazy
Satisfaction	Reward	Acceptance

Leadership defined only by climate or traits becomes nonfunctional, as characteristics alone cannot be made operational. Much research has been concerned with characteristics associated with the role of the leader. The successful administrator is commonly viewed as intelligent, possessing a well-balanced personality, assured of self-worth, accepting of others, a catalyst, responsible and accountable, having insight, imagination, and creativity, and exercising good judgment in problem solving and decision making.

Traits and climate are not mutually exclusive; therefore neither operates alone. The climate around an individual does not remain constant, nor do his circumstances remain the same. It is not possible to say of a person that he "is always cooperative" or that he "is always permissive." Perhaps Leo Tolstoy best expresses the fluidity of man:

One of the most widespread superstitions is that every man has his own special, definite qualities; that a man is kind, cruel, wise, stupid, energetic, apathetic, etc. Men are not like that. . . . Men are like rivers: the water is the same in each and alike in all; but every river is narrow here, is more rapid there, here slower, there broader, now clear, now cold, now dull, now warm. It is the same with men. Every man carries in himself the germs of every human quality, and sometimes one manifests itself, sometimes another, and the man often becomes unlike himself, while still remaining the same man.

Throughout life each individual establishes a definite life-style of his own. He develops response patterns that work best for him. The person will tend to repeat those experiences that bring satisfaction and to discard those that cause discomfort.

Employment of the trial and error method is a forfeiture or abdication of the leader's responsibility to deliberate choice in leadership. One must cognitively, consciously, and systematically develop those personal characteristics that will contribute to the advancement of the leadership role.

Traits, simply named, are in the first stage of theory building. They remain nonfunctional until they are developed through the theoretical pattern to actualization. To become effective or useful, each trait must be converted into behaviors that can be operationalized. For example, the leadership trait stated as "responsible" is described and depicted in the second level of theory as "functions within the framework of the employer or agency," "fulfills agreement for services," and "accounts for actions." The third level, then, is accepting responsibility for nursing care giving and promoting fulfillment of agreements made with clients for services. The fourth level of theory in actualizing leadership responsibility includes (1) assessment with client of his needs for care, (2) determination of alternatives, (3) identification of risks, (4) selection of alternatives for action, (5) establishment of schedule for implementation, (6) involvement of others, (7) setting criteria for evaluation, and (8) implementation.

AWARENESS OF SELF

Awareness of self is the ability to be sensitive to one's own needs, motives, and responses to stimuli. Self-awareness enables the nurse-leader to help followers understand themselves and to develop their potential. In turn, the more the nurse helps others to grow, the more self-growth will occur.

Traditionally, nurses are seen as self-sacrificing; their individual needs are viewed as unimportant. Even the struggle for economic security is more difficult because of the image of the nurse as a self-sacrificing and giving person. The nature of nursing draws people to the field who have a need to be useful to others. Recognition of the individual needs of nurses and finding ways to meet those needs free the nurse to meet the needs of the patient.

PREDICTIVE PRINCIPLE: Knowledge and understanding of factors that contribute to mental health permit self-assessment of one's state of mental health.

The nurse enters the leadership role with certain needs, drives, and motives and seeks satisfaction from the total work situation. Individual feelings are based on many variables depending on goals and the nurse's ability to reach these goals. A person who follows a normal developmental pattern progresses from dependence (mother-child relationship) to the independent role and on to interdependence (in which a productive and satisfying working relationship with others is established). The basic urge of a human being is toward a state of physical, mental, and social well-being.

Insight—self-awareness—does not come in a vacuum; other people are involved in the process. In an environment where there is mutual respect, adequate feedback will take place and the leader will grow in self-awareness. The leader will then be able to carry out tasks of leadership in a better way and may achieve wholly unexpected and sometimes unique accomplishments.

PREDICTIVE PRINCIPLE: Identification of the leader's own needs aids in the identification of needs of others.

Man expresses needs from birth to death; the degree of importance of each need depends on conditions and circumstances. The basic needs are physiologic—the desire for food, rest, exercise, shelter, and protection from the elements. When basic needs are reasonably satisfied, others begin to motivate man, for he is not static. Other needs include the necessity for love, status, and recognition. The leader who understands his own needs in perspective and realizes that they are constantly changing can better understand these same needs in others.

PREDICTIVE PRINCIPLE: Accurate appraisal of self promotes healthy emotional organization.

PREDICTIVE PRINCIPLE: Acceptance of self creates a climate for the acceptance of others.

In the book *Your Erroneous Zones,* Dr. Wayne W. Dyer offers the concept that the one who would move from the virus of low self-esteem to the positive feeling of self-worth must first love himself. Self-love means feeling one is important, worthy, and beautiful. The individual recognizes himself as a unique and good individual and does not need to have others reinforce personal values or to engage in conforming behavior contrary to one's dictates. The secret to accepting one's self as a worthy person is to love one's self as one is without complaint and to allow others the same consideration. Dr. Dyer believes that by choosing positive self-images, one is enabled to become a happy, effective person. He predicts that setting standards for one's self within this positive framework allows the individual to reach heights otherwise unthinkable and that the happier one chooses to make himself, the more intelligent one becomes. The reward for self-appreciation is two pronged. Personal satisfaction is realized through evidences of growth, and because self-acceptance and self-assurance are present, the individual can accept others as they are and challenge them to move into the realm of positive thinking.

The leader's acceptance of himself enables him to accept his followers. Self-acceptance is built on self-awareness; the leader who has achieved this status is likely to develop a sense of personal integrity and self-worth to the extent that he behaves constructively even when his authority is threatened. For example, when a care giver asks the leader, "Are you sure this is what we should do?" the leader may interpret the question as the follower's not feeling secure about the leader's judgment. The amount of anxiety the question creates and the leader's response depend on his self-image and self-awareness. If the nurse-leader believes the authority role is being questioned and feels threatened, he is apt to follow with a defensive response, such as "Don't you think I know what I'm doing?" or "What right have you to question my orders!" Such a response would bring about feelings of defense, hostility, and aggression in the questioner. If the nurse-leader has insight and self-awareness, the focus of interaction can be on activities that will clarify messages and produce better results. The leader's response to the member might be "Can you give me a better picture of your concern?" or "You don't feel comfortable about this plan of action?" The leader will then wait for the questioning person to elucidate his feelings. The results of this response are twofold: (1) the action in question will be reevaluated and (2) the nurse-leader will demonstrate acceptance of the member.

Self-understanding can be increased through evaluation of clinical conference processes. Members of the group can help the nurse-leader to expand self-understanding. Listening to tape recordings of meetings or conferences will help the nurse-leader develop insight and understanding regarding the effect of his behavior, attitudes, and methods on others. Assistance in the evaluative process can be sought from the group members involved.

Sensitivity training is another source of help for the nurse-leader. This training usually involves a series of meetings in which emphasis is placed on activities and interactions that develop greater awareness of a responsiveness to other's needs. The training group is designed to promote personal growth. It focuses on individual and group behavior, awareness of self, and social processes. The goal is to help members become more aware of the way they affect others and how others affect them, both consciously and unconsciously. Business and industry use this training extensively on the premise that leaders with greater insight into self have greater job potential and productivity.

Institutes and courses designed to assist in the development of increased self-understanding are often available to nurses through adult education programs, the community, professional groups, and colleges and universities. Occasionally, highly qualified people are willing to come to the agency if enough interest and action are generated. The nurse-leader can play an important role by becoming the facilitator and by requesting assistance in the task of self-development.

All methods for assisting the nurse-leader to increase self-understanding require an expenditure of time, effort, and money. The responsibility for seeking assistance lies with the recipient, but the provision of courses is an in-service educational activity.

If the nurse-leader is to develop to fullest maturity, avenues must be sought that assist in self-development. Just as cosmetics are used not because a woman is ugly but because she hopes that her best features will be accentuated and the less desirable ones will be subdued, the nurse seeks more complete self-understanding to minimize weaknesses and to maximize strengths.

The more the nurse knows about himself, the greater the likelihood of achieving healthy living. Attainment of conscious self-awareness is a difficult process. But personality may change, expand, and integrate even though the process is slow.

Every human being faces obstacles that thwart achievement of goals. The frustrations resulting from unsuccessful attempts to attain goals may elicit discomfort and feelings of inadequacy. When a goal is established, movement is in the direction of that goal. The individual tends to repeat those experiences that bring him satisfaction and to discard those that cause him discomfort. When an obstacle prevents goal achievement, aggressive reaction may occur either directly or indirectly. For example, a nurse-leader decides that a group meeting will be conducted to establish nursing care plans for the patients assigned. Plans for the meeting are announced to the group, and a time is set for early afternoon. During the course of the day, each of the members gives an excuse about why he cannot attend. The nurse-leader attempts to overcome the excuses but is alone at the time of the scheduled conference. The leader becomes frustrated and vents hostile feelings on the members throughout the remainder of the day. Nothing is accomplished except that the leader's reactions have been transmitted to others, who, in turn, act in the same nonconstructive manner.

The problem could have been resolved had the nurse identified feelings and attempted to determine the reasons for the resistance to the proposed conference. The most logical approach for gathering data in this situation is to ask those members involved the reasons for their resistance. At an ensuing session the leader could raise the issue by reviewing the incident of the previous day. For instance: "I realize that I must have done something to cause all members to stay away, but I do not know what the mistake was. In order for me to avoid another incident of this kind, I need to know what I did. Will you help me?" or "Could you tell me more about it?" "What feelings led up to your action?" If the leader is sincere in desiring to learn the facts, the group members will recognize these feelings and honor them with feedback concerning the incident. Successes and failures can be validated so that similar incidents will not occur; the leader is then better equipped to move on toward desired goals.

Ideals of achievement are a part of human makeup. Many factors influence the development of concepts about what kind of person an individual would like to be. Ambitions, aspirations, satisfactions, and rewards change with each life experience. The nurse may have entered the profession because of a desire to help others, or he may have wished to become a specialist doing vital and exciting work. Either of these ambitions may be achieved if the nurse assesses capabilities, recognizes limitations, and plans accordingly. For example, in the role of nurse-leader, planning, directing, and participating in the care-giving process provide the leader a feeling of self-worth and satisfaction from being able to serve others and a perception of accomplishment from achieving a personal goal.

When a nurse's ability is inadequate for achievement of ambition, frustration occurs; if uninterrupted, it may destroy his sense of well-being. If knowledge and experience are insufficient for reaching goals, constructive steps must be taken to make up the inadequacies.

Self-confidence can be developed as increased self-knowledge is acquired and some successes are achieved. If the challenge of leading is too great for the nurse's capacity, lack of self-esteem and feelings of insecurity will arise. When the nurse-leader feels inadequate, such feelings may be the cause of destructive behavior; the leader may become too demanding and critical of others in an effort

to maintain self-image. For example, the leader who feels incapable of understanding the cardiac monitoring system may assign a patient to be monitored to
another nurse. When the nurse asks the leader for assistance in interpreting
data, the leader may react with an angry statement, such as, "Don't you know
what you are doing? A nurse should keep up with what is going on!" Thus the
nurse-leader attempts to build self-esteem at the expense of another person.

The following would have been a constructive approach to the situation.
When the nurse-leader knew the group was to be responsible for the care of a patient requiring cardiac monitoring, the following steps could have been taken to
ensure safety and high quality of care for the patient:

1. Making it known to the head nurse that no nurse member had the specialized
   knowledge required to assume care for a patient who required cardiac monitoring
2. Taking steps to secure a person qualified to care for such a patient
3. Initiating plans to gain the necessary knowledge

When the nurse becomes more understanding of his own assets and liabilities, develops a basic understanding of personal and professional self, and feels
comfortable enough to share this knowledge with others, growth as a nurse-
leader will occur.

PREDICTIVE PRINCIPLE: Accomplishing goals through assertive behavior enables a nurse-
leader to exercise the rights of self without denying the rights and feelings of others.

PREDICTIVE PRINCIPLE: Consistent use of nonassertive behavior ignores personal rights of
the nurse-leader and leads to lowered self-esteem and maladaptive behaviors.

PREDICTIVE PRINCIPLE: Achievement of one's goals through aggressive acts violates another person's rights and results in feelings of domination, humiliation, and hostility.

Assertiveness is the ability to (1) express one's positive and negative feelings
and rights in a socially acceptable, respectful manner, recognizing other's rights
and feelings; (2) make requests and have needs met; (3) refuse unrealistic demands or requests one does not wish to comply with; and (4) initiate and termi-
nate conversations. Assertive behavior enables the nurse-leader to act in the best
interests of self, clients, and members of the health care team by expressing
honest feelings comfortably and without undue anxiety.

The first step toward becoming assertive is the development of increased self-
awareness aimed at helping the individual to become more aware of himself and
his relationships with others and to become more skilled in communicating with
his associates. Status, job attitudes, and interpersonal needs are reviewed. Very
often, nurses see themselves as second-class employees, as victims of the medical
staff or structure, unable to exert power and influence in strategic circumstances,
rather than as peers and colleagues, with the ability and right to act on their own
convictions.

The assertive nurse-leader practices the art of assertion by initiating contact
with others, making requests, and having needs met. There is need to state positively who the nurse is, if unknown, and the message intended. "I am Mrs.
Brown, the primary care nurse for Mr. Langley. I understand that he did not have
his midnight medication for pain as prescribed. Will you please explain the omission?" Or the nurse leader may state, "You have been late to work three days in

a row. I would appreciate your being on time tomorrow. I will expect you at 6:45." A nurse might counter an assignment assertively with the remark "I cannot accept the assignment without adjustment. Caring for these five clients is too much for me to accomplish with quality and safety. I will care for three, but not five."

Another skill of assertion is dealing with criticism, both in giving and in receiving. It is best to give criticism as near the time of incident as possible and to do so in a clear and forthright manner. "I observed you suction Mr. Turner. You did not give him enough time to rest between insertions of the catheter," or "Your nursing care plans are not up-to-date. Please correct this by the end of shift."

The proper way to receive criticism is to accept it, not necessarily as accurate or true but as a message. Next, one acknowledges the other's perception: "Thank you for telling me your opinion," "You don't like the way I did that," or "You'd like me to change." If more information is desired, questions are in order: "Could you be more specific?" "Will you tell me exactly what it is that I am doing that you do not like?" Then a self-disclosure statement may be made if it is important that the critic hear feelings. "I'm sorry you do not approve of what I am doing" or "I am frustrated when you seem to misinterpret my intentions" illustrate self-disclosing statements.

Of equal importance in assertion is giving and receiving compliments. Accepting a compliment with positive remarks such as "Thank you, that makes me feel good," or "Yes, I'm proud of that. I spent a lot of time on it," or "I'm glad you are pleased" indicates to the giver of the compliment that his opinion is valued and reinforces compliments to be given in the future. Rejecting a compliment has at least two underlying messages. One is that the receiver discounts himself or he discounts the giver of the compliment. "Oh no, that was a terrible job!" or "I was just lucky, I guess" imply that the person offering the compliment is too ignorant or insensitive to know the truth about what was done or who did it. The implication is that the receiver is not worthy of recognition or praise or positive regard.

Another component of assertive behavior is the use of nonverbal skills. These are discussed in detail in Chapter 4 on communication. Such things as physical distance, posture, body movements, eye contact, facial expressions, and voice inflections interface and play a significant role in outcome.

It is very easy for leaders to confuse aggressive behavior with assertive behavior, with regretful outcomes. With aggression, the individual acts or moves in bold and hostile ways, often accomplishing goals at the expense of others. People tend to respond in a manner corresponding to that to which they have been exposed. When, for example, the leader humiliates or embarrasses others by confronting them with their actions in public and by not being sensitive to situations, that leader will more than likely experience backlash from those dominated at their first opportunity.

Nonassertive behavior is practiced when the individual denies self, giving in to the wishes of others. The one who holds desires internally usually has a low self-esteem, is shy and reserved, and finds himself unable to assert individual rights or the rights of clients and staff under most circumstances. Behaviors familiar to the nonassertive nurse are apologetic speech, avoidance or withdrawal, hedging when asked to make a decision, and nervousness and anxiety. The nonassertive leader avoids direct confrontation, thus allowing people and circumstances to dominate him. Unable to speak thoughts or feelings in an appropriate manner, this kind of leader experiences feelings of helplessness and powerlessness that can lead to abdication of accountability in the leadership role. A usual outlet for the nonassertive nurse is to engage in self-pity, righteousness, and superiority and to spend time telling anyone who will listen how difficult his lot is. He may use the bureaucracy of the health institution as an excuse for failure to exercise his authority, power, and influence, but the truth of the matter is that the nonassertive behavior must bear the blame. Ironically, many who are nonassertive finally, after being frustrated repeatedly, explode into angry and vengeful aggressiveness in the form of inappropriate, emotionally honest, direct, and self-enhancing behavior at the expense of another.

Effective assertive behavior maintains a balance between totally assertive and nonassertive behavior. Criteria of openness and honesty in expressing one's beliefs and reactions without infringing on the rights of others provide a guide as to which kind of behavior is right for each situation. Assertion is not being in a constant state of confrontation. It is making choices about what to say, when, how, and to whom. There are times when a leader knows it is best to be nonassertive, as in a situation of extreme anger where assertive behavior would intensify the heat of emotions. The effectively assertive nurse would choose to react sensitively, remain issue-oriented, and delay resolution of the conflict until both parties are able to interact reasonably and responsibly. The nurse-leader who chooses assertive behavior as a plan of action will increase in self-confidence, maintain individuality, be accountable for quality health care to clients, and not hesitate to negotiate with those in control of organizations. Through the assertion process the nurse-leader will also feel freer to listen, to counsel, and to speak out appropriately in leadership situations. In this way the nurse's rights are recognized, and he becomes a more effective advocate of the rights of others.

KNOWLEDGE OF THE JOB

The nursing leadership role assumes certain basic knowledge and skills. These attributes are assured and perpetuated through accreditation of schools of nursing and hospitals, through the licensure of nurses, and through the system of rewards and punishments built into employment situations. Clients depend on the nurse's clinical judgment for giving the best possible service. The nurse-leader is expected to provide direction in all areas of planning, administering, and evaluating nursing care. The extent to which the nurse-leader is successful in role adaptation, perception, and response to leadership requirements directly relates to (1) the leader's ability to build theory and utilize it, (2) the range of conscious role learning, (3) role taking, (4) role enactment, and (5) a large role repertoire. An example of behavioral objectives that reflect this knowledge and ability is as follows:

1. Demonstrates a working knowledge of leadership theories and operational definitions that enable the nurse to move toward full maturity and to be

optimally useful in nurse leadership practices within the health care delivery system

2. Establishes plans to obtain desired and appropriate care with client and works with people and/or agencies that may enhance or inhibit care in the promotion of health
   a. Recognizes components of good health practice for each client and identifies rights being threatened
   b. Clarifies with client standard for good health practice, identifies risks involved, and allows patient to make an educated choice
3. Implements and evaluates planned change for the purpose of promoting optimal health in client and society
4. Exercises responsibility and accountability for self and others in nursing practice for the provision and/or promotion of quality health care
5. Collaborates, coordinates, teaches, and consults in diverse nursing settings
6. Demonstrates characteristics and values inherent in the leadership role
7. Assumes leadership in recognizing the need for adaptations as trends emerge and initiates or participates in research that will contribute to the body of knowledge necessary for judicious decision making

PREDICTIVE PRINCIPLE: The demands of the situation in which a leader is to function influence the qualities, characteristics, knowledge, and skills necessary for successful leadership.

It is impossible for a nurse to possess knowledge and skills necessary to function in all aspects of nursing today, for this career is multifaceted and complex. But the practitioner can influence the development of optimal leadership abilities by collaborating with other persons to (1) preassess leadership qualities, characteristics, knowledge, and skills for the job; (2) plan ways and means to acquire additional service tools viewed as necessary for the proposed managerial role; (3) obtain feedback to ascertain increased level of competence; and (4) secure an assignment commensurate with knowledge and ability.

Clinical competence is effectively rewarded by advancement. Hence competent nurses are often assigned to cardinal positions. This clinical expertise contributes to effective guidance but does not ensure that the nurse will possess leadership qualities. The value of technical knowledge or proficiency in facilitating leadership depends on the situation and the tasks to be accomplished. If technical knowledge is not relevant to the goals established, it will be of minimal service either to the leader or to the recipient of services.

Anxiety is generated in situations that make demands for clinical knowledge the nurse has not acquired; this in turn disrupts organizational behavior patterns even in highly skilled nurses. All too often nurses are placed in roles where they are novices, in jobs that depend on knowledge pertaining to policy, procedure, and routine with which they are unfamiliar or that require expertise in unaccustomed clinical areas. This practice generates false incompetence. For example, a nurse-leader fully qualified to function in a pediatric unit may render poor service in an obstetric unit. Clinical knowledge about separation anxiety in the 2-

year-old child does not enable the nurse to make good judgments about post-partum bleeding.

Problems beyond the ability of the nurse-leader cause a high anxiety level and an indulgence in activities that in reality only drain off the excess energy generated by such high anxiety. An illustration of this is demonstrated by the following:

A group is responsible for the care of an agitated patient who needs the constant presence of a care giver. The nurse-leader's energy and time are spent in trying to get the charge nurse to assign an extra person, attempting to get the nursing service office to send help, trying to get the physician to change his orders or to request a private duty nurse, or trying to get the patient transferred to a different unit or put into an isolated or maximum security room.

This nurse-leader spends time in fruitless efforts and activities that do not contribute to the solution of the problem. Admitting ignorance about the care of agitated patients would have damaged the leader's self-esteem; consequently, the nurse-leader avoided this by engaging in activities, such as trying to obtain aid, that were acceptable to the group. Any consequent difficulties with the agitated patient can conveniently be the fault of those who did not respond as requested.

The nurse who is secure and has the ability to care for this type of patient helps the care givers devise ways of handling this problem. This can be achieved through teaching those skills necessary to care safely and effectively for the patient and through planning a cooperative effort. The time and energy spent in teaching and planning for this emergency will profit the whole membership when a similar problem arises. Goal-directed activity generates self-confidence, which is transmitted to others and is reinforced by success. An example of behavioral objectives that reflect an effective teaching-learning process is as follows:

1. Applies teaching-learning strategy(ies) and develops plan most useful for each teaching-learning situation in the promotion of health for individuals and groups
2. Identifies own learning needs that are congruent with own strengths, limitations, and potential in the light of own life needs; identifies and evaluates own learning process and makes necessary adaptations; formulates behavioral objectives that are congruent, relevant, and realistic to fulfill self-needs and modifies according to outcomes
3. Seeks to establish a learning environment that will permit relationships of trust, security, and feedback and will allow for realistic goal setting, practice, and assessment
4. Serves as a role model in the practice of physical and mental health in nursing practice; is alert to the need and methodology necessary to effect change
   a. Reflects optimal physical and mental health in nursing practice
   b. Establishes goals for self, recognizing own physical and mental capabilities and stamina

    c. Develops adaptive measures for modifying behavior according to individual assessment of physical and mental condition and expectations of the work setting

  5. Uses predetermined criteria to evaluate the effectiveness of the teaching-learning process for self and groups

Self-confidence is born of success and reinforced by enough success to allow failures to be perceived, not as basic inadequacies, but as momentary or transient failures. Self-confidence enables the nurse-leader to identify areas of knowledge and ignorance and to instigate activities that will increase knowledge and expand professional expertise.

Continuing education through self-study, in-service programs, or formal programs (organizations and colleges) will enable the nurse-leader to keep pace with professional technology. Part of the solution to the need for an increase in quality care is in utilization: better use of employees through on-the-job training for specialized skills. Policies that encourage continuing education will help to achieve the goals. Because of increased efficiency and fuller utilization of individual productivity potential, the professionally knowledgeable nurse is an economic asset to the public and to the employing agency.

The energy output utilized in attempting to circumvent a nursing situation decreases when the nurse can cope with a situation; energy can be directed toward achievement rather than circumvention.

The recent trend to offer nursing services at the colleague-peer relationship level, as with the primary care nurse who works in contractual agreement with the client, and other special nursing roles—described as extender, expander, assistant, associated, clinical specialist, and practitioner—necessitates preparation beyond that normally provided in nursing curricula.* Whatever the label and however the functions are described, an expanded role requires a corresponding increase in knowledge and skills to meet the challenge. Schools of nursing, particularly baccalaureate and graduate programs, are deluged with requests from federal, state, regional, and local commissions, as well as from individuals, to prepare the nurse with primary skills to provide better health care to increased numbers of people. Major content areas that have been largely absent from nursing curricula in the past are those of physical and developmental assessment and health history. For the practicing nurse, consistent acquisition of new knowledge requires aptitude and an investment of time and money. The nurse-leader committed to assuming a new role will seek and complete programs of study that will provide the necessary supplementary preparation.

PREDICTIVE PRINCIPLE: The degree to which the leader is clinically knowledgeable and competent directly influences feelings of security about the appropriateness of nursing activity.

Nurses have a responsibility to the client (Chapter 1), to their employers, and to those being led to be clinically proficient. Clinical competence gives the nurse self-confidence, which is communicated in both tangible and intangible ways to

---

*Management and supervision of patient care, Nurs. Clin. North Am. **8**(2):entire issue, June 1973.

clients, employers, and co-workers. Nurses who have sound basic knowledge and clinical expertise save time and energy for themselves and others. They understand when procedures are correct, and they are more innovative in devising better ways to accomplish a given task. Clinically knowledgeable nurses use the nursing process to discuss with clients and care givers the validity of established goals, the appropriateness of planned activities, and the work schedule necessary for achieving those goals. Individuals who turn to the knowledgeable leader for help and advice are rewarded by having their needs met. This reinforces trust in the leader's competence and frees care givers to rely on themselves and on each other in cooperative efforts. An example of behavioral objectives in the utilization of nursing process through the model of adaptation is as follows:

1. Extrapolates and applies relevant knowledge from nursing and related fields to the adaptation process with the individual client(s) and/or groups
2. Utilizes holistic approach in assessment of needs and implementation of care with each client
3. Assesses the position of clients and groups on the health-illness continuum
4. Assesses the adaptation of individuals in each of the three modes of adaptation—intrapersonal, interpersonal, and environmental—in a complete and logical manner; uses appropriate resources for data gathering; identifies significant relationships between modes and draws justifiable conclusions from data relationships
5. Identifies focal, contextual, and residual stimuli that influence the behavior of client; identifies and utilizes relationships between stimuli in planning care
6. Establishes priorities for provision of nursing care in concert with client
7. Implements nursing interventions designed to promote and support client adaptation
8. Explores opportunities for innovative nursing interventions; encourages clients and nursing staff to exercise initiative and creativity in goal realization

MUTUAL RESPECT

Maximum productivity results when consideration and respect are given to a health care giver's total personality; this means that recognition and utilization of the employee's desires, attitudes, interests, and motives are as important as attention to his physical efforts.

As consideration for worth and respect of the individual has progressed in health agencies, many current practices have developed. These include a recognition of the following: individuals vary in their personal aptitudes and interests; different jobs require different abilities; the emotional makeup of the individual influences job performance; and the prevailing spirit or feeling of the work force affects productivity. The need for mutual respect between employer and employee is gradually being recognized. Both have an interest in the well-being of the other, and the relationship between employer and employee must be harmonious if they are to work together toward their common objectives. This same philosophy applies to nurse-leaders and co-workers.

PREDICTIVE PRINCIPLE: Understanding and practicing the basic elements of mutual respect facilitate effective leadership.

Maximum utilization of personnel is influenced by the mutual respect between group and leader. Determination of basic elements inherent in respect is a difficult task in a society where people from varied backgrounds, free to develop their own philosophies of life, compose the work force.

In 1951 the National Education Association published the results of a survey to determine if there was a core of spiritual and moral values for operation in a free society on which all people could agree. The following values were agreed on*:

1. There is significance in the individual personality. (This was the basic assumption from which all others were formulated.)
2. The individual has the capacity to assume moral responsibility.
3. Institutions are the servants of men; men are not the servants of institutions.
4. Common consent is a basis for social action.
5. Devotion to truth is necessary for open, trusting human relationships.
6. Excellence in human achievement should be respected.
7. Moral equality is mandatory. No one in a democratic society has the moral right to injure the growth and development of another personality.
8. There should be brotherhood among people. This means the concern of one person for another—the interest of all people in relation to one another.
9. The pursuit of happiness is a legitimate goal.
10. Spiritual enrichment is desirable.

These points were the consensus of representatives from all ethnic groups, creeds, and religions in America as values that could serve as a basis for interrelationships. If the nurse-leader accepts these values and believes there is significance, worth, and dignity in the human personality, behavior, and attitudes, this belief will be indicated to others, and respect will be reciprocal.

Members invest authority in their nurse-leader with the expectation that their worth will be recognized and that the leader will attempt to meet their needs in the work situation and will support their values.

PREDICTIVE PRINCIPLE: Expressions of respect for others by the leader precipitate acts of mutual respect among members.

Nurse-leaders who care for others enter into relationships with co-workers that have significance and create feelings of mutual satisfaction and respect. When the practitioner's attitude indicates concern for co-workers, a respect model is provided. Knowledge of members' personal problems requires the nurse-

---

*Educational Policies Commission: Moral and spiritual values in the public schools, Washington, D.C., 1951, National Education Association, pp. 17-34.

leader to express feelings of concern and understanding and to construct a work environment that fosters the growth and potentialities of the members.

Situations can be structured that will enable members with problems to find ways within the work situation to deemphasize personal problems. However, it must be recognized that the nurse-leader's role is confined to prescribed activities within the work situation.

Admiration and respect for others can be expressed in many ways and still be in keeping with commitment. Sometimes the nurse-leader is hesitant to share feelings of esteem for others because of a fear that intentions will be misinterpreted or effectiveness as a leader will be lessened. The mature leader will realize the value of expressing feelings for others on appropriate occasions and will not deprive himself and others of the opportunity for successful reinforcement of the positive relationships that come from such expressions. A leader who respects another person will become involved in that person's development, and mutual growth will result.

Attitudes concern feelings and opinions and are revealed in both overt and covert ways. Those who are led expect the leader's attitudes to be constructive. They expect such attitudes as warmth, acceptance, objectivity, empathy, compassion, and respect to be exhibited by the leader. When the nurse-leader demonstrates to co-workers that others are held in high regard, a pattern of behavior for that group (feelings of trust) will be nurtured and mutual respect will follow. The nurse-leader and members will accept and respect one another as peers and work together to minimize weaknesses and maximize strengths.

When the concept of mutual respect is learned by the nurse-leader, constructive attitudes among members will be promoted. The extent to which co-workers adopt the nurse's attitudes toward others is a measure, to some degree, of the effectiveness of the leader.

OPEN CHANNELS OF COMMUNICATION

Many nurse-leaders feel unaffected by the environment in which they work. They are preoccupied with clients, audience, other members of the health team, or the administrative staff of the area. Authority figures are frequently equated with punishment and discipline. No previous personal contact with a specific managerial person or position is necessary for the authority figure to cause anxiety in some nurses. Effective utilization of the administrative staff in an agency, of an independent practitioner, or of a primary care giver presumes knowledge of the position and the function of each job and a broad understanding of the channels of communication. An example of behavioral objectives that reflect open channels of communication is as follows:

1. Selects, applies, and/or promotes appropriate interpersonal theories that positively affect the communication pattern(s) in health care delivery system
2. Assesses behaviors in self, client(s), and community that promote and block communication; develops, actualizes, and/or promotes alternative behavioral patterns

3. Assesses, plans, implements, evaluates, and revises communication strategies on an ongoing basis

PREDICTIVE PRINCIPLE: Knowledge of appropriate channels of communication facilitates efficient utilization of line organization.

The purpose of independent practitioners and health agencies is to provide quality health service to patients. This purpose is sometimes lost in the bureaucracy that has evolved in the struggle to meet rapidly expanding demands for health services, and the operation becomes an end in itself.

Nurses who know the lines of communication within and without formal health organizational structures can cope with the setting and can devise ways to facilitate and expedite nursing practice.

Studying the line organizational chart from an agency policy manual will not necessarily describe the responsibilities of each position. The nurse-leader needs to acquire knowledge not only of the line organization but also of job descriptions, if the organizational structure is to be useful.

The line organizational chart and the de facto organizational structure may not be the same; some people in the authority structure may be assuming roles and responsibility that have been officially prescribed to others. This can happen by incorrectly established custom or as a result of power struggles. The nurse-leader who participates in such practice reinforces the habit of working through inappropriate administrative personnel and is placed in a difficult and sometimes untenable position. When the nurse-leader finds that such conflicts exist, clarification should be sought from the nurse-leader's immediate superior in written form. Written memos empower the staff nurse to function more securely by providing a record of clarified channels for future reference.

Confusion, wasted energy, and decreased service to the patient as a result of poor use of the organizational structure can result in a situation such as the following:

The nurse-leader asks the supervisor of the unit for permission to hold a class with the ancillary staff about colostomy care. The supervisor gives permission and encouragement. The staff nurse asks the director of central supply to demonstrate use of the equipment. The nurse then posts a notice in the dining room inviting all interested nurses to attend. The in-service education director becomes upset because in-service education is his area of authority and he should have been consulted about the class.

The nurse-leader could have prevented problems in this situation by using the appropriate chain of command. Casual perusal of the organizational chart and job descriptions would have indicated to the nurse-leader that the in-service education director was a necessary person to consult before proceeding with plans involving other departments and people from other nursing units.

PREDICTIVE PRINCIPLE: The nurse working in an expanded role provides leadership initiative in establishing channels of communication congruent with the role.

The nurse engaged in collaborative interprofessional relationships, as in the practice of primary nursing care and/or expanded roles, will establish relevant and expedient channels of communication between employer, client and related individuals, or other implicated members of the health team. The expanded role includes people and/or functions that contribute to the nurse's care-giving repertoire. The practitioner establishes avenues of communication with these resources so that combined knowledge, skills, and support will be immediately assessable in routine or critical health giving situations. The expanded role requires the independent nurse to be conversant with contributing sources of communication and enables him to function appropriately in a given circumstance.

The nurse practitioner who functions beyond ordinary discipline boundaries performs without the structure often attendant with regulations of advisory councils, committees, and other direction-giving bodies. An expansion in role does not imply that the nurse is absolved from accountability to organizational framework whether casual (as with a verbal agreement between client and nurse) or highly structured (as in a complex health agency). Seeking suitable resources, guidance, and other assistance that accrue from established policy and procedure, either within or without the health agency, contribute to the client's welfare and the nurse's professional development.

KNOWLEDGE OF PARTICIPANTS' CAPABILITIES

Since World War II, nursing has been deluged with ancillary workers, each with a different background and preparation. These workers enter the nursing field to perform selected tasks under the supervision and direction of professional nurses. They bring to the job a wide variety of sociocultural and educational backgrounds. Nurse-leaders who assess the capabilities of each individual with whom they work can delegate tasks and responsibilities appropriately and assist each worker in developing his potential.

PREDICTIVE PRINCIPLE: An understanding of sociocultural backgrounds of members helps the leader assess job capabilities.

The recent advent of educational and training programs aimed at the unemployed and cultural and racial minority groups has brought large numbers of workers from various ethnic backgrounds into nursing. Race, English language skills, economic level, and the cultural experiences of these workers vary from the middle-class, white, third- and fourth-generation Americans who comprise the bulk of professional nurses. It is necessary that the nurse-leader be able to communicate clearly and relate effectively with these workers if their skills and knowledge are to be fairly assessed and their attitudes understood. This assessment helps the nurse-leader to understand the value systems (Chapter 3) of group members, to know how best to motivate them, and thus to know how to communicate with them effectively. A value system is brought to the job as a part of each person's personality. An understanding of value systems enables the nurse-leader to use the entire work force to full advantage and to promote effectively the development of individual and group potential.

Barriers to understanding and rapport, such as race and class, are not insurmountable. Prejudice, caste, and class conflicts exist in nursing, as in society, both openly and subtly. However, because of the changing self-image of subcultural groups and the legal protection of individual rights and dignity, racial and class prejudices are discussed more freely today than ever before. Nurse-leaders who ignore the presence of a group member from a subculture or avoid talking about differences in cultural or ethnic background do not prevent conflict; they only drive it underground. The critical problems of today's society will be reflected in each small group and must be faced.

Open discussions about individual differences or similarities will enable a leader to recognize how cultural, class, or ethnic characteristics influence individual value systems and behavior patterns within the nursing group. Talking openly and directly about class, color, and culture is difficult for the average middle-class white nurse; however, success in this area will come with practice. An observant nurse-leader who is sensitive to others can remark on incidents and solicit comments that help promote understanding of members. If a nurse-leader does not understand an individual's feelings, openly admitting the lack of understanding invites further exploration and leads to trust. Relationships based on understanding and insight promote the assessment of capabilities and the development of potential in individuals.

English language differences can influence how the leader perceives the care givers and can influence assessment of capabilities and potential. Dialects, poor grammar, foreign accents, and colloquial expressions along with unusual diction can mislead the unwary nurse-leader. Language differences are environmental, cultural, geographic, and educational; they have little to do with intelligence, ability, and job training. The effective nurse-leader will assess the worker's knowledge, maturity, skill, and experience and avoid assumptions based on language alone.

PREDICTIVE PRINCIPLE: Reactions to stress influence efficiency of performance in the work situation.

Job capabilities are influenced by many factors other than ability, knowledge, and skill. Personal crises absorb energy and drain resources that would normally be utilized in work functions. Thought patterns and observational skills are interrupted or inhibited by preoccupation with personal crises. The skillful leader will observe departure from normal work patterns and try to ascertain the reasons for the altered performance. This knowledge enables the leader to change work assignments or supervisory habits to conform to the demands of the new behavior pattern until the personal crisis is past.

Stressful job situations, such as patient emergencies, unexpectedly heavy work assignments, breakdowns in communications and interrelationships, nursing errors, and conflicts with physicians or supervisors, elicit responses from the nurse-leader and other care givers that are not normally seen in daily routine behavior. The nurse-leader who knows each worker's behavioral patterns not only can help to prevent disruptions of client care but also can anticipate how best to help the distressed member. Opportunity for members to discuss stressful work factors and their feelings about them as soon after the incident as possible decreases the accompanying anxiety and allows the daily work to progress smoothly. Such discussions while impressions and feelings are fresh give all participants a truer picture of what actually happened and furnish insights that contribute to the leader's knowledge of individual capabilities, increase job satisfaction, and save time and energy.

PREDICTIVE PRINCIPLE: Knowledge of a care giver's preparation and experience promotes fullest use of skills and provides a basis for continued growth.

The nurse-leader needs specific information about the education and work experience of each group member to delegate the work load appropriately and to determine the amount of supervision and teaching necessary to develop personnel potential. Some of the necessary information may be in employment records, but frequently the personnel files are not open to staff nurses. The nurse often must depend on personal interviews and observations for information necessary to proper utilization of all personnel. The following is an example:

Mrs. Pedersen, a skilled nurse-leader, had worked with Mrs. Williams, an aide, for six months. Mrs. Pedersen discovered during a conversation at lunch one day that Mrs. Williams had worked in a home for the aged for 15 years. The aide stated that she had always loved aged people and liked to work with them; she derived satisfaction from getting them to eat and drink and from contriving ways to motivate them. On working with Mrs. Williams, Mrs. Pedersen observed that the aide was very knowledgeable and creative with elderly patients and was able to learn much from working with her. As nurse-leader, Mrs. Pedersen utilized this aide to help other ancillary workers who were assigned to geriatric patients.

A formally planned assessment interview would have revealed Mrs. Williams' strength much earlier and would have benefited both patients and personnel.

Sources of information

Two basic sources of information are available to the nurse-leader: the assessment interview and observation. The following outline is designed as a guide to activities that will provide the nurse-leader with needed member assessment data.

    I. The assessment interview
      A. Establishment of a time and place that provide privacy and freedom from interruptions
      B. Introduction of purposes of interview and how information will be used
      C. Establishment of rapport conducive to an exchange of information; inquiring about the following to obtain the specific information desired:
        1. Educational background—amount of formal education (grade completed, high school diploma, education after high school, extent of college work)
        2. Formal job training
          a. Length of program and when completed
          b. Formal classroom content (anatomy and physiology; bacteriology and aseptic technique; talking with patients; procedures—list common ones encountered on present job; organizations of work; observations—recording and reporting)
        3. Clinical practice
          a. Real or simulated situation (patient care or practice on dolls or fellow students)
          b. Experience in systems of care (primary, case, functional, team)

        c. Type of patients included in experiences (medical, surgical, obstetric, psychiatric)

        d. Nursing setting (home, convalescent hospital, acute hospital, outpatient clinics)

        e. Opportunity for practice of nursing procedures

        f. Amount of supervision

        g. Who supervised (teacher or nurse on unit or others)

        h. Nursing activity preferences and type of patients preferred

    D. Conclusions

        1. Brief summary of notes taken regarding content and tone of interview

        2. Structure for follow-up at later date as necessary

  II. Observation

    A. Observation of work in progress during normal workday activities

    B. Survey of work results

        1. Assignments completed as directed

        2. Patient appearance

        3. Content of reporting to group and nurse-leader and/or charting

    C. Observation of relationship with other personnel and group

    D. Participation-observation

Assessment interview. Time and place for the assessment interview must be mutually convenient to both parties. A well-planned and structured interview does not take long. A prior explanation of what will occur in the interview should be given to the care giver so that he will come prepared and thus reduce the time required for the conference. Fifteen to twenty minutes should be sufficient for such an interview. Keeping appointments punctually and terminating the conference on time are important. Punctuality helps convey the value of both the worker's and the leader's time.

Setting an atmosphere for the interview occurs both during the preliminary discussions about the interview and within the interview itself. Openness and sincerity are behavioral messages that put the interview on an honest, productive basis. Subterfuge, hesitancy, and lack of candidness elicit responses with the same characteristics.

Nurse-leaders who ask co-workers, instead of the individuals involved, about fellow workers' abilities, problems, attitudes, and preparation are engaging in a practice that will create distrust among the members. Often the leader who follows such a practice not only receives fallacious information but also loses the trust and support of the group.

A relaxed atmosphere is helpful to the establishment of rapport. Relaxed informality is not lack of structure; it is naturalness. Any activity, posture, or attitude that helps both parties behave in a normal way helps establish rapport. Both interviewee and leader should feel free to smoke or take refreshment. These are socializing activities that promote naturalness. A room where there is privacy and, if possible, comfort is helpful. Job responsibilities of both persons should be assigned to other care givers for the duration of the interview; this enables the devotion of attention to the subject and prevents interruptions.

The nurse-leader who begins an interview with a well-defined plan for achieving objectives is likely to reach those objectives. Having a specific and topical list for discussion will produce the best results. Keeping the list in view and making notes as the interview progresses will be helpful to the interviewer by keeping attention focused on the subject and giving a brief record for future reference.

Evaluation of interview data requires sensitivity to nonverbal responses and interpretation of verbal responses. The nurse who fidgets, fusses, or verbally hedges may be attempting to say what he thinks the interviewer wishes to hear, to mask his true feelings, or to cope with anxiety. The interviewer must weigh all the responses (verbal and nonverbal) of the worker and attempt to evaluate them. Clarifying remarks can take the form of statements, observations, or questions, such as "Will you describe what you learned in your classes on aseptic technique so that I understand a little better?" Statements calling for further descriptions, elucidation, and information help the nurse-leader to clarify and evaluate responses.

Observation. The leader must have practical and real knowledge of a group member's ability gathered from firsthand observations of the nurse at work. Assessment of the worker's ability can be made through several observational methods. Observing work in progress gives the leader insight into the worker's effectiveness, safety, and efficiency. Patients who appear clean and comfortable when care is completed and nursing care plans that have been carried through are indicators of worker ability. The content of written or oral reports can also be used by the nurse-leader as assessment data.

Participation-observation is probably the method of observing most effective for nurse-leaders. It will prove useful in assessments, which are done for the purpose of providing a basis for optimal utilization of personnel and encouraging professional growth. Participation-observation is observing another's conduct while participating with him in job performance, for example, observing how sheets are handled and how a bed is made while helping to make the bed. Participation-observation must be explained to ancillary workers to enable the nurse-leader to observe without usurping the worker's role. Participation-observation experiences provide the following opportunities:

1. An opportunity for the nurse-leader to assess the member
2. An opportunity for the nurse-leader to teach and learn
3. An opportunity for the nurse to observe the nurse-leader in the care of patients (role modeling)

Plans for participation-observation can be arranged in a group meeting with the client or family in which the purposes for the observations are discussed. Arrangements can be made for the nurse-leader to work closely with each member at a convenient time. It is essential that the members have a clear understanding of the purposes of the participation-observation experiences.

Observational assessments help the nurse-leader make assignments that enable the full utilization of each person's capabilities. Working together fosters mutual respect and mutual assessment. Since the nurse-leader has prescribed activities, plans must be made for short participation-observations on a daily basis so that observations can be made of routine work, as well as of special assignments or new procedures.

The ability to function is dynamic and changes with the variables of conditions, environments, and associations with people. The nurse-leader can only try to assess and reassess each worker. This continuous assessment process enables the nurse-leader to delegate responsibility and supervise work appropriately while promoting the greatest development of personnel potential. The outcome of this approach will improve the quality and safety of nursing care.

ENVIRONMENT

The nurse-leader concentrates on human motivation and group behavior and takes into consideration the work environment, which in part determines the scope and limitations of activity.

Technical environment includes the physical geography, organizational layout, equipment, system of supply, scheduling, and methods of administering services. The nurse-leader's work environment includes all technical aspects and the conditions, circumstances, and pressures that influence administrative processes.

The findings of much of the research in executive behavior support the conclusion that effective performance of leaders is directly related to the organizational environment.

An alert and interested nurse-leader will find ways to meet personal needs in the work environment, protecting client, employees, and self from harmful environmental factors, taking advantage of desirable aspects, and changing the environment in ways that make it a better source of need satisfaction. To accomplish this, the nurse-leader understands and is able to apply those principles that contribute to a satisfactory environment.

PREDICTIVE PRINCIPLE: A work environment that is open and amenable to valid change assists in personal and professional growth and development.

Work experiences that allow the nurse-leader to satisfy intellectual curiosity enable an acquisition of skills and knowledge necessary for intelligent, efficient work and informed living.

Each leader and participant needs opportunities to engage in experiences that promote ongoing motivation to grow professionally. Work environments can make provision for the expression of personality through creative activities. Identification with the results of one's own activity and taking pride in personal achievements promote professional productivity. Creativity is seen at all levels and can be applied to the most ordinary tasks. Creativity that is utilized can increase efficiency. With imaginative design and innovation, job activities may be completed in less time, with less energy expended, and with less equipment used.

Originality of thought can result in increased service to patients and greater job satisfaction. Creativity flourishes in an environment where each worker believes that his ideas and opinions are received by leaders and peers and are given the same consideration as every other group member's. Henry Ford believed that if a lazy man is given a job to do he will find the quickest and easiest way to perform the task. In the same vein, give a well-prepared nurse-leader a job, and he will devise the best possible way to perform the assignment.

It is possible to pursue the goals of individuals, organizations, and agencies without destroying human values in the process. The organization has a great stake in developing its people and thus in serving human values and organizational ends. Individual or small employers and management of health agencies that take specific steps to ensure the work environment give nurse-leaders an opportunity to grow and develop will have more stable and productive personnel. The achievement of emotional maturity in the leader depends on an environment that provides him with opportunities to express independence and autonomy, to have a part in determining the outcome of efforts, and to participate in significant relationships with others. Innovations that promote desired changes in environment can support optimism and the freedom to be productive.

APPLICATION OF PREDICTIVE PRINCIPLES OF LEADERSHIP BEHAVIOR

In the role of primary care giver, the nurse assessed the geriatric, bed-rest client to be suffering from respiratory insufficiency.

Problem	Principles	Prescription
The need for reduction or alleviation of respiratory insufficiency	Knowledge of theory levels and ability to formulate valid predictive principles promote the leader's ability to identify the levels on which members are functioning to facilitate growth in problem solving and goal attainment. Knowledge of a care giver's preparation and experience promotes fullest use of skills and provides a basis for continued growth.	Proceed through four levels of theory building: 1. Name and categorize the problems (complete with assessment of problem). 2. Relate the factors (signs and symptoms) to normal base lines. 3. Relate to situation, that is, recumbency and immobility lead to systemic tissue hypoxia and venous stasis; gravity makes mechanical resistance to breathing greater in the supine than in the erect posotion. 4. Prescription: check laboratory results of blood gas measurements, reorder if necessary; assess level of orientation, extent of knowledge, and willingness to participate in the development of a problem-oriented care plan; teach patient necessary knowledge and skills; plan with him times to elevate head; auscultate lungs for rales; cough, turn, and deep breathe; observe rate, depth, and quality of respirations; passive range of motion exercises to extremities. Enlist support of client's family and other involved persons in carrying out care plan.

BIBLIOGRAPHY
Books

Alberti, R., and Emmons, M.: Your perfect right: a guide to assertive behavior, San Luis Obispo, Calif., 1974, Impact Publishers.

Argyris, C.: Management and organizational development, New York, 1971, McGraw-Hill Book Co.

Auld, M. E., and Birum, L. H.: The challenge of nursing: a book of readings, St. Louis, 1973, The C. V. Mosby Co.

Barrett, H. H.: Individual goals and organizational objectives, a study of integration mechanisms, Ann Arbor, Mich., 1970, Institute for Social Research, The University of Michigan Press.

Bower, F. L.: The process of planning nursing care: a model for practice, St. Louis, 1977, The C. V. Mosby Co.

Brown, E. L.: Nursing reconsidered: a study of change. Parts 1 and 2, Philadelphia, 1970, J. B. Lippincott Co.

Carlson, C. E.: Behavioral concepts and nursing intervention, Philadelphia, 1970, J. B. Lippincott Co.

Chenevert, M.: Special techniques in assertiveness training for women in the health professions, St. Louis, 1978, The C. V. Mosby Co.

Combs, A. W., Avila, D. L., and Purkey, W. W.: Helping relationships, basic concepts for the helping professions, Boston, 1971, Allyn & Bacon, Inc.

Dolan, J. A.: Nursing in society, a historical perspective, Philadelphia, 1973, W. B. Saunders Co.

Drucker, P.: Management: tasks, responsibilities, practices, New York, 1973, Harper & Row, Publishers.

Dyer, W.: Your erroneous zones, New York, 1976, Funk & Wagnalls, Inc.

Galassi, M., and Gallasi, J.: Assert yourself: how to be your own person, New York, 1977, Human Sciences Press.

Ganong, J., and Ganong, W.: Nursing management, Germantown, Md., 1976, Aspen Systems Corporation.

Herman, S.: Becoming assertive: a guide for nurses, New York, 1978, D. Van Nostrand Co.

Jourard, S. M.: Disclosing man to himself, New York, 1964, D. Van Nostrand Co.

Jourard, S. M.: The transparent self, New York, 1964, D. Van Nostrand Co.

Kramer, M., and Schmalenberg, C.: Path to biculturalism, Wakefield, Mass., 1977, Contemporary Publishing, Inc.

Loye, D.: The leadership passion: a psychology of ideology, San Francisco, 1977, Jossey-Bass, Inc., Publishers.

Mager, R. F.: Goal analysis, Belmont, Calif., 1972, Fearon Publishers, Inc.

Maslow, A. H.: Motivation and personality, New York, 1954, Harper & Row, Publishers.

Stevens, B.: First-line patient care management, Wakefield, Mass., 1976, Contemporary Publishing, Inc.

Stevens, W.: Management and leadership in nursing, San Francisco, 1978, McGraw-Hill Book Co.

Tead, O.: The art of leadership, New York, 1935, McGraw-Hill Book Co.

Periodicals

Bradner, P.: A matter of identity, Nurs. Outlook **21**(5):332-334, 1973.

Fagin, C.: Accountability, Nurs. Outlook **19**(4):249-251, 1971.

Hall, D. T., and Nougaim, K. E.: An examination of Maslow's need hierarchy in an organizational setting, organizational behavior and human performance, Nurs. Outlook **16**(3):12-16, 1968.

Helmann, C.: Four theories of leadership, J. Nurs. Admin., pp. 18-24, June 1976.

Huckabay, L., and Arndt, C.: Effect of acquisition of knowledge on self-evaluation and the relationship of self-evaluation to perception of real and ideal self-concept, Nurs. Research **25**(4):244-251, July-Aug. 1976.

Krueger, J.: Utilization of nursing research: the planning process, J. Nurs. Admin., pp. 6-11, Jan. 1978.

Lindeman, C.: Nursing research priorities, J. Nurs. Admin., pp. 20-21, July-Aug. 1975.

McClure, M.: The long road to accountability, Nurs. Outlook **26**(1):47-50, 1978.

Miller, D. I.: Leaders march to a different drummer, J. Nurs. Admin. p. 3, Jan.-Feb. 1971.

O'Donovan, T.: Leadership dynamics, J. Nurs. Admin., pp. 32-35, Sept. 1975.

Pierce, S., and Thompson: Changing practice: by choice rather than chance, J. Nurs. Admin., pp. 33-39, Feb. 1976.

Reres, M.: Tapping human resources, J. Nurs. Admin., pp. 18-19, July-Aug. 1975.

Styles, M.: Dialogue across the decades, Nurs. Outlook **26**(1):28-32, 1978.

Thomas, L. A.: Predicting change in nursing values, J. Nurs. Admin., pp. 50-58, May-June 1971.

White, H.: Perceptions of leadership styles by nurses in supervisory positions, J. Nurs. Admin., pp. 44-51, Feb. 1972.

APPENDIX

DERIVATION OF PREDICTIVE PRINCIPLES FROM
SEVERAL AUTHORITATIVE SOURCES

Principles are derived from events. People observe events and record the logical serial order of the occurrence of the event. A theory is established about the cause and effect of the event, which then must be tested for validation. If a theory or hypothesis can be validated, it becomes a law; if it cannot be validated, but evidence seems to support the theory, it is still a usable tool.

The nurse-leader is seldom the originator of a completely new fact, concept, law, or principle. In most instances the nurse-leader depends on the published work of authorities to provide the sources from which predictive principles may be extracted. Those who would compile predictive principles of any given topic must search the literature for pertinent material, critically evaluate the validity of the material, and convert the concepts gleaned from the literature into predictive principles. This process can be described in nine steps. The following are the operational steps in extracting predictive principles from the literature:

1. Determine the topic or area to be considered.
2. Search the literature for books, articles, or pamphlets germane to the subject.
3. Read extensively in the field; keep a list of frequently recurring concepts (and include the source of each concept for reference).
4. Identify in the literature statements about how concepts influence or are related to each other and make appropriate notations on the cumulative list.
5. Select from the accumulated list material relevant to the concept of the circumstances, conditions, or behaviors (CCB) triad.
6. Determine from the authoritative sources on the accumulated list the predicted outcome of the CCB triad concept selected.
7. Determine the appropriate active verb phrase that will connect the concepts selected.
8. Add the qualifiers that will precisely indicate the specific delineations necessary to make the predictive principle valid and relevant.
9. Repeat steps 5, 6, 7, and 8 for each additional predictive principle for the determined topic until all major concepts on the list have been formulated into predictive principles.

The following is an example of the extraction of one predictive principle from an authoritative source using the first eight steps.

Problem: To make progressive changes in the nursing team routine.

1. *Determine the topic or area to be considered.* The topic is determined by the problem to be solved. In any given problem it will be necessary to use predictive principles from several areas. In this instance the nurse-leader would draw on a variety of topics or areas for predictive principles to use to accomplish the desired goals. Some of these areas would be leadership, teaching-learning, group dynamics, and interpersonal relationships. From each of these areas the nurse-leader would select or formulate the appropriate predictive principles for the task and designate them as "principles for making changes." This topic then becomes the area of desired predictive principles.

2. *Search the literature for books, articles, or pamphlets germane to the subject.* The objective for the review is to identify and extract those concepts that will form the basis for activities and behaviors that will stimulate and enable group change. The searcher seeks any resources that he postulates will be helpful in the determined subject area. For the objective given the nurse-leader would search the literature of such fields as psychology, sociology, business and industry, education, and nursing.

3. *Read extensively in the field; keep a list of frequently recurring concepts (including sources).* Certain topics or concepts recur with frequency in the literature of any given subject. A list of the recurring concepts enables the nurse-leader to determine the salient themes in any given subject with minimum effort and maximum speed. A list for the selected topic would contain such concepts as the objective of change, motivation, need, problem identification, group involvement, group commitment, individual security, careful planning, design and sequence for change, and optimum pace.

4. *Identify in the literature statements about how concepts influence, or are related to, each other, making appropriate notations on the cumulative list.* These notations are for the purpose of clarifying concept relationships and will readily facilitate the formulation of principles. The following is a cumulative list of concepts with notations that clarify concept relationships.

Concepts	Notations about predicted outcome and relationships
1. Clearly establish objectives of change	1. Direction, evaluation, minimum sidetracking
2. Group involvement	2. Related to commitment to outcomes of change
3. Group commitment	3. Grows with increasing participation in planning and decision making
4. Individual security	4. Providing individual with knowledge and skills and right to err with ego support during change
5. Careful planning	5. Logical order, central authority
6. Design and sequence	6. Purpose, focus, pace, progress, individual security, limitations
7. Optimum pace	7. Imposed by time and available materials
8. Motivation	8.
9. Need	9.
10. Problem identification	10.

The list is incomplete, as there are no notations for concepts 8, 9, and 10. The investigator need only follow the prescribed outline. Bibliographic data must be kept during the task so that credit may be given to the sources used.

5. *Select from the accumulated list material relevant to the concept of the CCB triad.* If the concept list and notations are complete, this step requires only that the appropriate concept be selected from the list. For example, "design and sequence" might be selected as the CCB triad concept.

6. *Determine from the authoritative sources or the accumulated list the predicted outcome of the CCB triad concept selected.* Again, as previously, if the concept list and notations are complete, this step requires only that the appropriate predicted outcome be selected from the notations on the list. For example, the principle formulator selects "purpose," "focus," and "progress" from the alternatives on the compiled list.

With the CCB triad and the predicted outcome concepts selected, all that remains is to relate them in some logical, meaningful way.

7. *Determine the appropriate active verb phrase that will connect the concepts selected.* The active verb is important because it determines the extent and degree of the relationship between the CCB triad and the predicted outcome. The writer of the principle could choose words such as *ensure, influence,* or *promote* for the active verb.

The principle formulator has found evidence in the literature that **purpose, focus,** and **progress** are influenced by many factors in addition to **design and sequence.** With this evidence in mind, the formulator selects "promote" rather than "ensure" as a more valid active verb.

At this point in the construction of a predictive principle the components appear as follows:

CCB triad	Active verb	Predicted outcome
Design and sequence	promote	purpose, focus, and progress

Although stated as a principle, qualifiers are needed to give the concepts context and limitations.

8. *Add the qualifiers that will precisely indicate the specific delineations necessary to make the predictive principle valid and relevant.* This is the final step in constructing a single principle. The choice of articles, adjectives, adverbs, and other parts of speech that set its limits is important because qualifiers affect the predictive principle's validity and clarity and may be necessary to make the predictive principle a complete sentence. A predictive principle using the selected components complete with qualifiers could read as follows:

Carefully predetermined **design and sequence** for change **promote** work that is **purpose focused** and **progress** that proceeds as rapidly as possible.

DERIVATION OF A PREDICTIVE PRINCIPLE FROM A SINGLE AUTHORITATIVE SOURCE

The writer of predictive principles may find a paragraph in an authoritative source clearly stating a predictive principle within the text itself. The predictive principle formulator will find it expedient to identify the parts of the predictive principle and extract it directly from the literature. Such a paragraph is quoted here, and the components of the predictive principle are identified within the text.

Attaching the label of evolutionary to change might be viewed by some as an opportunity to forestall any real innovation or as an excuse for lack of progress. To the contrary, although the suggested pace is less rapid, *evolutionary change requires a carefully predetermined* **design with definite sequence,** *pace and substance. These considerations are necessary to* **insure** *that* **purpose** *is always centrally* **focused** *and* **progress accomplished** *with all deliberate haste.**

In this quotation the concept of the CCB triad stands out clearly as **"design with definite sequence."** The predicted outcome appears within the text as **"purpose . . . focused and progress accomplished."** The critical principle formulator will find **"insure"** unacceptable as a valid active verb and will substitute a more realistic one such as *promote*. The result is a predictive principle derived directly from an authoritative source. It will read as follows:

A carefully predetermined design and sequence for change promotes work that is purpose focused and progress that proceeds with deliberate haste.

COMMON PREDICTIVE PRINCIPLE FORMULATION ERRORS

Blunders or errors in predictive principle formation have some similarity to principles and are often confused with predictive principles. Discriminating between predictive principles and nonprinciples is often difficult. Familiarity with common errors in predictive principle formation can prevent misconceptions, reinforce valid examples, and help the beginner avoid errors. Most common errors in predictive principle formation take the form of directions, descriptions, statements of fact, or pseudoprinciples. Examples of common errors in principle construction using the predictive principle stated previously are listed here.

Directions. Directions either state how to do something step by step or contain the words *should* or *ought to*. These are actually level IV situation-producing theories.

The effective leader should do the following:

1. Gather data pertinent to the current situation
2. Decide which data are applicable
3. Use data to make decisions

Descriptions. Descriptions state how a person behaves or what an activity is like. Descriptions often take the form of characteristics; there is no *active* verb.

A good leader will always have knowledge pertinent to the current situation on which to base decisions and judgment.

Facts or valid statements. Facts or valid statements are usually about the circumstances, conditions, or behaviors, or about the predicted outcome; however, they do not show relationship.

Knowledge is of use only if it is pertinent to the current problem.

---

*From Beggs, D. W.: Team teaching, Indianapolis, 1964, Unified College Press, Inc., pp. 102-103. (Italics and boldface added.)

Weak predictive principles take the form of principles in that they have a CCB triad connected to a predicted outcome; however, the active verb lacks the quality of certainty. Such words as *apparently, might, may,* and *perhaps* make the predictive principle so weak that it is almost useless as an action base.

Leaders who have knowledge pertinent to the current situation might make valid judgments and decisions.

Invalid principles. Invalidity is the most common form of error. Predictions that use erroneous material or fail to use modifiers appropriately often produce invalid predictions.

INDEX